14

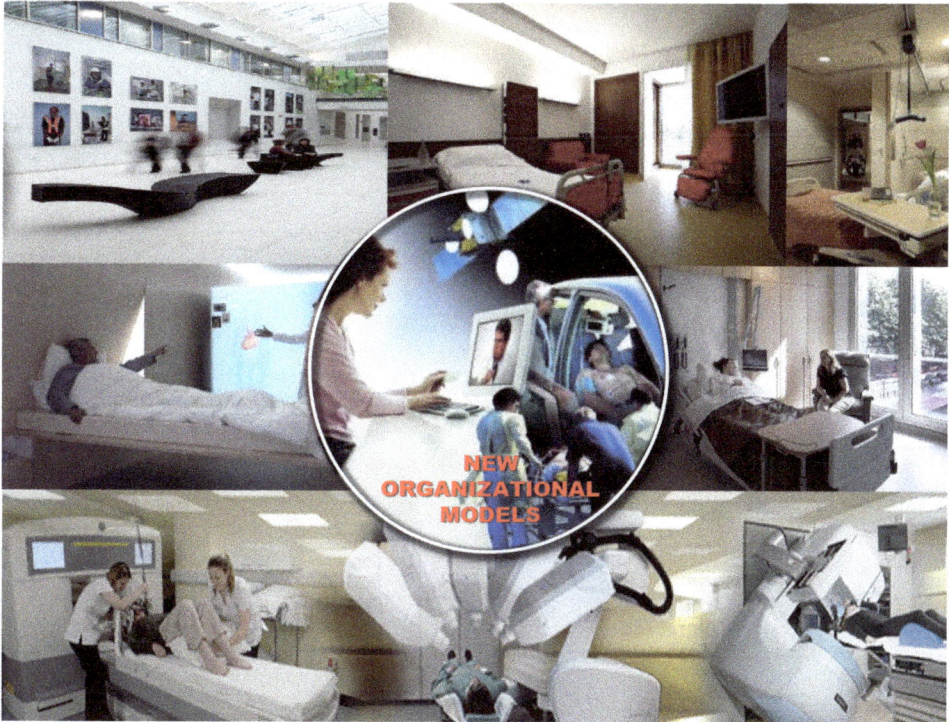

7. New organizational models advocated by the hyper-accelerated dynamic of biotechnological innovations.

tributions: from business to design, up to technical construction, not excluding the use of incentives in the form of sharing the achieved savings/benefits of the process: in other words, the importance of placing emphasis on the management of transdisciplinary decisions in real time and throughout the entire development of an intervention programme.

In Britain and North America, prestigious institutions such as the AIA (American Institute of Architects), the UKOGC (United Kingdom Office of Government Commerce), the world of big business and some large public commissions (V.A. — Veterans Health Administration) converge on the need to focus on "design approaches" in which the coordination of design strategies and operational solutions sees the involvement, in equal measures and from the initial stages of the decision-making process, of the client, design engineers and businesses with logic and tools that are well beyond the traditional "tender" procedures, highlighting how, in numerous experiences that have been developed and monitored, these models have produced unexpected results.

Intervention programmes developed in accordance with the principles of the integrated global approach for the construction of somewhat complex hospitals have seen all the parties involved fully satisfied in terms of compliance with budgets, the dramatic reduction in disputes, the prompt resolution of technical and design problems, the sharing of risks

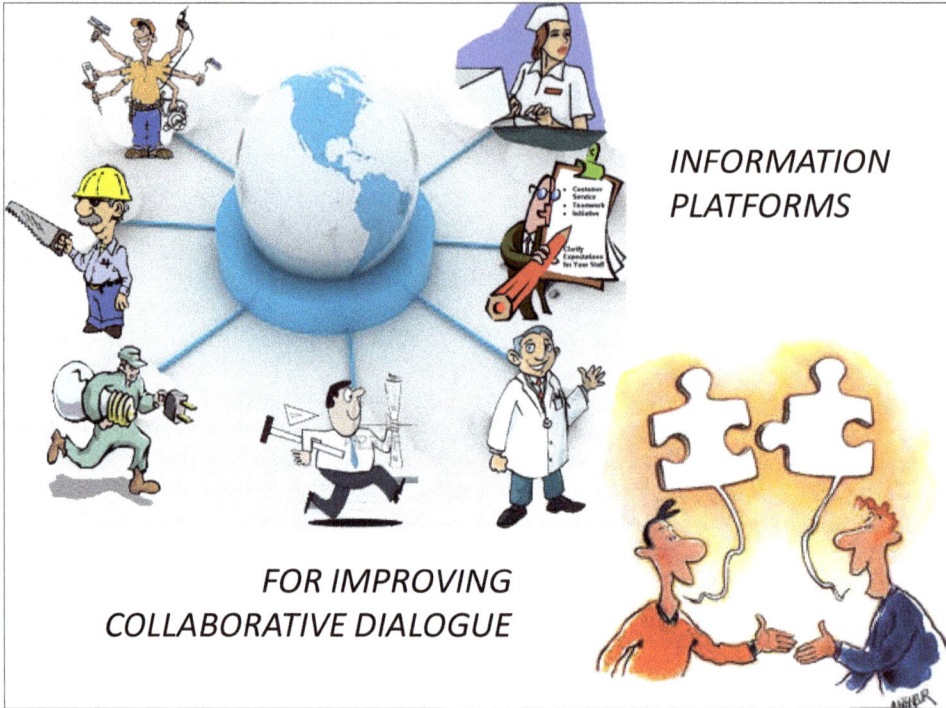

6. The use of common advanced information platforms improves collaborative dialogue.

the need for all parties to recover an ethical dimension that recognizes the mutual usefulness of the contributions with respect to the legitimate interests of each party: the performability of the work for the client, a fair profit for the builder and professional gratification, with satisfaction in terms of creative sensibility, for the architect. To encourage contribution from all parties concerned, contractual and procedural forms could be used that allow risks and profits to be shared in the knowledge that everyone is working towards the same goal.

With the spread of NTs in the construction sector, the progressive establishment of LEAN and IPD (Integrated Project Delivery) models and the spread of interoperability, the objective of an informed consultation on project deci-sions becomes increasingly viable and tangible.

In the international context the afore-mentioned problems have for some time stimulated reflections, proposals and feedback of considerable importance, highlighting a kind of convergence on the reasons for the distortions and the methods to overcome them. The trend that is pushing the international hospital construction market towards "integrated design approaches" highlights how, in order to respond to the critical issues, we must act on organizational process models that enhance collaboration principles among all the players involved in the process "from the earliest moments of the decision-making choices", recognizing the high level of added value that can be derived from integrating all the con-

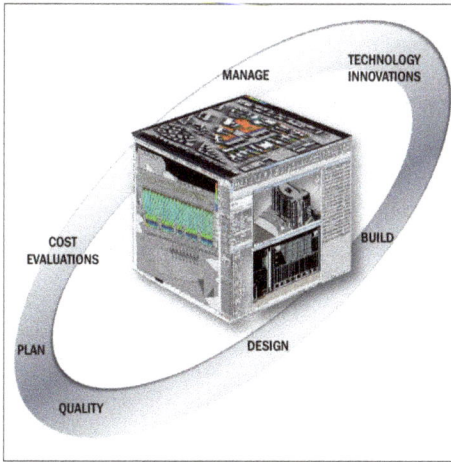

4. BIM (Building Information Modeling).

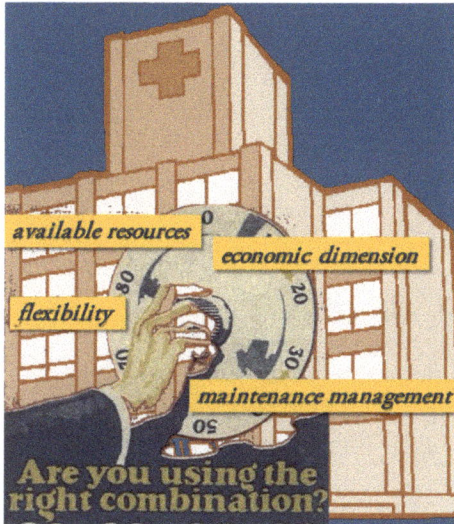

5. The evaluation of alternative solutions in the design of hospital facilities.

12

ways to encourage interaction between all those who help to define the conditions for the effective feasibility of the hospital, there are still significant inefficiencies in the process.

This confirms, once again, that a culture where all the players fully share mutual responsibilities with respect to the objectives has not yet been created.

What conditions, then, are required to overcome the aforementioned critical situations?

The answers can be different, and different in nature.

In the meantime we should be aware that when the principles of "competitiveness" are – rightly – stressed in order to achieve the objectives for the improvement of quality and the containment of costs and time frames in the construction of hospital facilities but – alas – continuous failure is experienced on account of the mechanisms that regulate the same competitiveness, then perhaps it is necessary to expand the spectrum of ideas and have the courage to recognize the errors made so as to propose suitable solutions.

If, in all the complex decision-making processes, like those that concern hospital architecture, the continuous and progressive sharing of choices on the part of all operators is considered a strategic condition for the success of the planned initiative and if the design process can in any case be likened to a complex system of conscious decisions taken by all the operators, then we cannot underestimate the importance of the techniques and procedures designed to facilitate sharing.

The basic assumption is still, of course,

suitably commensurate to the economic dimension of the available resources. The same could be said for the evaluation of alternative solutions in relation to the economic implications concerning the maintenance management and the efficiency of the same.

With regard to the second issue, namely

lutions. Whether in relation to problems of actual perceived quality or unjustified increases in the implementation costs and time scales for hospital works, the reasons for the critical situations can, in any case, always be attributed to the inadequacy of operational models, the poor technical culture of the decision-makers and operators, discrepancies between the decision-making areas and the lack of tools for informed consultation on the solutions.

This transpires, for example, from the very limited importance given to pre-planning briefings and the thorough formalization of applications, despite the fact that their strategic importance is now recognized with respect to the quality of the design.

The progressive development of the BIM (Building Information Modeling) techniques, advanced simulations systems and techniques for the structuring and implementation of technical economic databases, if managed with computationally integrated techniques, may allow designers and commissioning bodies to visualize, knowingly and reliably from the early design stages, the economic performance effects resulting from each of the alternatives they intend to hypothesize and evaluate. These kinds of trends produce, as an effect, the necessary rethinking of how the feasibility projects and corresponding preliminary design documents should be developed which, along with more frequent and widespread competition procedures, form the basis of the decisions on which the implementation projects of the complex works are then developed.

Purely to demonstrate the effectiveness of these tools we can refer to the level of marked awareness that may characterize the decisions taken by the commissioning bodies in assessing the degree of "appropriate flexibility" to be conferred to the design solution so that it can be

3. *The dynamic briefing process.*

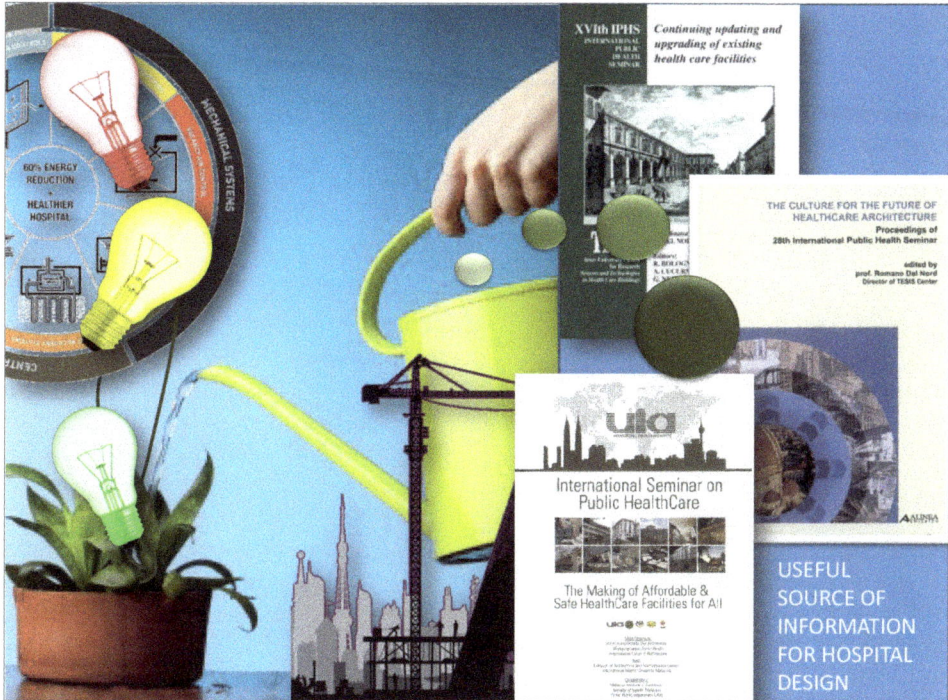

2. UIA /PHG seminar proceedings affecting decision making actions.

extremely profitable insights to guide the future decision-making actions of the various categories of operators concerned in the world of healthcare.

The numerous and diverse Proceedings produced to date represent an extremely useful source of information not only to document the evolution of the principles and methods used to design the works but also to understand the level of importance attributed to the issues that most frequently drive the members of the PHG to address their resolution.

The issues most frequently explored include those related to the impact produced by innovations on the tools and techniques to produce quality designs, the methods for encouraging interaction between those who make the decisions and the new methods of treatment made

possible by the biomedical resources.

As regards the former, attention is highly focused on automatic control tools that can make the objectives of quality compatible with those of containing spending within predetermined limits during all the phases of the progressive in-depth analysis of the design, from the preliminary design phases to those of the detailed project of the construction site. In this context the greatest difficulties and efforts lie in the early developmental stages of the design process, knowing that any errors made in these phases have a strong impact on the actual feasibility of the works and their effective economic sustainability, with detrimental effects on corrections and alterations introduced at the later stages of the technical development of the so-

Cultural Issues on the Complexity of Hospital Design

Romano Del Nord
Professor University of Florence
Director of TESIS Inter-University Research Centre

The international debate on the critical factors that result in an increasingly complex approach to the design of hospital facilities aimed at meeting the inevitable objectives of social, economic and environmental sustainability mainly focuses on the topics of flexibility, humanization, the right economic investment, integration between the hospital macro-functions, managerial efficiency, technological and biomedical innovation, the relationship with the city as well as ways of achieving greater economies.

For each of these themes attitudes and interpretations are encountered that do not always converge but that certainly stimulate reflection on the decision-making choices that complexify the task of the hospital designers.

The UIA/PHG - International Union of Architects/Public Health Group seminars, as previously scheduled on an annual basis, associate the discussion of current topics with the comparison between contributions from operational experience in the field which can provide

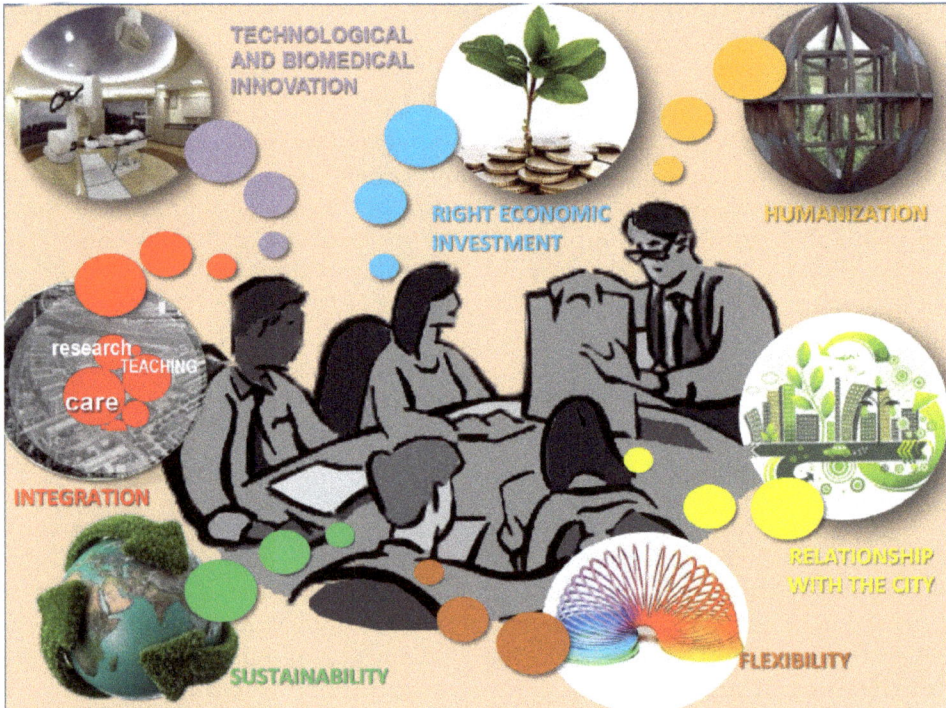

1. *The topics of hospital planning and design.*

TESIS Inter-University Research Centre "Systems and Technologies for Social and Healthcare Facilities"
University of Florence, Italy

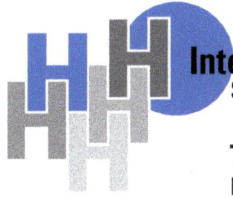

International Hospital Projects
Session introduction

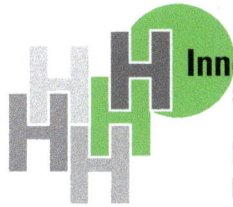

Innovative Technologies
Session introduction

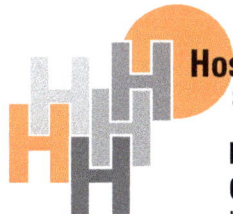

Hospital Planning Evaluations
Session introduction

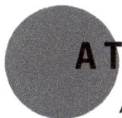

A Tour Through the Hospital

FOREWORD

On behalf of all the members of the UIA / Public Health Group I wish to express our deepest appreciation to our senior longstanding member, Prof. Romano Del Nord and Ms. Francesca Nesi for all their great efforts to assemble and edit the proceedings of the UIA Public Health Group's 32nd annual meeting in Oslo, Norway, in March 2012.

In addition we wish to express our very deepest appreciation to Hans Eggen, Director of the UIA Public Health Group for his excellent leadership and innovations during his 5-year term. Thank you Hans, and thank you for all your great assistance in making the transition into leadership.

Congratulations to all the members of the UIA Public Health Group for their excellent papers that were presented at the Oslo conference.

It is indeed an honour to have been elected as the new Director of the UIA Public Health Group. I look forward to working closely with you, to further advancing the state of the art of Health and Hospital Facility Research, Planning and Design, and to furthering the contributions our group can make.

We look forward to each member's participation in the UIA Public Health Group's 33rd annual meeting in Toronto, Canada: "Taking Aim at Health Care Quality through the Design of the Environment of Care".

The pursuit of better health, better healthcare, and lower per capita cost will be addressed at the UIA-PHG 2013 Annual Seminar at IIDEX CANADA 2013 Toronto, Ontario, Canada, 24-28 September 2013, a collaborative conference between the International Union of Architects – Public Health Group (UIA-PHG), the Royal Architectural Institute of Canada RAIC, Health+Care Group, Interior Designers of Canada, and Global University Program in Healthcare Architecture (GUPHA).

Tuesday 24 September 2013 GUPHA Meeting
Wednesday 25 September 2013
Opening Evening Reception
Thursday 26 September 2013
Seminars Social Dinner
Friday 27 September 2013
Seminars UIA Dinner
Saturday 28 September 2013
Facility Tours UIA Meeting

We urge each of you to recruit and encourage the participation of younger new members. Thank you and see you in Toronto in 2013.

George

George J. Mann, AIA

The Ronald L. Skaggs FAIA Endowed Professor of Health Facilities Design; College of Architecture, Texas A&M University; College Station, Texas 77843, USA; tel 979 845 7856, fax 979 8621571; email: gmann@arch.tamu.edu; manngj1@yahoo.com;
First Holder of the Skaggs - Sprague Endowed Chair of Health Facilities Design;
Director of the UIA / PHG - International Union of Architects / Public Health Group
President and Co-Founder, GUPHA (Global University Programs in Healthcare Architecture)
Founder and Advisory Board Chairman, The RPD (Resource Planning & Development) Group

INTRODUCTION

A learning Work Programme based on regional and international experience Oslo 2012

1. Who is the Public Health Group?

It has 62 members from all continents and others can participate as guest members too. Information about our activities and future intentions is available on the web.

2. International seminars

Conferences combined with hospital visits held each year in another UIA member country seem to be very effective. The focus has to be adapted continuously and actual topics must be set, also bearing in mind sustainability, the lifecycle economy and the healing environment. Time is also reserved for all those actually present during the few days.

3. Success with partner organisations

For the 2012 conference we took the opportunity of creating a joint venture with the national organisation of all Norwegian Hospitals (NSH) and the Norwegian Architects Forum for healthcare buildings. It became clear once more that the success of such a conference is based on the combination of a regional network and an international group.

4. Topic themes

First of all we were interested in understanding the specific healthcare situation in the country being visited and then examining examples and experiences had in other continents. The aim was to discuss different aspects of topical subjects examined in the sessions and to learn from the experiences of others. What all countries have in common is that we are all faced with a growing population and growing healthcare costs, but under completely different climatic, demographic, social and financial conditions. A challenging title for everyone is:

Keeping up hospital quality in an era of financial problems and cost control
The sessions were entitled:
- Nordic Hospital Projects
- Flexibility
- International Hospital Projects
- Innovative Technologies
- Hospital Planning Evaluations

Hans Eggen
Director of the UIA Work Programme Public Health

Index

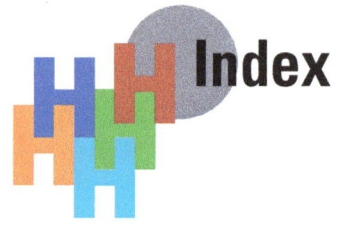

Index

and profits, and the effective prior understanding of the implications underlying the design solutions implemented. All this confirms the importance of acting on procedural logic rather than on the consequent and in any case necessary specific innovations.

In a futuristic scenario in which the "design" can really assume a dimension where it expresses and represents the synthesis of multiple decisions that are coordinated, conscious and shared in terms of all performance, economic and social aspects, it becomes strategic to provide developed contributions on operational methods and the tools through which this integration of knowledge and desires can become a reality.

The process through which the decision-making choices take shape during planning seriously conditions the quality of the decisions themselves just as the finalization of the hard and soft innovative techniques necessary to encourage co-operation on all levels, through the use of information platforms that facilitate the real acquisition of knowledge, opens up large areas of scientific interest specifically relevant to us. The same building information models which, in their most advanced form, create dialogue between the project and information databases that substantiate their physical and functional characteristics and the technical-construction, performance and economic content, can transform into platforms to facilitate collaborative dialogue and support conscious decision-making extending to a foreshadowing of the impact on the management phase of the planned works.

In this kind of environment it becomes important to know how to renew the process leadership profile in the awareness that it may become a success factor if it takes on the role of facilitator rather than controller, promoting the collaborative atmosphere that encourages the

15

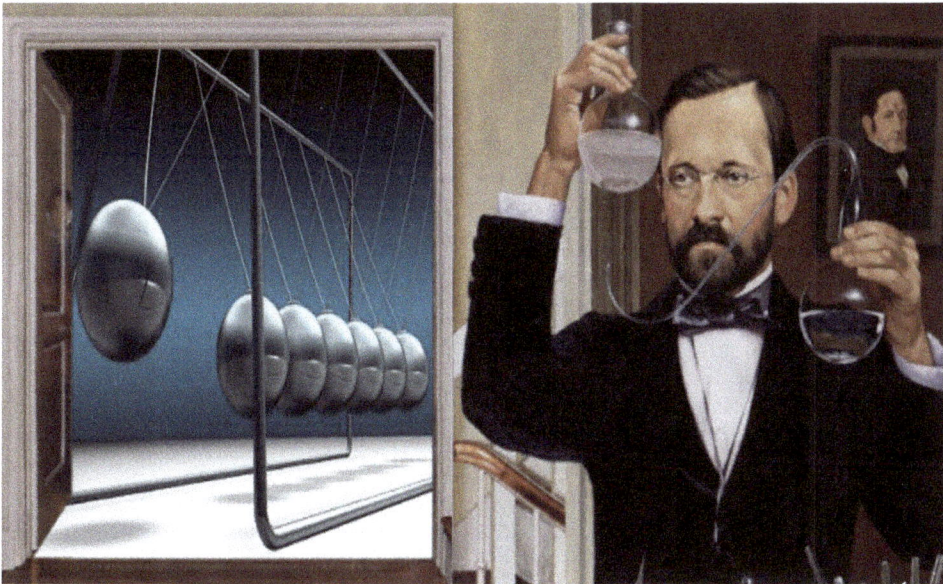

8. *Technology transfer.*

TESIS Inter-University Research Centre "Systems and Technologies for Social and Healthcare Facilities"
University of Florence, Italy

TESIS

16

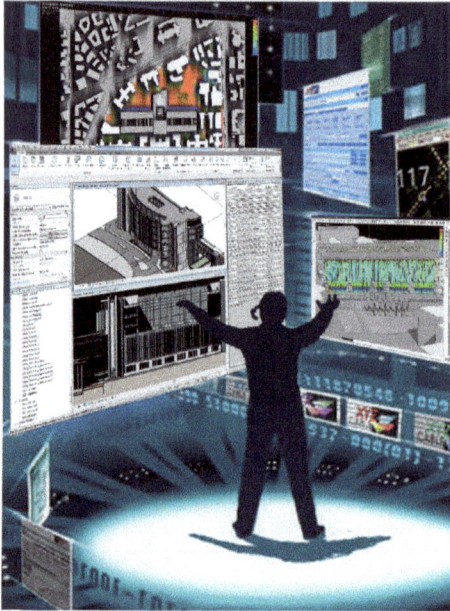

9. Virtual laboratories as advanced tools for the simulation of models for the use and enjoyment of the hospital spaces.

formation of truly integrated partnerships.

In relation to the third issue, namely the new treatment and organizational models advocated by the hyper-accelerated dynamic of biotechnological innovations, attention tends to be focused on the structural and technological requirements of the hospitals of excellence aimed at encouraging the widespread use of the results of translational research, that is on the physical-spatial and organizational conditions necessary to facilitate integration between the functions of care, hospital-related experimental research and the training of technicians and healthcare professionals capable of competently manipulating what has emerged from the applied research, both at the level of sophisticated tools and at the level of "treatment procedures".

To achieve these objectives the most advanced situations propose aggregative models for very different functions and spaces even though they are all geared towards maximizing the benefits of multidisciplinary integration within the hospital. The most important differences concern the reciprocal location of the main macro-functions, and the systems of connection and interdependence between them.

Other central topics in the cultural debate — addressed in the following documented presentations — concern the "different interpretations" of the concept of "hospital quality", the contribution to the redevelopment and renewal of the urban fabric that the hospital can offer in the event of the renovation of existing buildings, the increasingly enhanced interdependence between the hospital, nature and green spaces with an emphasis on the importance of the environmental landscape requirements, the growing significance of the energy component in the research and experimentation of technological innovations in hospital design, the new forms of industrialization and prefabrication that alter — as much in terms of products as construction processes — the way of understanding hospital architecture and, not least, the growing support for virtual laboratories as advanced tools for the simulation of models for the use and enjoyment of the hospital spaces.

The discussion of these issues highlights not only the level of increasing complexity that hospital design must face but, as already mentioned, the multidimensionality of the ideological and cultural contrasts that substantiate it through the wealth of ideas and reflections.

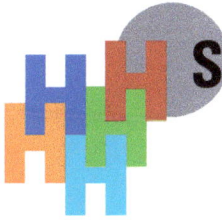

Seminar Sessions

TESIS Inter-University Research Centre "Systems and Technologies for Social and Healthcare Facilities"
University of Florence, Italy

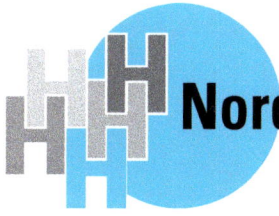

Nordic Hospital Projects
Session introduction

The Nordic hospital projects illustrated in the course of the session highlight how the patient-centered design approach must necessarily be applied in the next few years in close connection with two other emerging issues: on the one hand the need for integration between research activities, education and assistance, and on the other the theme of environmental sustainability understood not only as a reduction of energy consumption at the building scale but also as the hospital's relationship with the surrounding environment at the urban scale.

Ragnhild Aslaksen's lecture is a reasoned overview of the quality and new trends of hospitals in the north of Europe. Starting with the design experiences of the early nineties, the author describes the best practices of buildings constructed by applying the patient-centered design approach. The comparative analysis of selected healthcare environments highlights the practical application of design principles that provide an active contribution to improving the wellbeing of users (healing environments).
Future challenges in hospital design are the need to promote user participation in the design process and the requirement to integrate environmental quality with design strategies aimed at environmental sustainability.

Ragnhild Aslaksen p. 21

The new campus and university hospital project of Nya Karolinska Solna described in Christine Hammarling and Charlotte Ruben's paper is a significant example of best practices in healthcare planning and design. The main concept of the project is based on the integration of the three main activities of assistance, education and research in order to ensure the mutual exchange of knowledge among health professionals and researchers. The design solutions help to improve the quality of the healthcare settings through the optimization of functional distribution, the connection between the indoor and outdoor environments, the choice of a transparent envelope and the application of Scandinavian design principles.

Christine Hammarling and Charlotte Ruben p. 35

The case study of the New Hospital in Gødstrup, presented at the session by John Arne Bjerknes, is an example of the design of healthcare buildings in which the morphological and typological choices made are geared towards integrating the hospital complex with the surrounding environment.
The building spaces are designed to improve the humanization of the environment and to find a balance between the beauty and functionality of the facility. The hospital shape as well as the materials used for the façade were selected with the aim of linking the hospital to the environment: the building is composed of an ordered sequence of arms that generate an articulated profile open to nature; the building envelope is composed of large windows and balconies that allow users to look out and see the landscape.

John Arne Bjerknes p. 47

TESIS Inter-University Research Centre "Systems and Technologies for Social and Healthcare Facilities" University of Florence, Italy

1. Aarhus Universitetshospital.

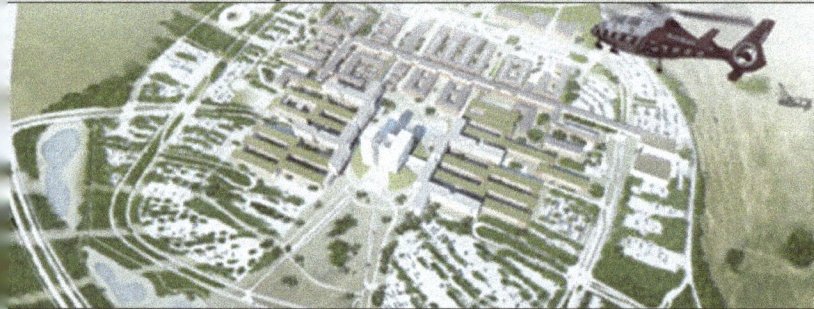

2. Regionshospitalet Gødstrup.

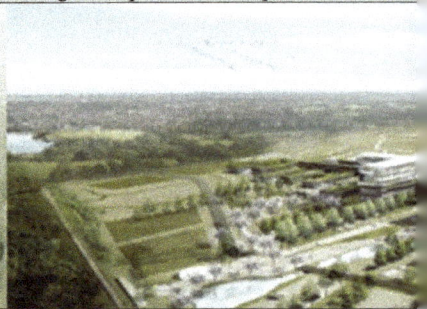

7. Nyt Universitetshospital, Odense.

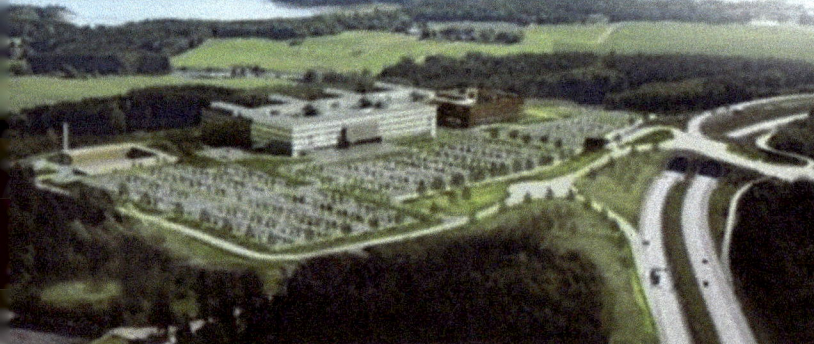

5. Kolding Hospital, extension.

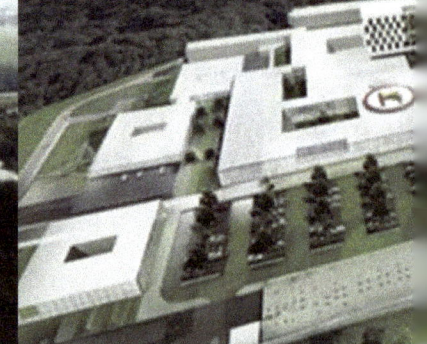

4. Nytt Østfoldsykehus.

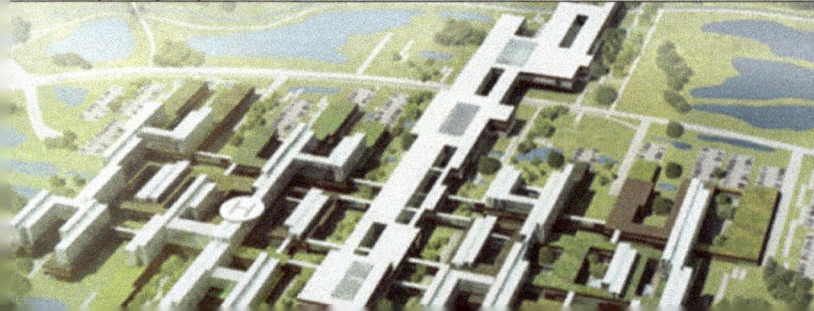

8. Nytt Rikshospital, Oslo.

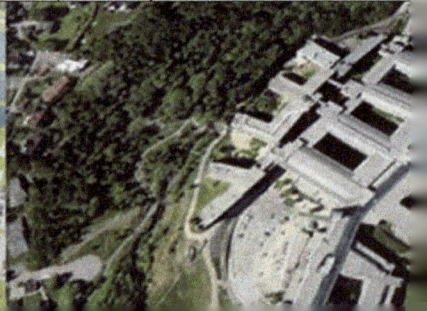

The Qualities and Tendencies of New Nordic Hospitals

Ragnhild Aslaksen
Associate Professor NTNU
Chief Architect Helsebygg Midt-Norge

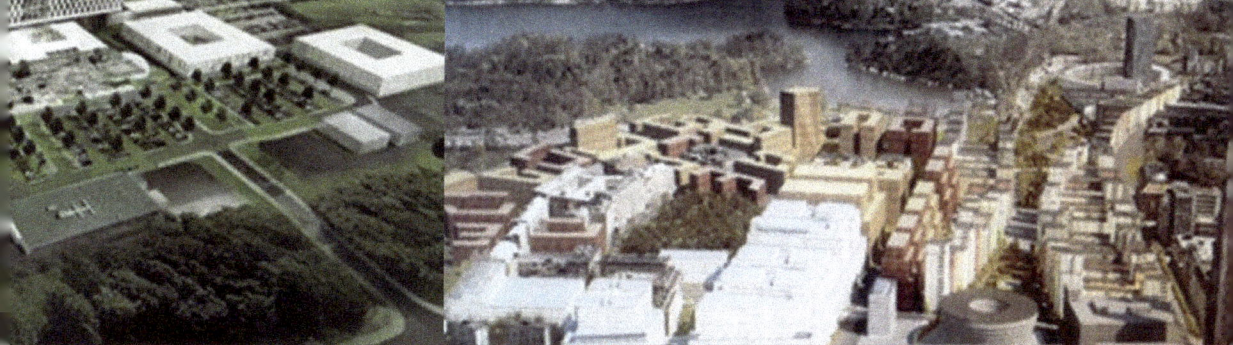

3. Nye Ahus, Akershus.

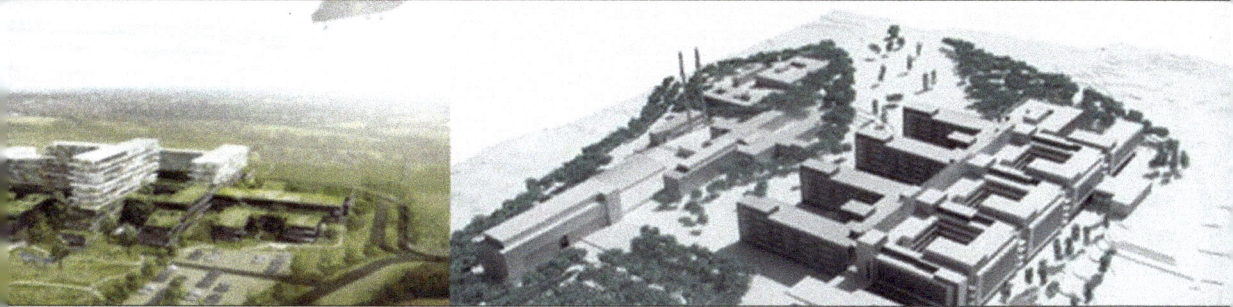

6. Nya Karolinska Solna, Stockholm.

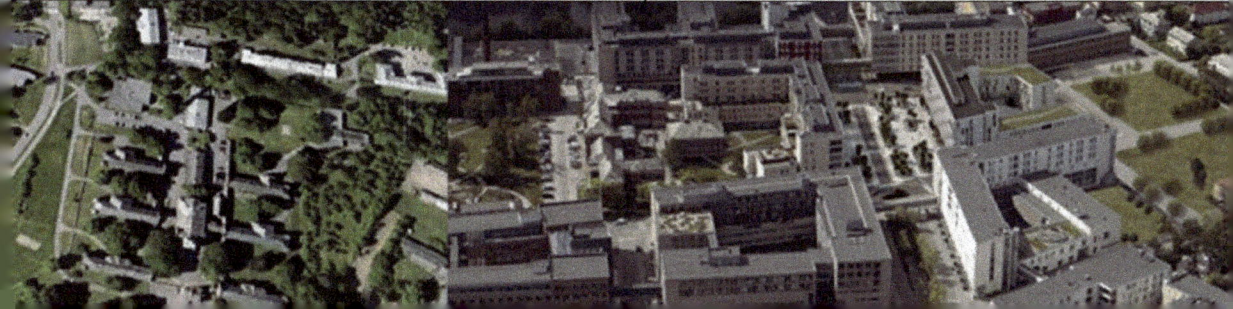

9. St. Olavs Hospital, Trondheim.

Rikshospitalet in Gaustad, designed by Medplan Architects (completed in 2000

Rikshospitalet in Gaustad, designed by Medplan Architects (completed in 2000), marks the starting point of the discussion on qualities and tendencies in new Nordic hospitals.

The characteristic and innovative features of the project are:

• megastructure – the combination of a strong concept and a relaxed expression;
• colocation of the university and psychiatry;
• green environments and landscape adaption; low rise – 4-floor buildings, views, nature, daylight;
• urban qualities – entrance square with a tower and (curved) indoor street;
• clinical concept – central block with radiology, theatres and a "horizontal" ward block;
• technology – technical floors, a new level of technical quality in equipment and installations, "luxurious" theatres in terms of space and technology;
• new standards for the use of space in Norwegian hospitals, mainly concerning technical spaces;
• art – the first large-scale systematic art project in a Norwegian hospital, integrated in most public areas in order to strengthen place identity, help wayfinding and generally raise quality.

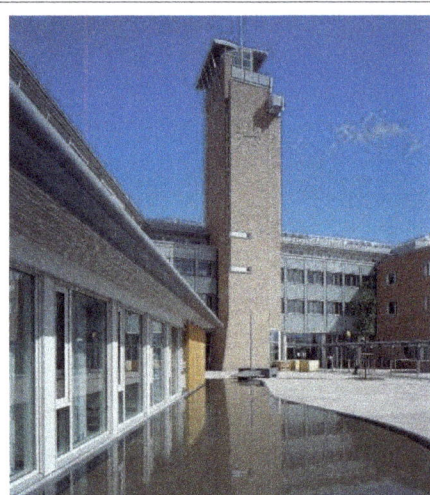

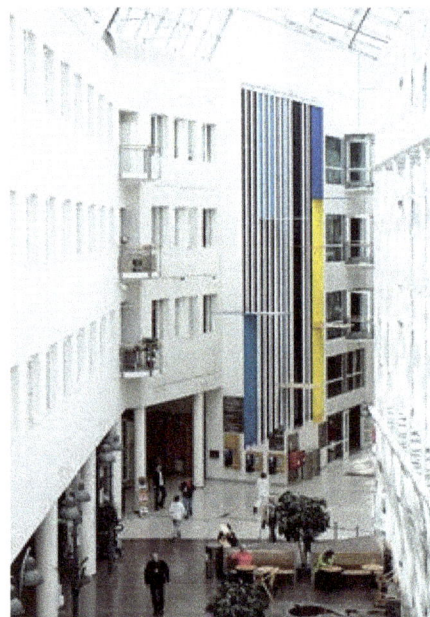

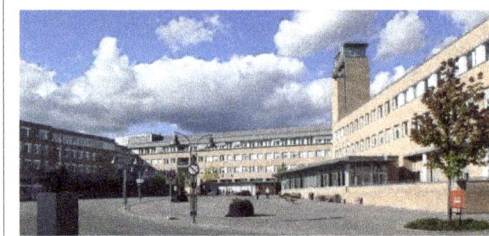

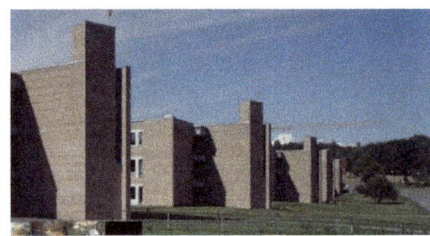

22

10. Nytt Rikshospital in Gaustad, Medplan Architects (completed 2000).

The vision for Rikshospitalet was to create a "humanistic hospital", and in architectural terms this meant, among other things:
• "human scale" – low rise, daylight, views, green environments, art;
• landscape adaptation and a high quality public space; indoor street, tower and central square;
• inherent quality – not "humanized"; the quality occurs as a result of the main structure;
• a sense of care and coherence; meaningful variations not endless repetitions;
• overall better and more "normal" quality architecture.

Rikshospitalet was designed too early to take into account aspects that were later developed in subsequent projects and had great influence in terms of concepts and solutions:
• patient focus, single occupancy and ward clusters;
• clinical clusters and central structure;
• extensive integrated ICT systems;
• strict energy use regulations.

St. Olavs Hospital, Trondheim University Hospital, was designed by Frisk, Medplan, Trondheimslaget and Team St. Olav.
St. Olavs Hospital represents a new step in the evolution of the new Nordic hos-

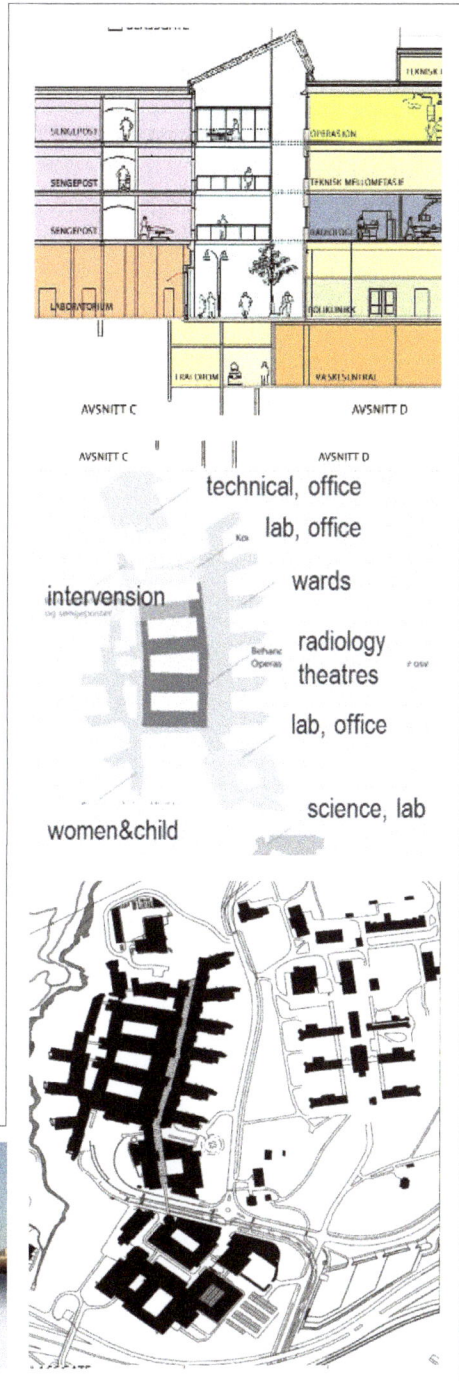

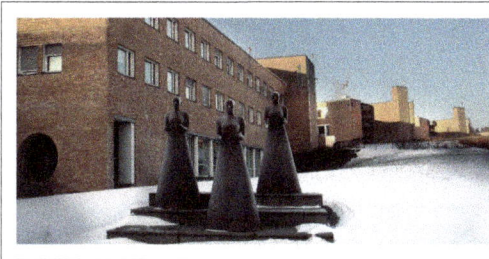

23

11. *Nytt Rikshospital in Gaustad, Medplan Architects (completed 2000).*

TESIS Inter-University Research Centre "Systems and Technologies for Social and Healthcare Facilities"
University of Florence, Italy

24

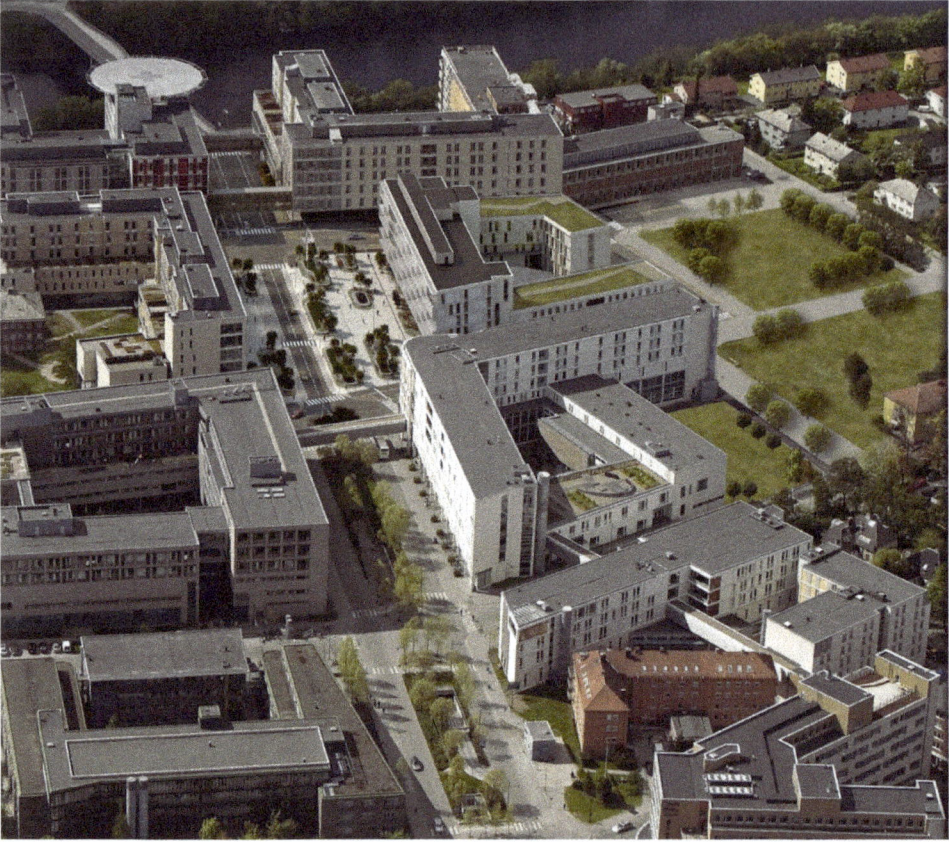

12. St. Olavs Hospital, Trondheim University Hospital. Architects: Frisk, Medplan, Trondheimslaget, Team St. Olav.

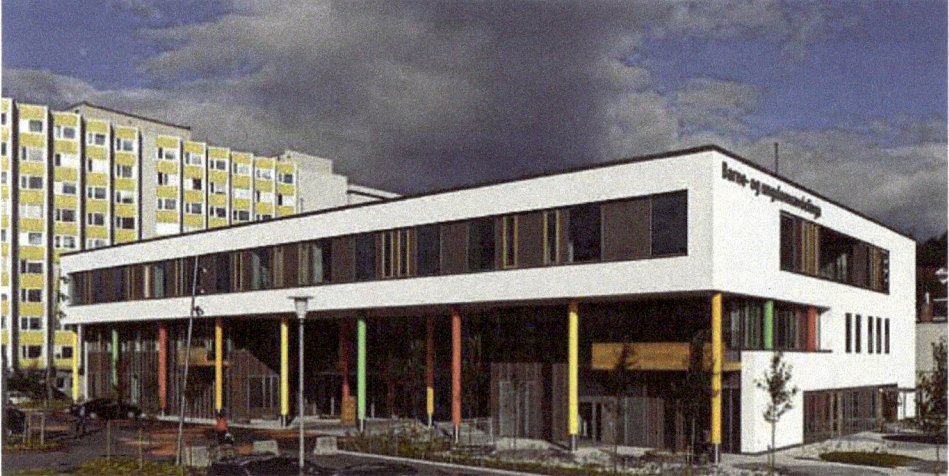

13. New Children's Hospital, Ålesund. Architect: C. F. Møller Architects.

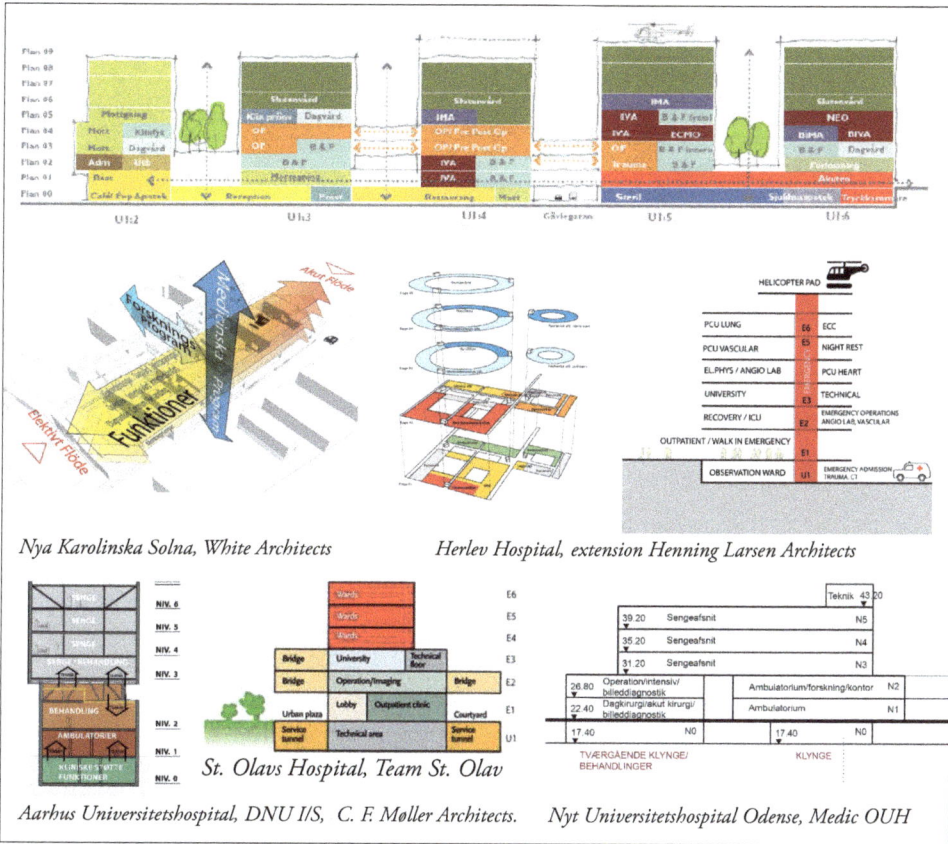

Nya Karolinska Solna, White Architects

Herlev Hospital, extension Henning Larsen Architects

St. Olavs Hospital, Team St. Olav

Aarhus Universitetshospital, DNU I/S, C. F. Møller Architects.

Nyt Universitetshospital Odense, Medic OUH

14. Hospital concepts: sections.

pitals. The project is based on a patient-centered approach and green design principles, such as:

• an integrated university clinic; the hospital and university intimately integrated in each building complex;

• the patients' perspective; formalized patient participation in all levels of planning and design;

• single occupancy for most patients including intensive care;

• "Sengetun" – new ward clusters that provide a combination of privacy and close staff contact;

• healing environments – nature/daylight/art integrated on all design levels;

• advanced and highly integrated ICT; "everything on the internet";

• automatic transportation systems, pneumatic tubes, AGW, waste handling;

• phase 3 – low energy – passive house standard.

The new children's hospital in Ålesund, designed by C. F. Møller Architects, offers an example of excellence in the design of single occupancy children's and neonatal units.

It is possible to observe how the design of the new Nordic hospitals has developed in different directions due to the

26

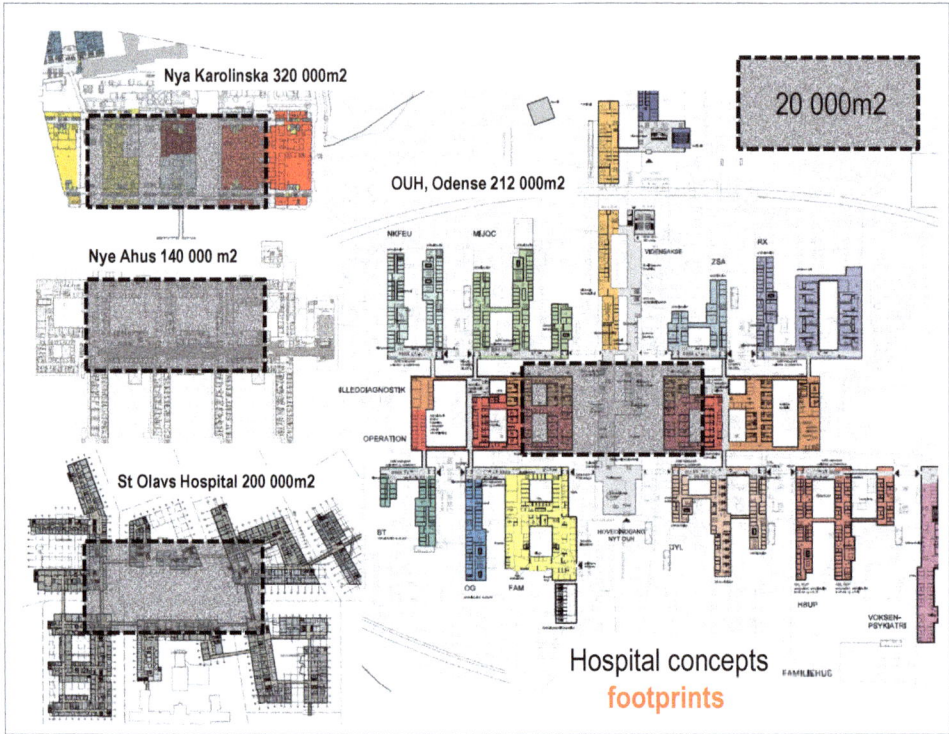

15. *Hospital concepts: footprints.*

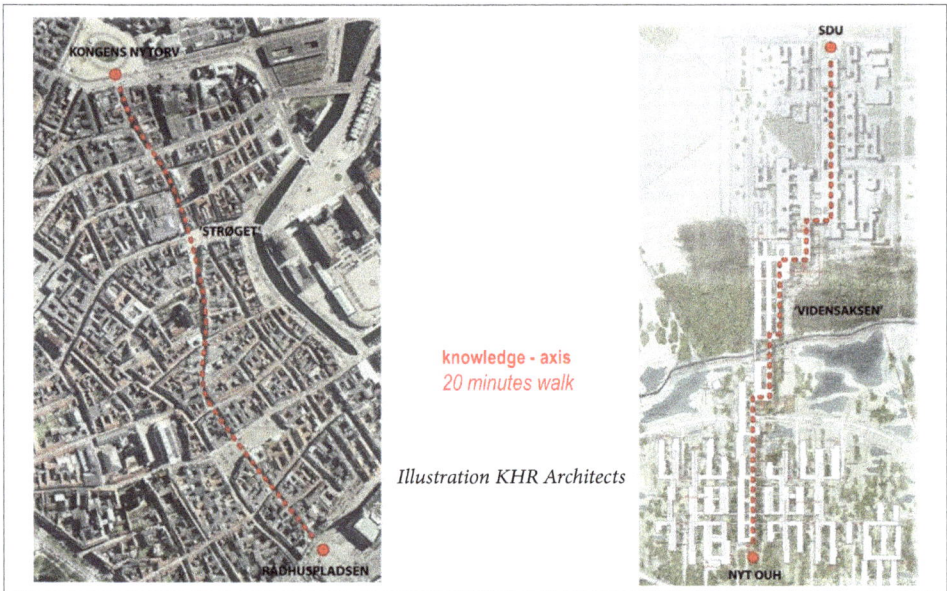

16. *Hospital concepts: knowledge axis.*

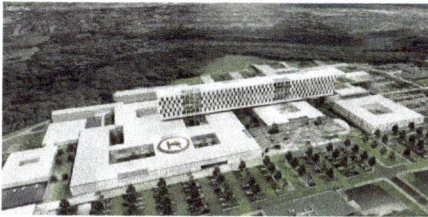

Kolding Hospital, Schmidt Hammer Lassen Architects

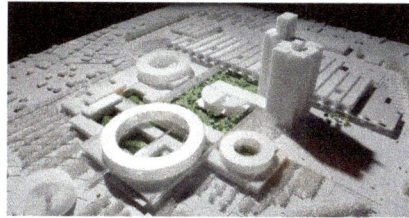

Herlev Hospital, Henning Larsen Architects

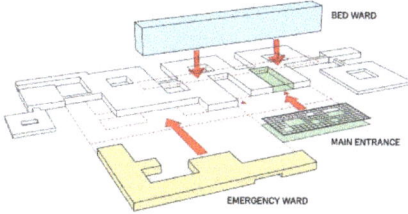

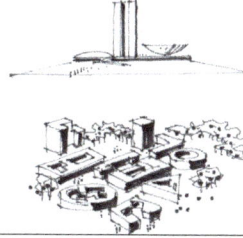

17. *Hospital concepts: extensions.*

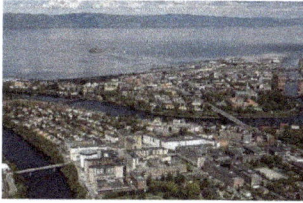

St. Olavs Hospital, Trondheim, Frisk, Medplan, Team St. Olav

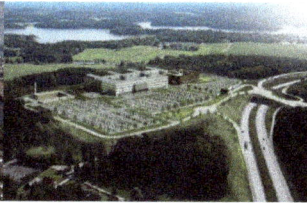

Nytt Østfoldsykehus, Eliassen og Lambertz –Nilssen, Architema, A.A.R.T

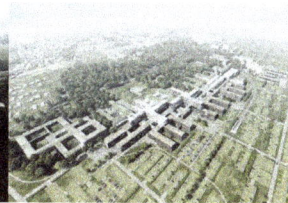

Aalborg Universitetshospital , competitionproject, Indigo

18. *Hospital concepts: location.*

choice of concepts and local priorities. Looking at a selection of footprints and sections, some tendencies become apparent.

Hospital concepts: sections

Three main tendencies appear – combined or alone:
• horizontally connected and vertically divided clinical clusters or central structure;
• wards located above hot floors and ambulatory care units;

• vertically organized acute axis or acute patients flow concentrated or/and separated from the elective patients flow.

Nya Karolinska Solna, Herlev Hospital (with extension), Nyt Universitets hospital in Odense, Aarhus Universitets hospital and St. Olavs Hospital are examples of these tendencies.

This organization has proven to be relatively flexible in adapting to the change in treating inpatients to treating outpatients. It is relatively simple to refurbish wards into outpatient clinics without disturbing patient logistics.

Hospital concepts: footprints

Two main tendencies appear, which are developing into extremes in both directions:
• concentrated high-rise buildings with minimized footprints, often in urban settings;
• horizontally organized structures with "maximized" footprints, mostly on free land.

This is where the tendencies differ the most. The extremes are demonstrated by Nya Karolinska in Stockholm, which is the most concentrated, and Odense University Hospital, which is the most spread out.

The Norwegian Hospitals, St. Olavs Hospital in Trondheim and Nye Ahus

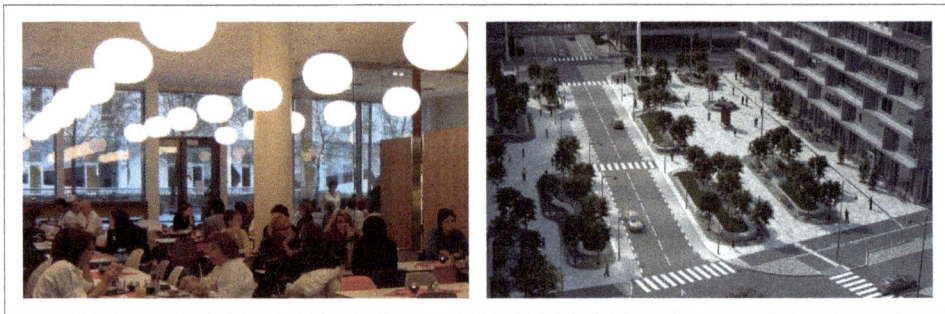

19. *St. Olavs Hospital, Trondheim, Frisk, Medplan, Team St. Olav.*

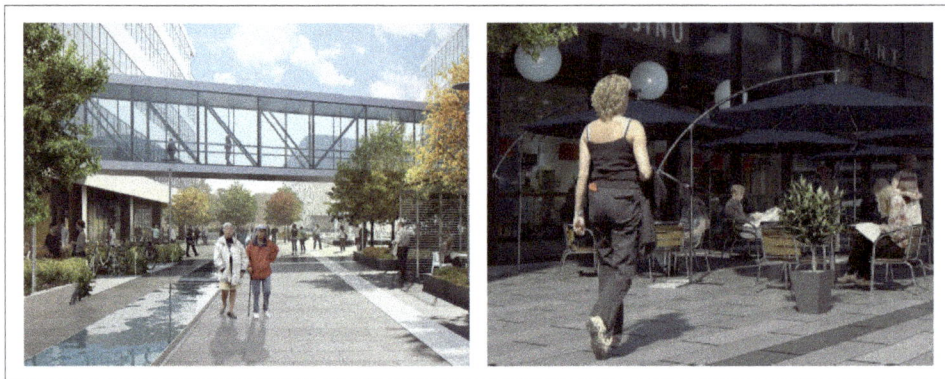

20. *Nya Karolinska Solna, Stockholm, White Architects.*

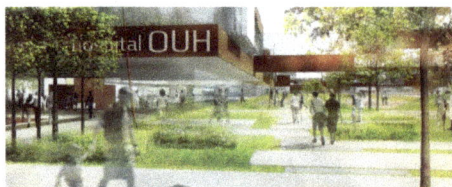

21. *Odense.*

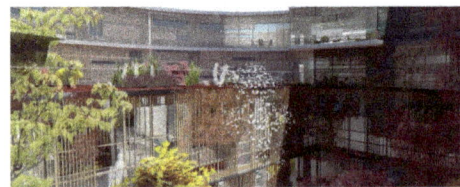

22. *Herlev.*

28

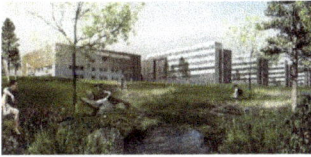
23. Østfold.

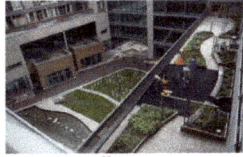
24. Trondheim.

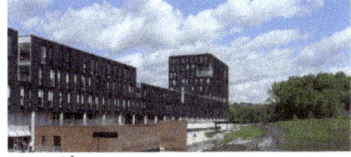
25. Ahus.

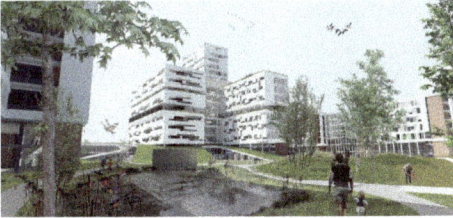
26. Aarhus.

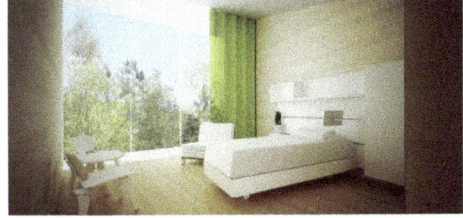
27. Espoo, K2S.

29

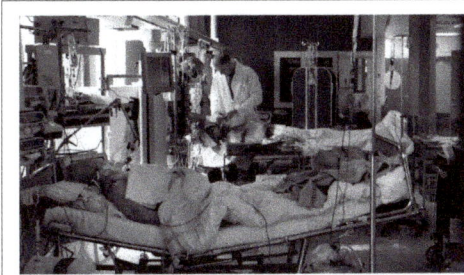
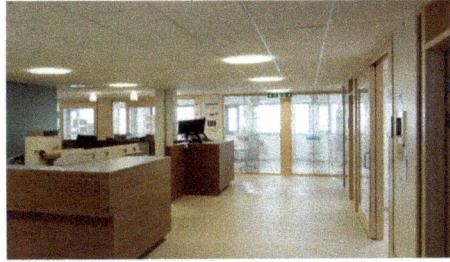
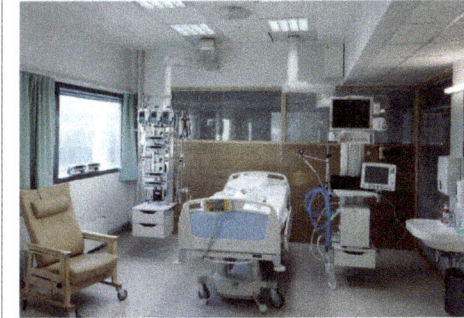
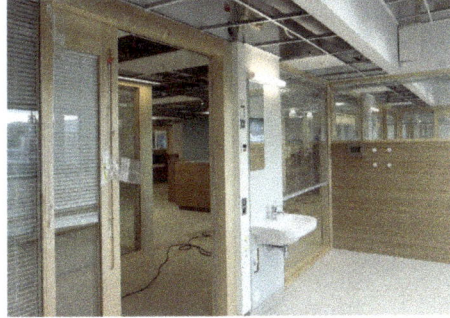

28. Traditional ICU versus St. Olavs Hospital, Central ICU.

in Oslo, both with suburban and central locations, represent the middle ground.

The illustration 15 compares footprints from some of the new Nordic hospitals:
• Nya Karolinska (320,000 m²);
• Nye Ahus (140,000 m²);
• St. Olavs Hospital (200,000 m²);
• OUH, Odense (212,000 m²).

Hospital concepts: knowledge axis

The theme of the knowledge axis, in which treatment, research and landscapes are tied together, was developed by KHR Arkitekter in the Odense University Hospital project. To walk the knowledge axis from one end to the other takes a good 20 minutes.

Hospital concepts: extensions

Kolding Hospital, designed by Schmidt Hammer Lassen Architects, and Herlev Hospital, designed by Henning Larsen Architects, offer two different examples of how it is possible to expand a horizontal hospital with vertical and horizontal expansion and transform it into new functional and architectural concepts.

Hospital concepts: sustainability and location

Green design principles should also cover the hospital location and urban integration. Hospitals are highly transport-intensive with thousands of daily encounters (staff, services, patients, visitors).
Specific locations should take into account the influence on car traffic and carbon dioxide emissions.

Where is the most sustainable location for a hospital? There are also two design issues to consider: how much green do we need in order to create a healing environment, and how do we improve the quality of urban integration, as in the case of two hospitals, St. Olavs and Karolinska.

Hospital concepts: healing environments

Aesthetic – (the opposite of unaesthetic) is what we experience with our senses. From this point of view the "Hospital of the Senses" comprises extensive knowledge about how hospital architecture influences our health and wellbeing though stimulation of the senses ("Sansernes Hospital" was written by

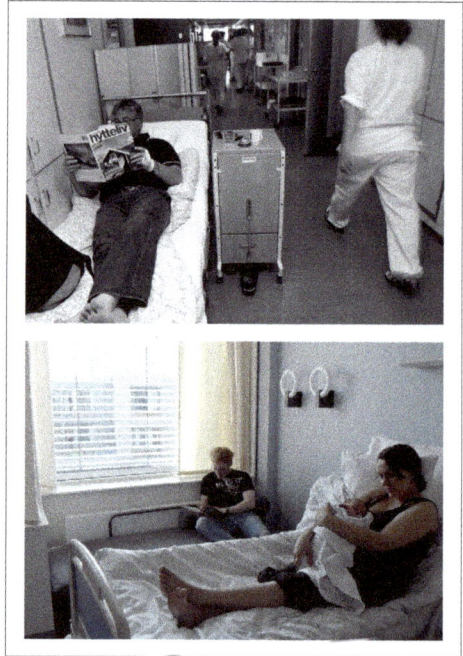

29. Space for privacy – single occupancy.

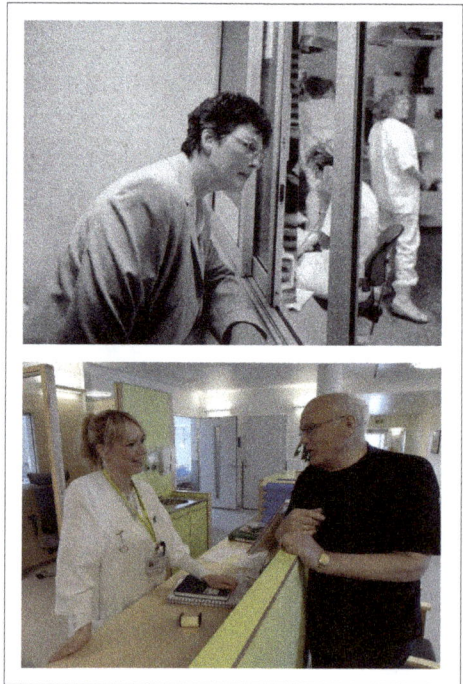

30. Space for contact – open workstations.

30

Lars Heslet and Kim Dirknick-Holmfeld, Arkitektens Forlag 2007). The book claims that the future Hospital of the Senses will bypass the Technological Hospital, not by replacing it but by including it.

Healing Environments are characterized by the presence of aspects like nature, natural materials, daylight, views, normality, and art.

The new Nordic hospitals are now designed with these qualities to a greater extend. Some recent examples in Odense, Gødstrup, Herlev, Østfold, Trondheim, Ahus, Aarhus and Espoo K2S (images 21-27) show the application of this design approach.

At St. Olavs Hospital, the Central ICU is designed with single occupancy, natural materials, daylight and views. These environments differ from traditional ICUs which, on the contrary, are characterized by multi-occupancy and focus on technology. Single occupancy ensures privacy and open workstations provide areas for contact.

New requirements often create a pressure for space expansion: single occupancy, work environment requirements, separated flows, universal design, new equipment and technology, technology-driven sustainable solutions and energy saving. As a result more energy-using spaces and longer travel distances were created. It is essential to challenge the tendency to create "more of what we have" with innovative design.

Due to single occupancy requirements new hospitals need innovative solutions

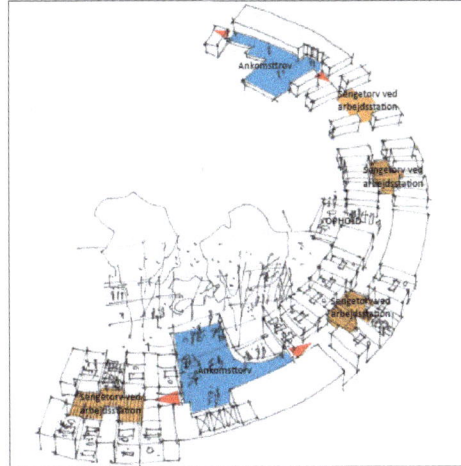

31. *Herlev Hospital, extension.*

31

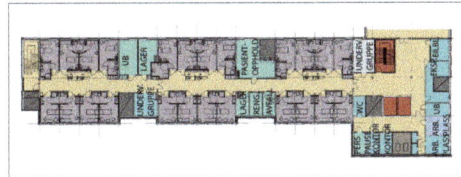

32. *St. Olavs Hospital.*

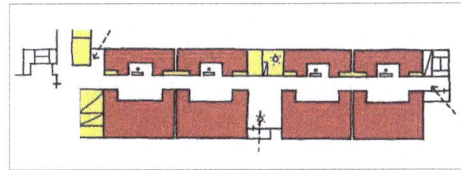

33. *Nye Ahus.*

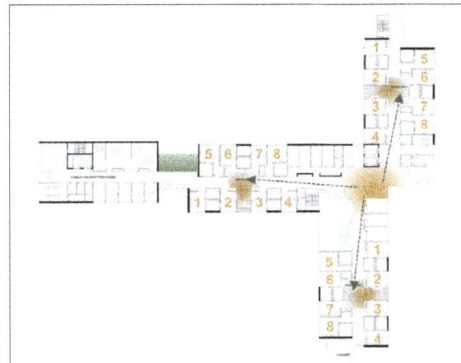

34. *Aarhus Universitetshospital, DNU I/S, C. F. Møller Architects.*

TESIS Inter-University Research Centre "Systems and Technologies for Social and Healthcare Facilities"
University of Florence, Italy

TESIS

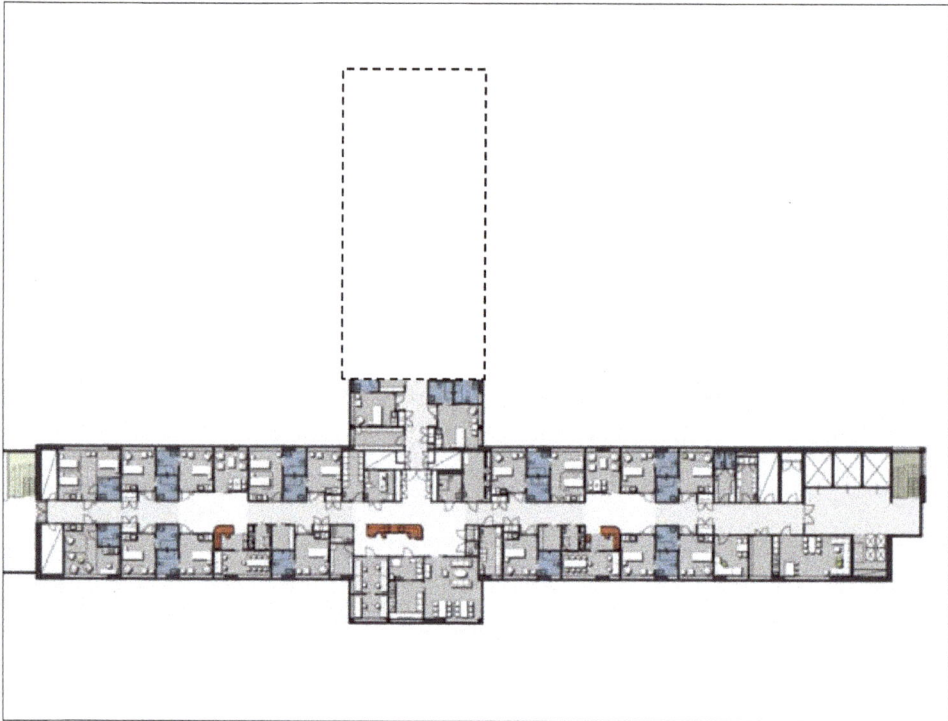

35. Tehuset, Borås, extension, Sweco Architects.

to avoid isolation and increased travel distances, costs and use of space.

The new bed clusters are designed to avoid isolation and minimize staff walking distances in single occupancy areas. At St. Olavs Hospital this solution was created without space expansion.

Hospital staff and planners have a blind spot concerning patient views and needs. If the goal is to create a patient-oriented hospital, the patient must be represented as an equal in all parts of the planning and design processes, representing patient perspectives and priorities.

This is often neglected and other less challenging solutions are chosen with lesser results:

- political visions of patient focus;
- non-binding ideas workshops, public meetings, etc;
- non-binding involvement in parts of the planning process;
- the adoption of evidence-based design criteria in planning;
- patient security reports and representatives.

These are good but not sufficient to secure new patient-oriented solutions. Priorities often change when under pressure, but patient experiences and views are necessary all the way. Some main patient concerns include increased protection of privacy during hospital stays (among other single patient rooms), easy

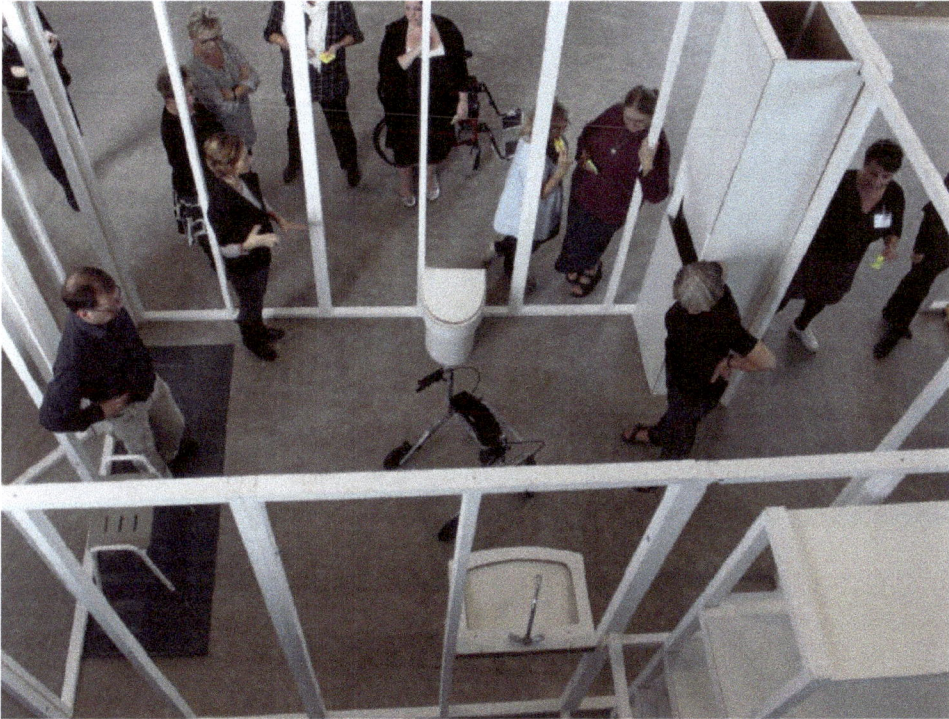

36. *Centre for user-focused innovation.*

access to staff (open receptions, open ward stations, etc.) and accessibility for all users/patient groups by applying universal design. Just as for staff participation, training is needed for patient participants so they can act professionally in representing the patient perspective.

In the last 15 years it has been possible to assist and witness a great rise in the quality of technology, the understanding of patient perspectives and the value of the hospital environment. In conclusion, the future challenge for hospital design is how to include and integrate broader perspectives of hospital buildings, from the macro environment (sustainability) to the micro environment (senses).

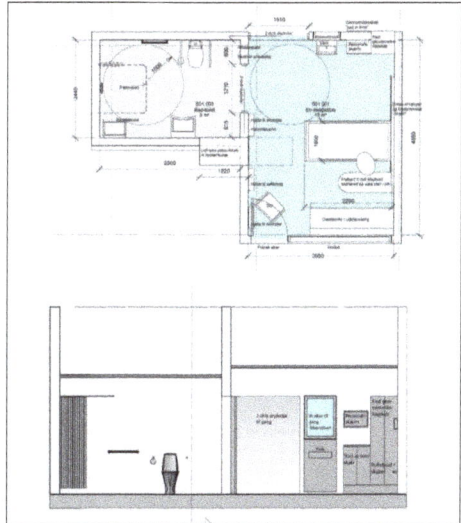

37. *Centre for user-focused innovation, plant and section. New Karolinska, Stockholm 2017.*

1. *New Karolinska Solna, aerial view.*

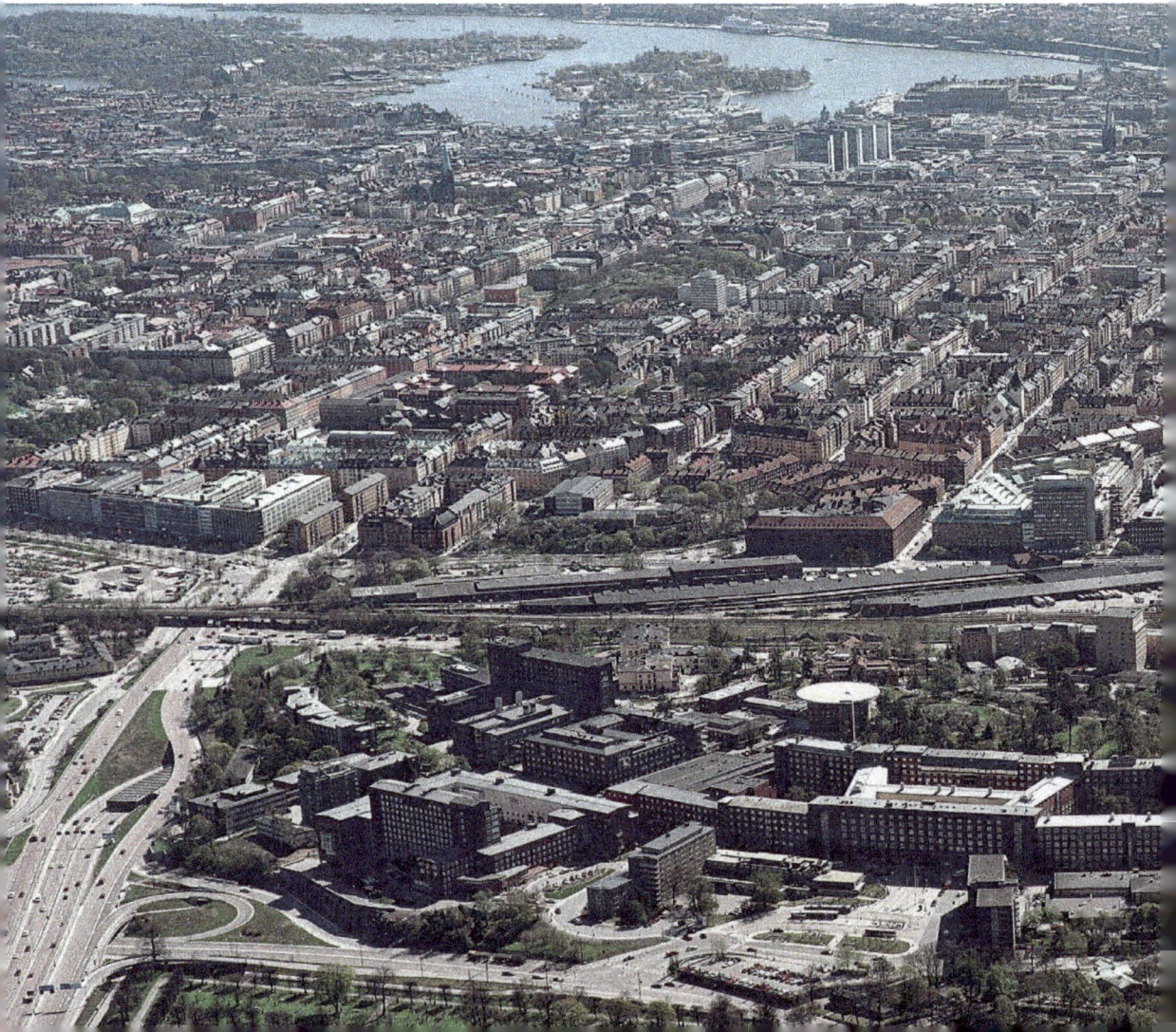

Nya Karolinska Solna - Sweden

Christine Hammarling and Charlotte Ruben
Healthcare Architects White Tengbom Team

35

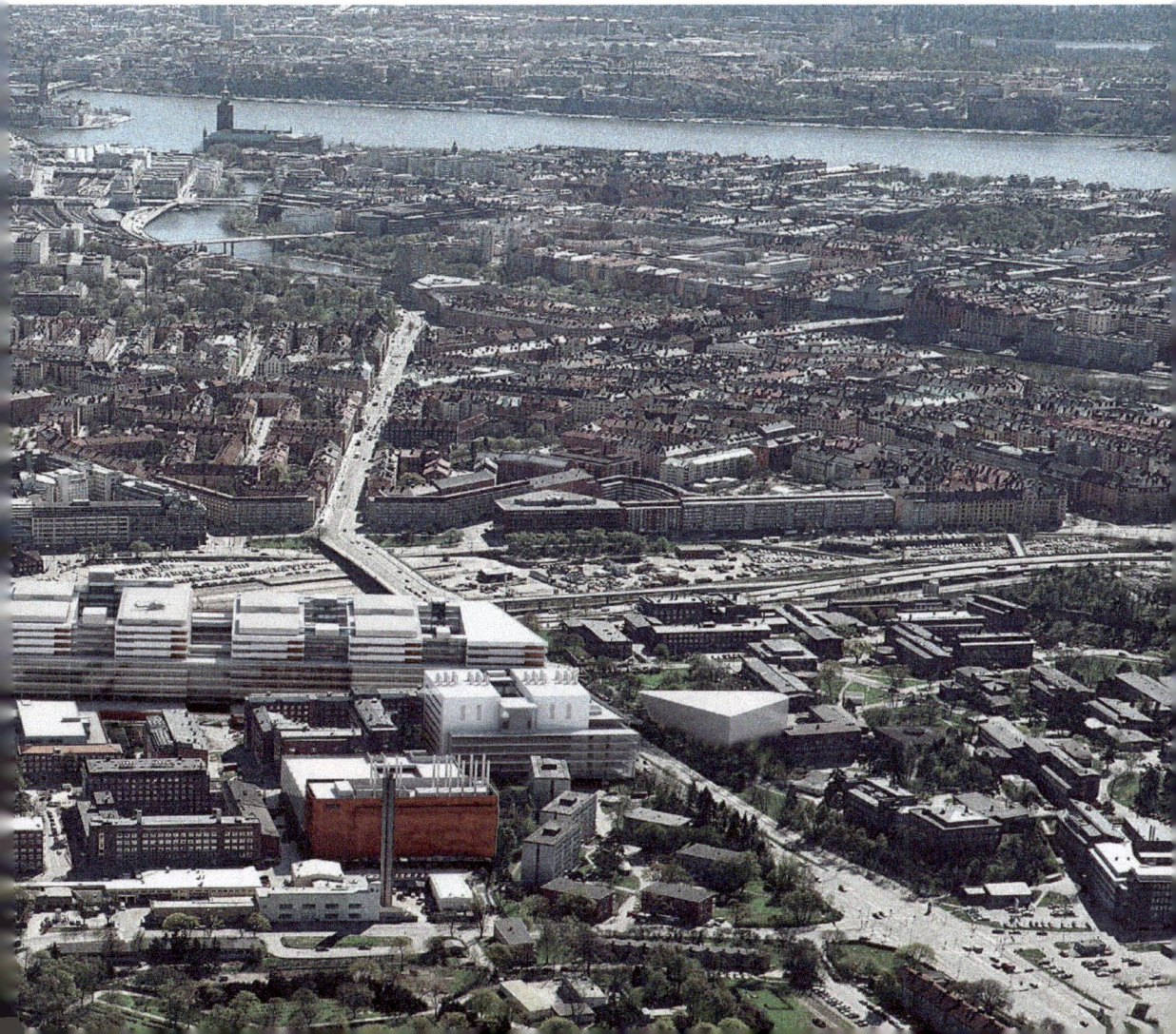

The design of the Nya Karolinska Solna[1] is in line with the Swedish Healthcare objectives which provide for easily accessible local healthcare, qualified specialized care and efficient acute care.

The Swedish Healthcare system serves 9 million inhabitants and operates through 7 university hospitals, 70 regional hospitals and 1000 local healthcare centers.

Stockholm, with its 2 million inhabitants, is the area with the highest concentration of people across the country.

The Nya Karolinska Solna is a part of a larger project entitled Stockholm Life Science, which provides for the integration of four centres of knowledge around Karolinska Hospital: Stockholm University, the Royal Institute of Technology, the School of Economics and Karolinska Institute.

The Stockholm Life Science project consists of a new hospital of 320,000 m², 5,000 apartments and 36,000 workspaces.

36

1 Client: Stockholm County Council
Building Proprietor: Swedish Hospital Partners
Building Contractor: Skanska Healthcare AB
Facility Management: Coor Service Management
Architect: White Tengbom Team
Structural Engineer: Skanska Teknik / Ramböll
Mechanical/electrical/plumbing: SWECO / ÅF

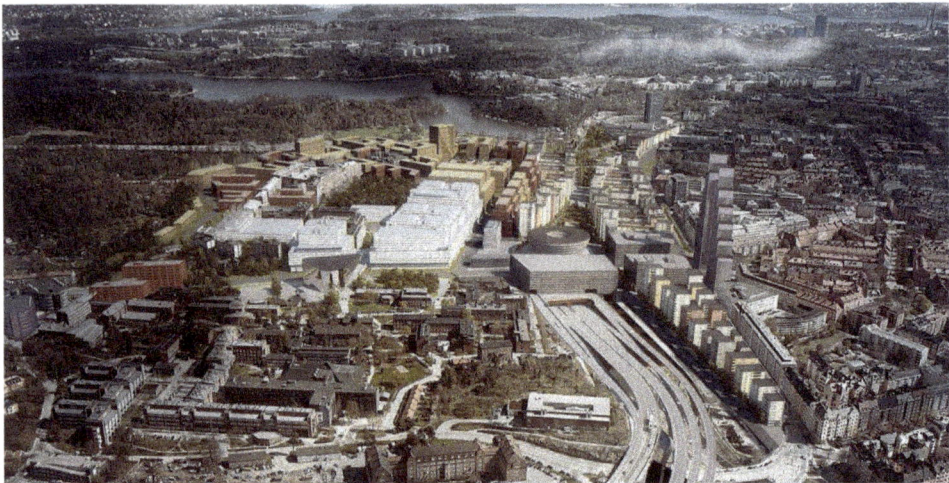

1. New Karolinska Solna, aerial view.

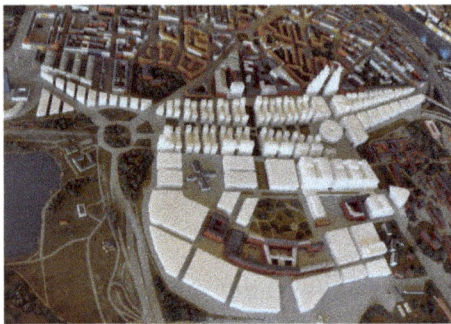

2. Stockholm Life Science.

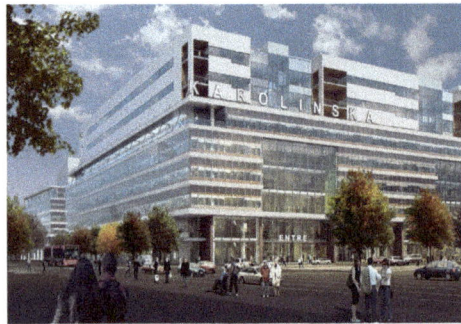

3. Karolinska University Hospital.

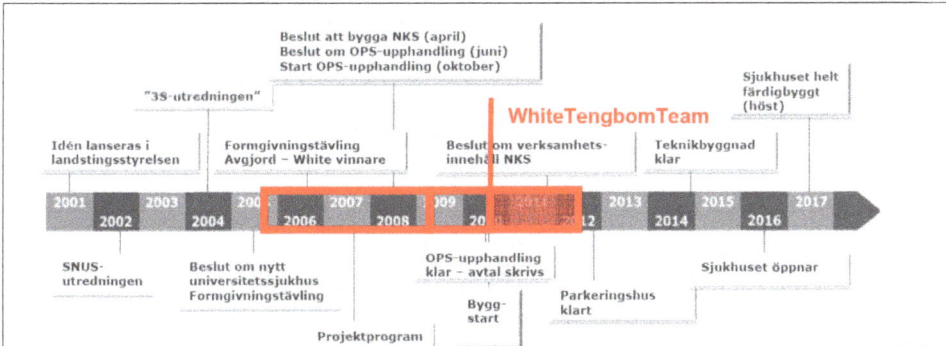

4. The building process.

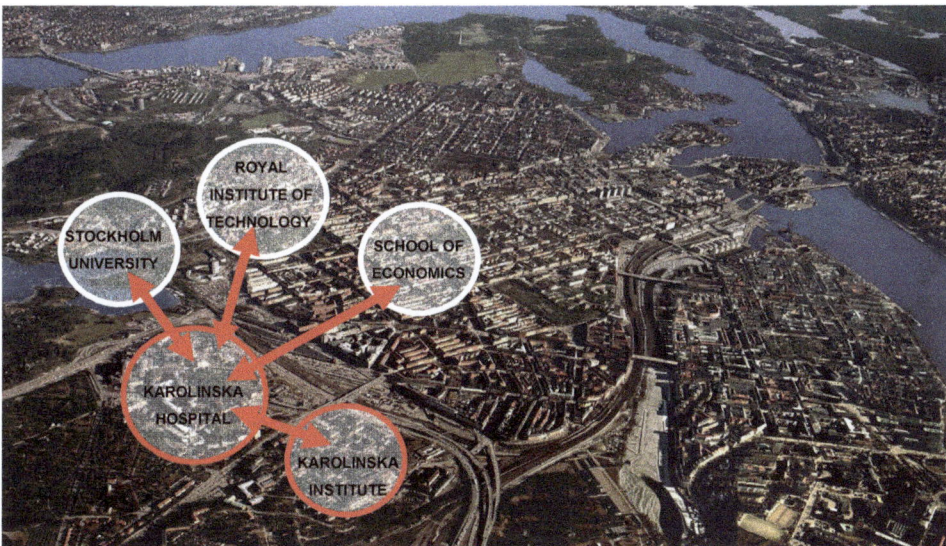

5. Stockholm Life Science.

The project for the New Karolinska Solna aims by 2025 to provide 228,000 m² for treatment areas, 41,000 m² for laboratories, 17,000 m² for technical support, 7,000 m² for a patient hotel, 27,000 m² for parking, for a total of 320,000 m²; furthermore there will be 170 outpatient rooms.

In the Nya Karolinska Solna project the client is Stockholm County Council and the building contractor is Skanska Healthcare AB; the project covers a total floor area of 320,000 m² at a cost of SEK 14.5 billion (USD 2.4 billion). The work is scheduled to be carried out in 2016-17. The Nya Karolinska Solna is the world's largest PPP hospital (25-year contract) and Sweden's first.

The White Tengbom Team was involved in the construction process from 2005 to 2012 with the main aim of creating a sustainable structure.

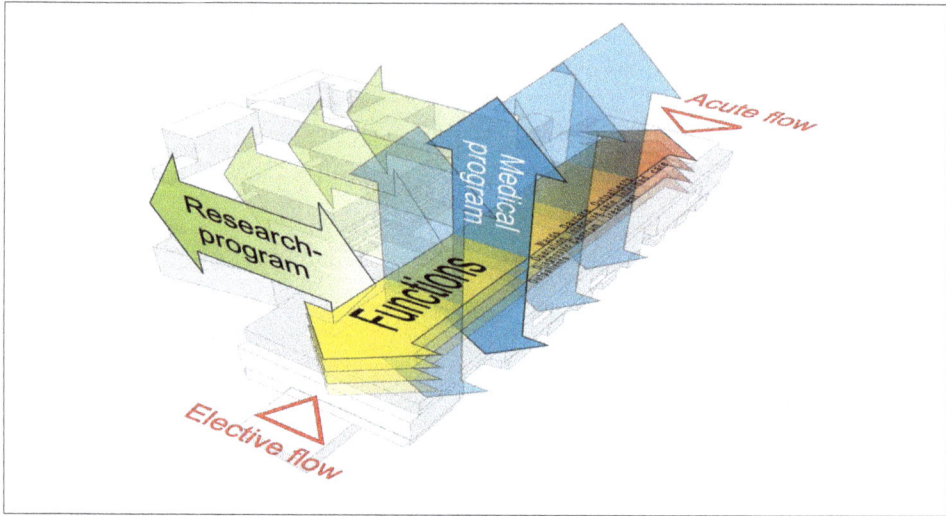

6. Organization.

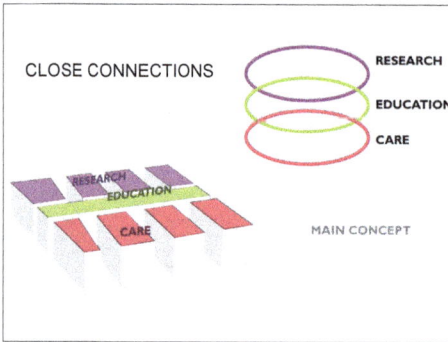

7. Close connections.

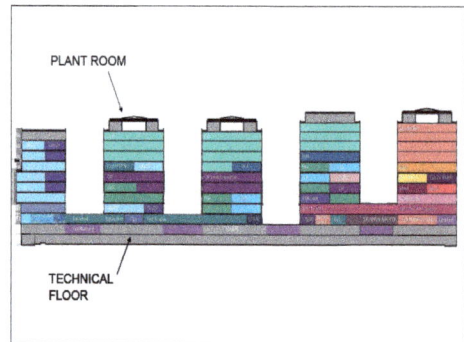

8. Vertical organization.

The main project goals were:
1. integration between medical care, research and education;
2. attractive human environments with high architectonic values;
3. efficient care processes and the optimized utilization of resources;
4. general solutions that permit the continuous development of activities;
5. a clear role in the city;
6. sustainability perspective on all levels.

The main concept is close connections between research, education and care, and this is expressed through close relationships and a high level of integration.

The scope of the project is:
- +100 daycare beds, +100 beds in a patient hotel;
- 600 care units (400 inpatient single rooms, 100 daycare units, 100-125 outpatient units, 100 beds in a patient hotel);
- 125 ICU beds;
- 35 operating theatres;

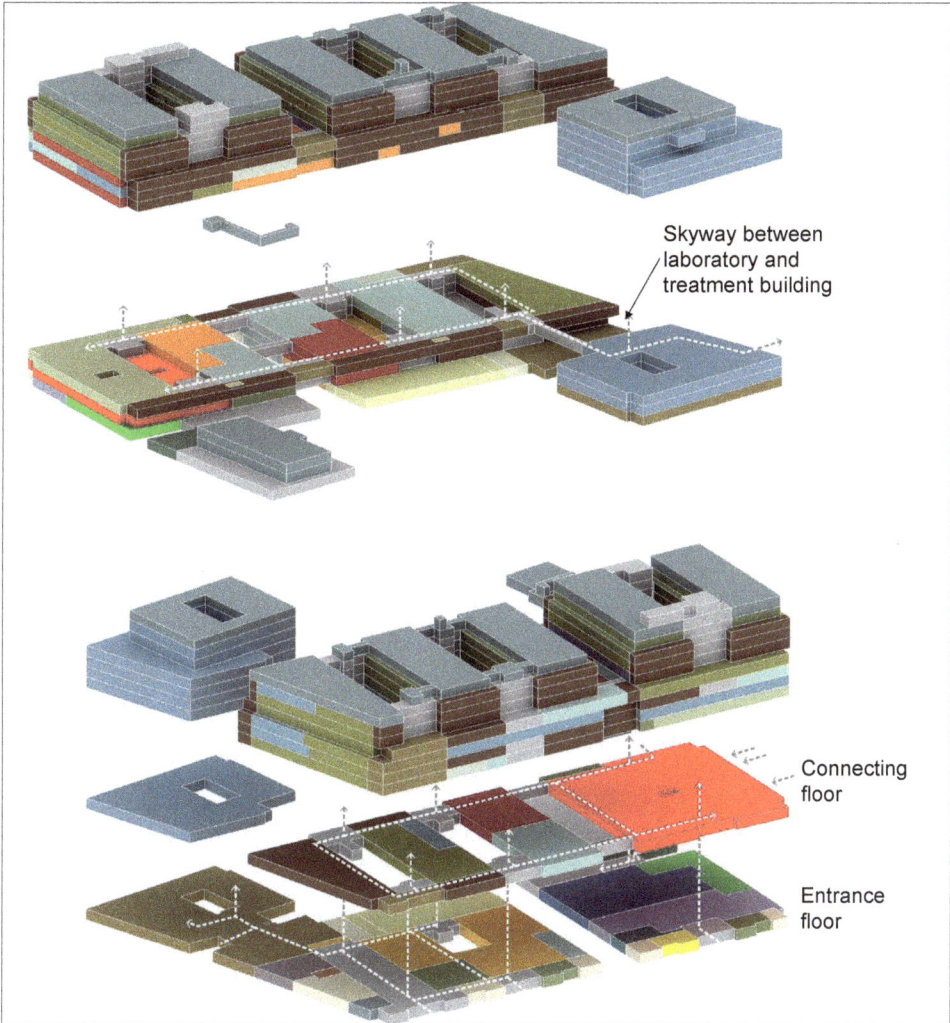

Skyway between laboratory and treatment building

Connecting floor

Entrance floor

9. Organization.

- 8,600 m² for diagnostics;
- 8 bunkers (radiology);
- accident and emergency department (175 patients/day);
- 50,000 m² for research (laboratories);
- 1,200 car parking spaces (with the opportunity to expand).

The buildings are organized in three main directions: horizontal, vertical and crosswise. In the horizontal direction the areas are arranged to accommodate the elective flow at one end and the acute flow at the other.

Functions organized in the horizontal direction include: wards, daycare and outpatients; operations, intensive care and intermediate care; diagnostic centrum / treatment; and outpatients.

TESIS Inter-University Research Centre "Systems and Technologies for Social and Healthcare Facilities"
University of Florence, Italy

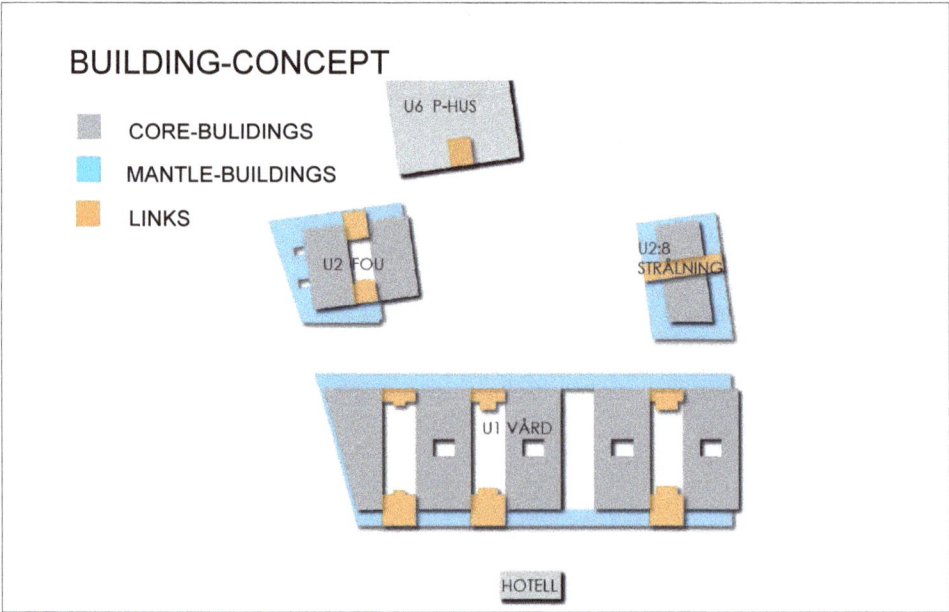

10. *Building concept scheme.*

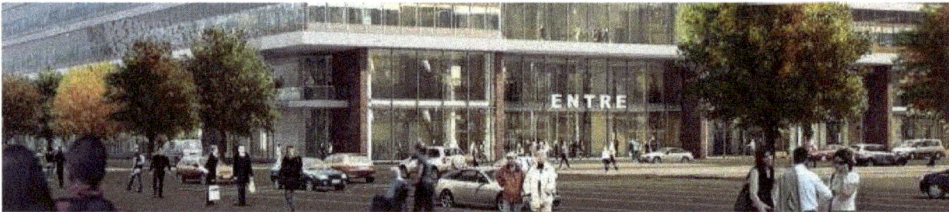

11. *Main entrance.*

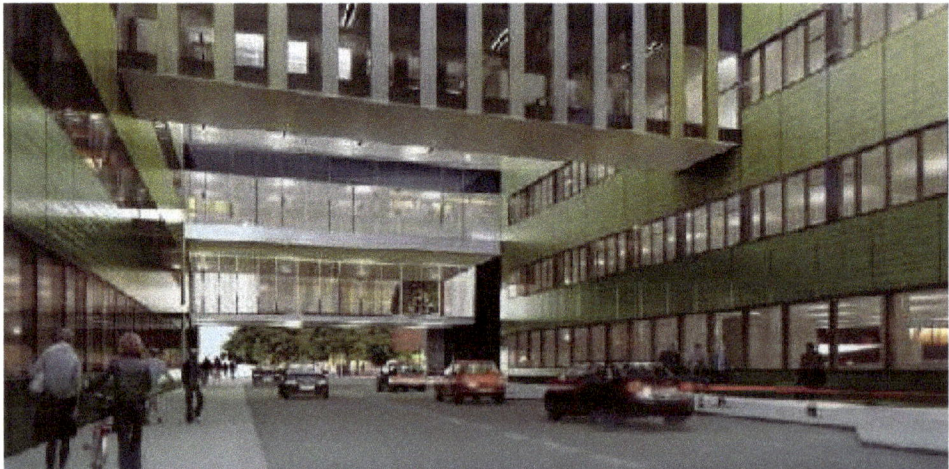

12. *Gävlegatan.*

The vertical direction is dedicated to the medical program and the crosswise direction to the research program. The top floor is used as a plant room and the basement as a technical floor. Above the entrance floor is a higher-level connecting floor with a skyway between the laboratory and the treatment building.

The project is characterized by a close connection between the exterior and the interior. The architecture enhances the natural light with its transparent surfaces and project features include the presence of inviting spaces and urban integration with a typical Scandinavian design approach. The hospital is part of the city and therefore it is accessible and has many entrances, as well as an improved and diversified street level.

The buildings are composed of three parts: core areas, mantle areas and linking areas. The cores contain "hot floors" (treatment and research); the mantle areas are support zones (admin/education), and the linking areas connect the hospital with public environments (entry hall, waiting lounges).

A general and flexible structure was de-signed through the creation of multidisciplinary environments. The buildings are designed to maintain a separate flow of elective and emergency patients.

Base building

A general and standardized structure provides flexibility in how the areas are used; the base building module is repeated and constitutes the invariable and constant part of the building. It is composed of shafts, staircases, AGV-stations, an environmental room, MEP, pneumatic tube systems, toilets, and has a baring capacity of 10kgN/sqm and a floor-to-floor height of 4.9 m.

Buildings are organized into efficient and separate flows: the ambulatory and emergency areas have different elevators and staircases from the visitor and staff flows.

Interior design is 100% patient-focused with single-patient rooms, mobile diagnostic equipment and multidisciplinary teams.

Daylight and views are aspects that connote the public environment. Scandina-

41

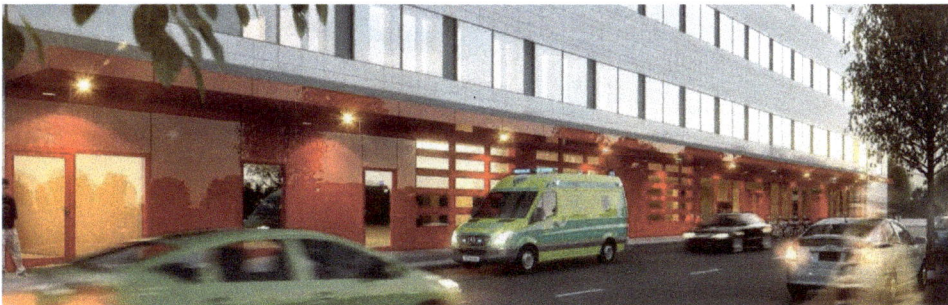

13. *Emergency entrance.*

TESIS Inter-University Research Centre "Systems and Technologies for Social and Healthcare Facilities"
University of Florence, Italy

42

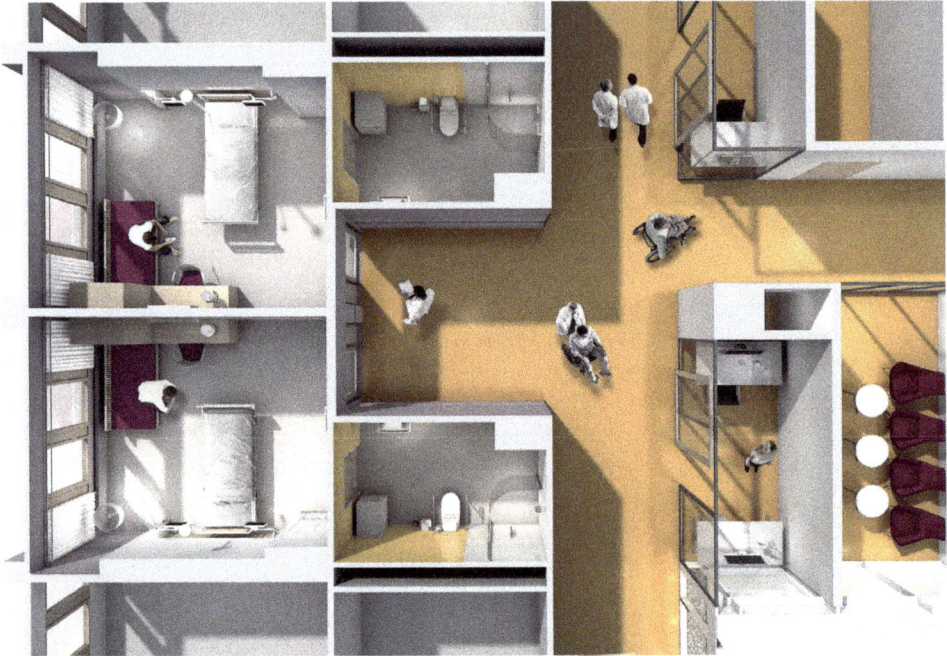

14. General and flexible structure in a multidisciplinary environment.

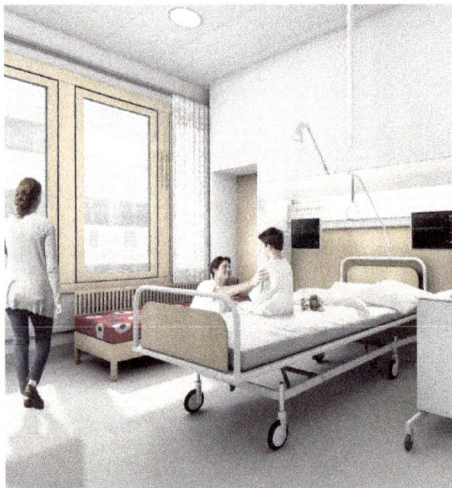

15. The ward.

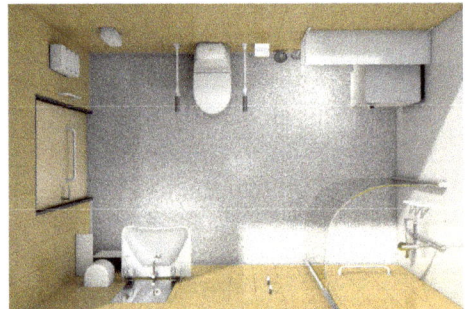

16. Individual hygiene room/unit.

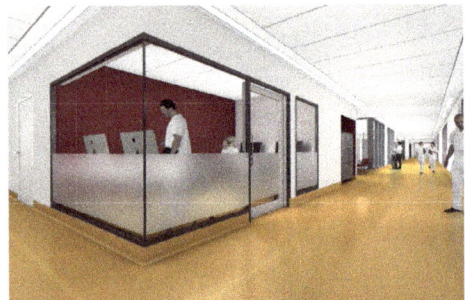

17. Reception.

vian sustainable design is applied using natural materials such as glass, steel, wood and stone, and the project is inspired by typical landscapes and changing seasons.

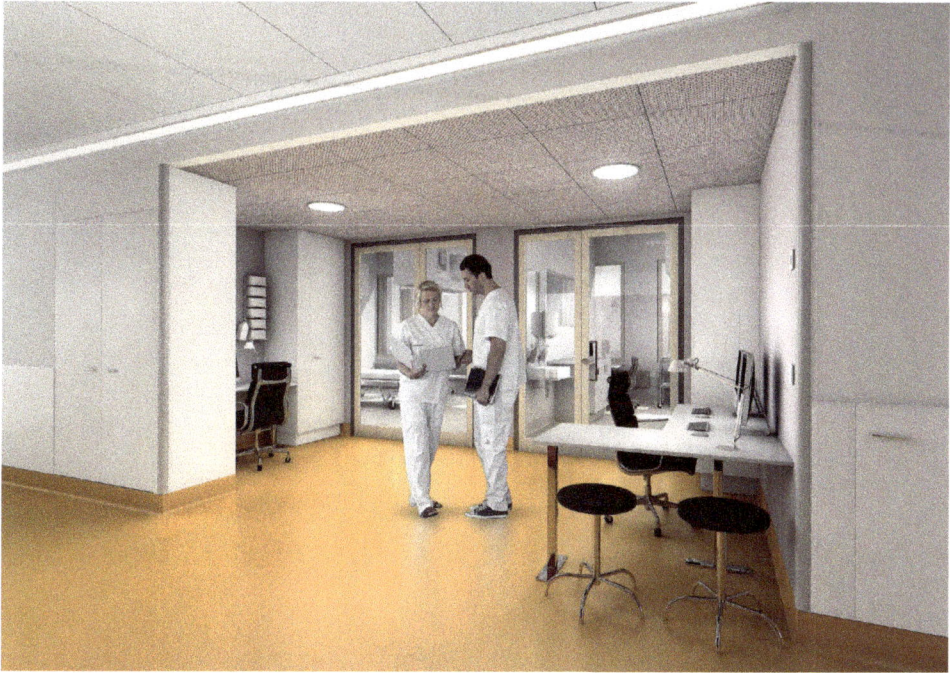

18. *Workstation.*

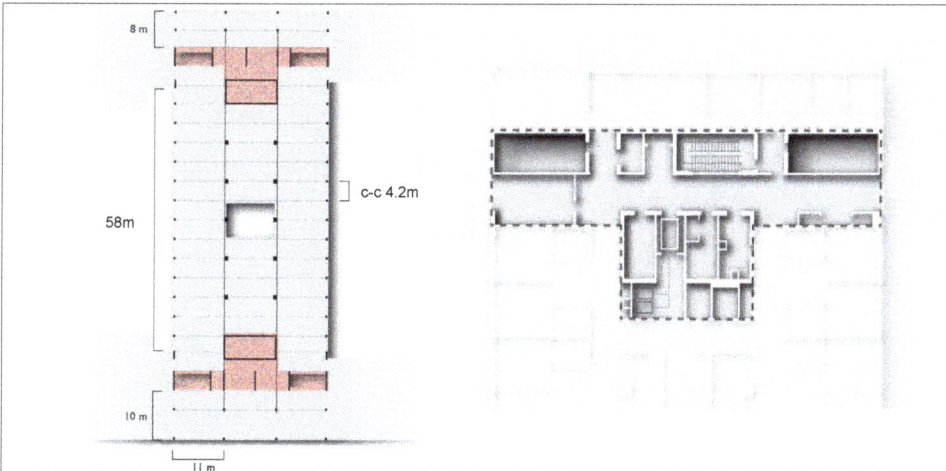

19. *A general and standardized structure, base building.*

The project aimed to create a sustainable hospital, and to this end the following strategies were applied: sustainable site (public transportation system); climate neutral (100% renewable energy); local energy production (120 boreholes); energy efficient buildings (110kWh/kvm); gold classification for energy, the indoor environment, materials and thermal heating.

44

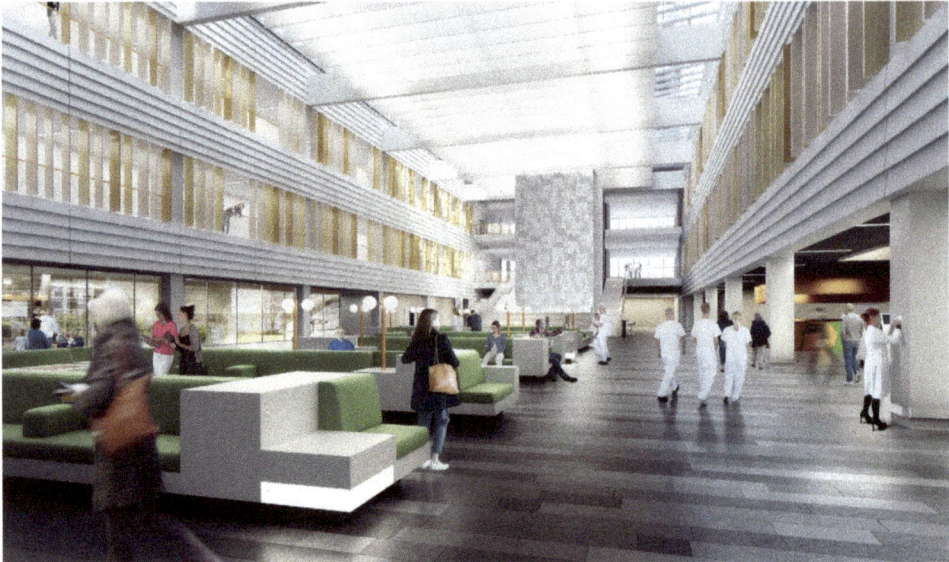

20. *Public environment: atrium.*

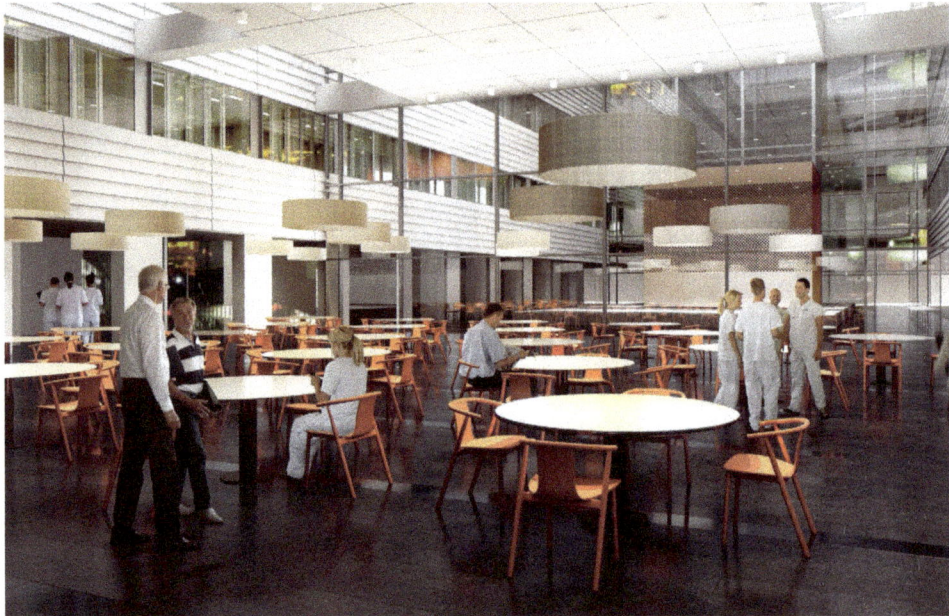

21. *Public environment: restaurant.*

The White Tengbom Team believes in the importance of the health-promoting effects of architecture and in a holistic mindset – urban planning and clinical design, by designing general and flexible buildings with attractive environments for patients and staff and providing efficient and sustainable solutions.

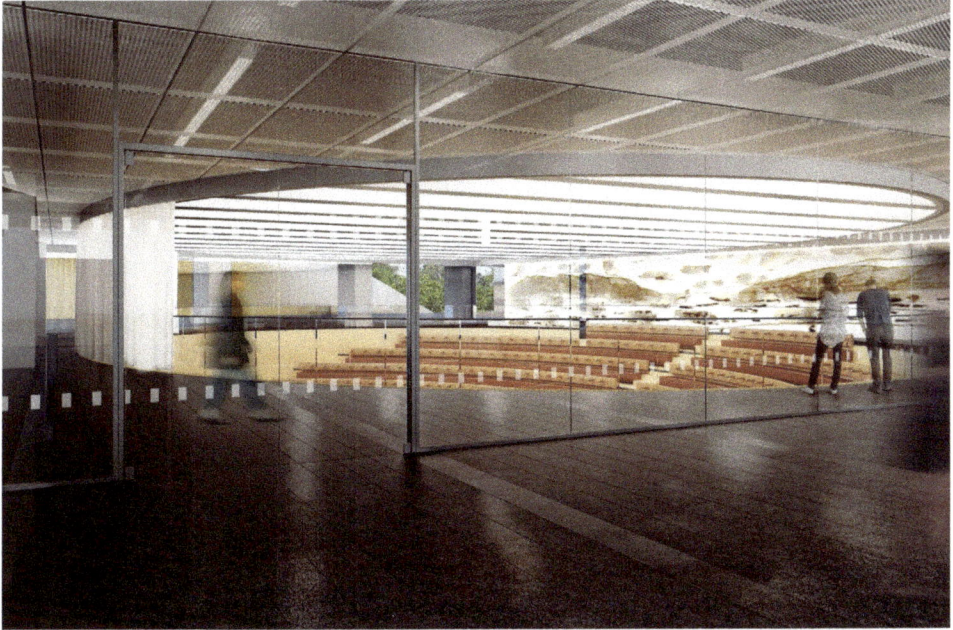

22. *Public environment: auditorium.*

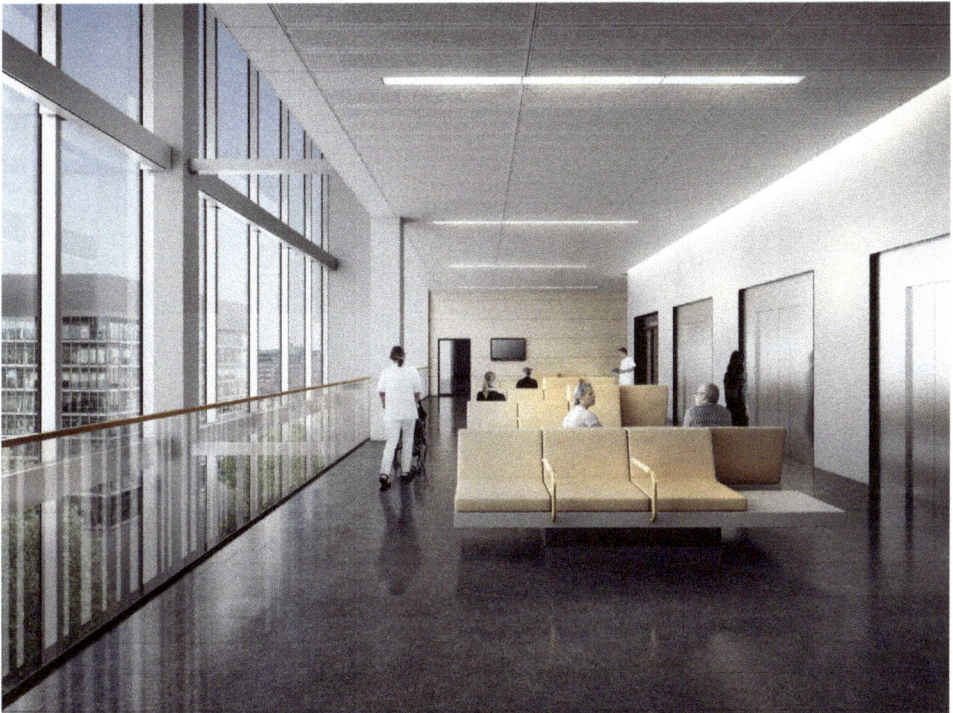

23. *Public environment: waiting area.*

TESIS Inter-University Research Centre "Systems and Technologies for Social and Healthcare Facilities"
University of Florence, Italy

1. *New hospital in Gødstrup - Denmark.*

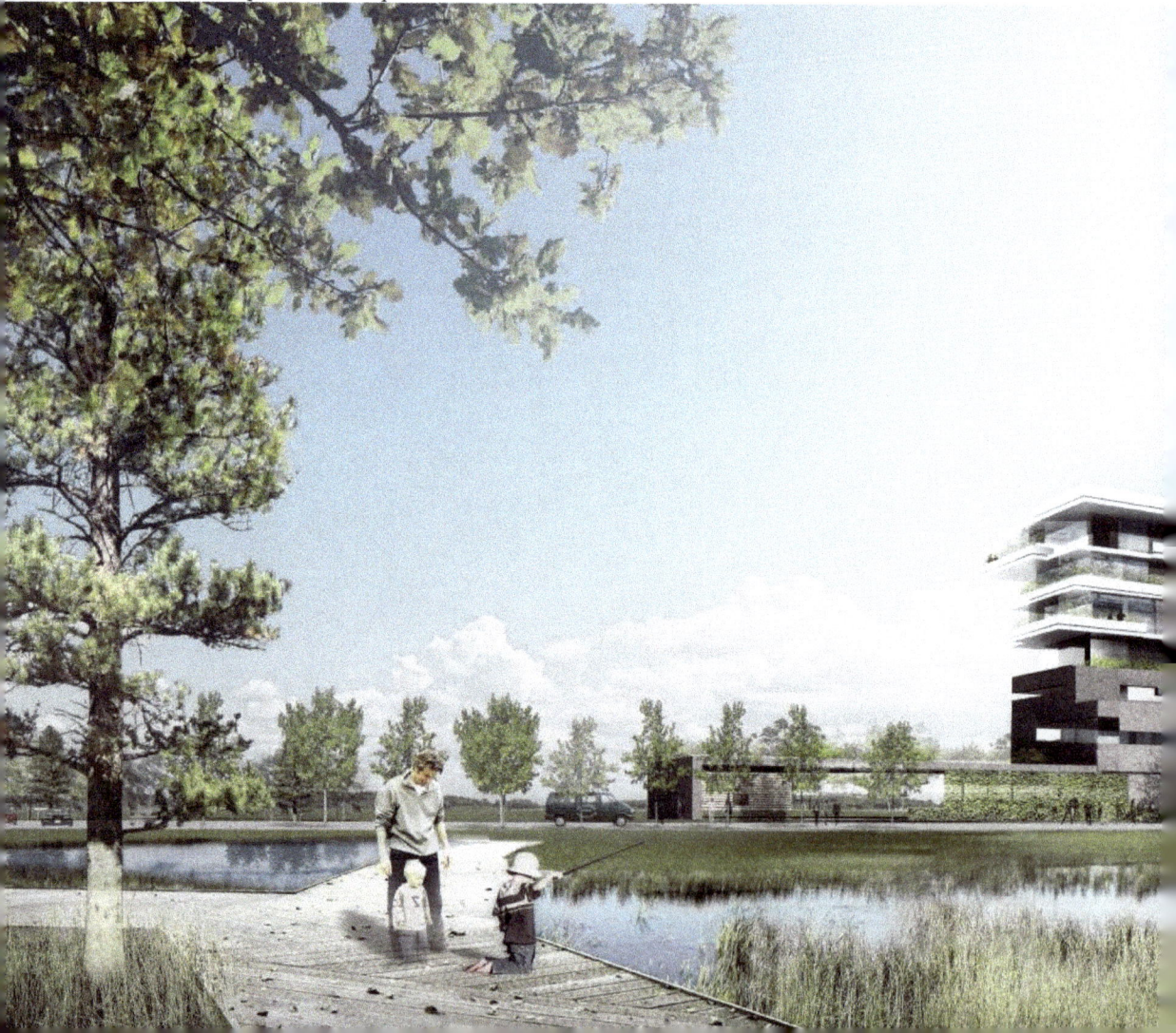

New Hospital in Gødstrup - Denmark

John Arne Bjerknes
Partner NSW Arkitekter & Planleggere

47

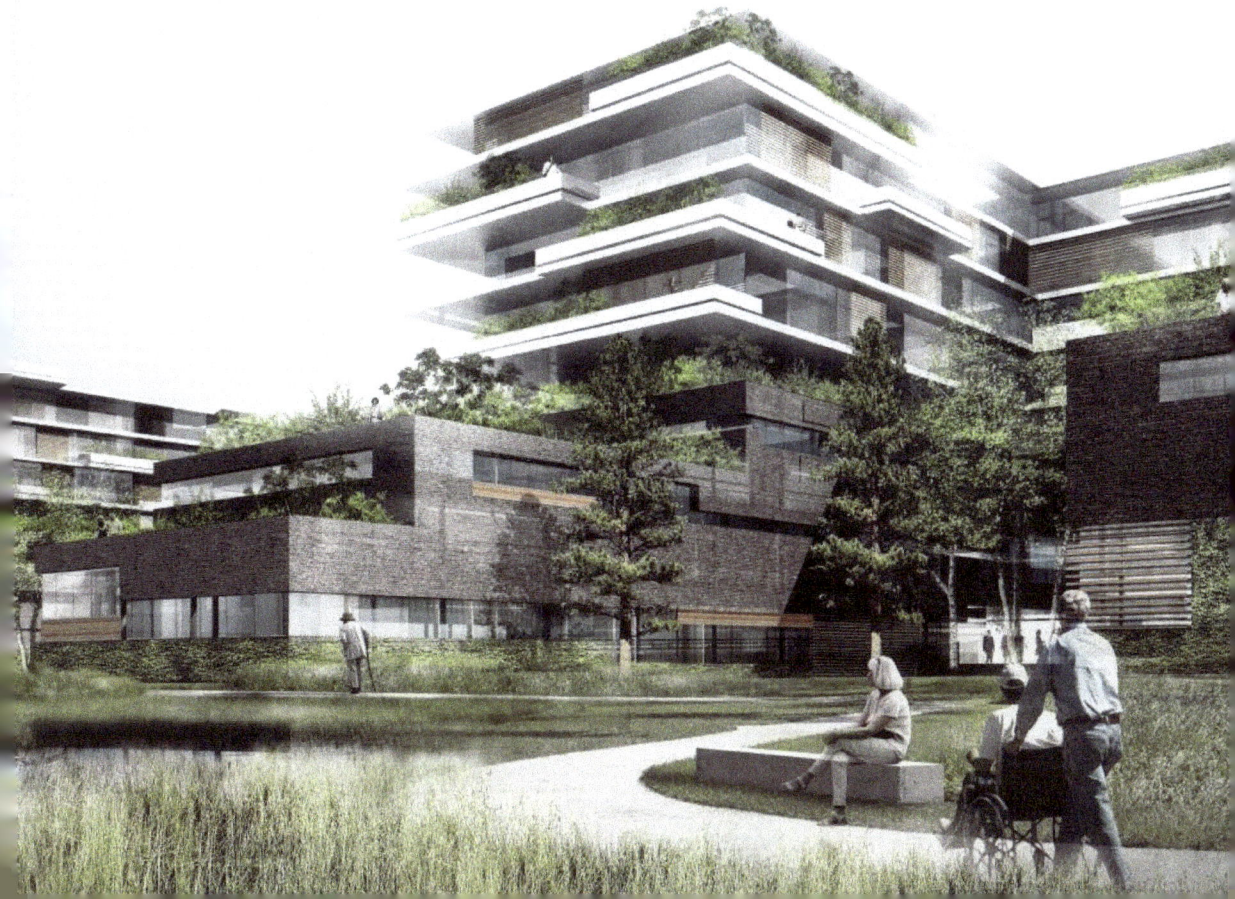

In November 2010 the Central Denmark Region launched a competitive program for 6 prequalified consortia. The competition was held in 2 stages, with the first phase in the spring of 2011. Two projects went ahead and the 2nd phase of the competition, the final, was held over the summer. The winning project[1] is described in this paper: a tough and highly exciting competition process that lasted a whole summer.

The theme of the competition was to design a very complex hospital in large building lots. The competition raised issues related to the pragmatic and functional distribution of the areas. At the same time the need for humanized environments was expressed in relation to form versus function. The design issue was how to create functionality and beauty at the same time and therefore

1 DNV Gødstrup – architecture, functionality, logistics
John Arne Bjerknes, partner, CEO – Johannes Eggen, partner,NSW Arkitekter & Planleggere AS
CuraVita consists of the architectural companies AART Architects, NSW Arkitekter & Planleggere, Grontmij, Moe & Brødsgaard and Hospitalitet.
Arup is also associated as a sub-consultant

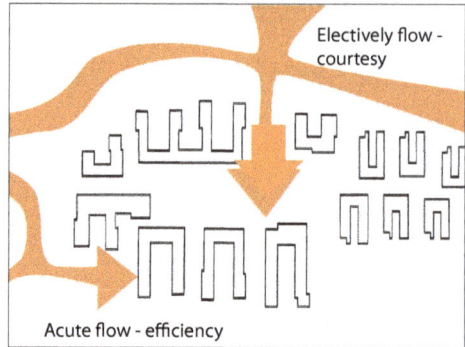

2. The hospital layout is simple and straightforward: there are different entrances for acute and elective patients.

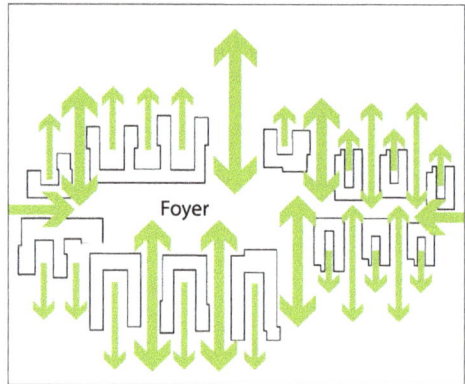

3. The base edge is constructed in a north-south direction with respect to the landscape; fingers radiate into the ground.

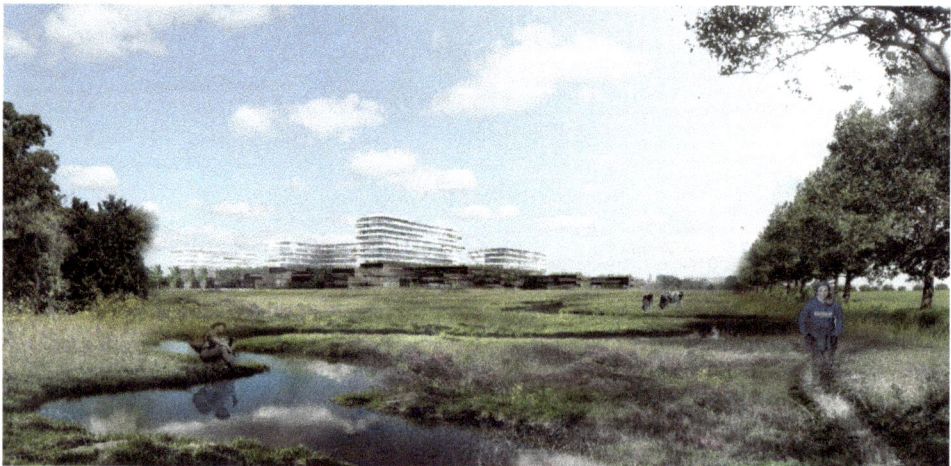

4. Architectural concept: integration of the hospital with the landscape.

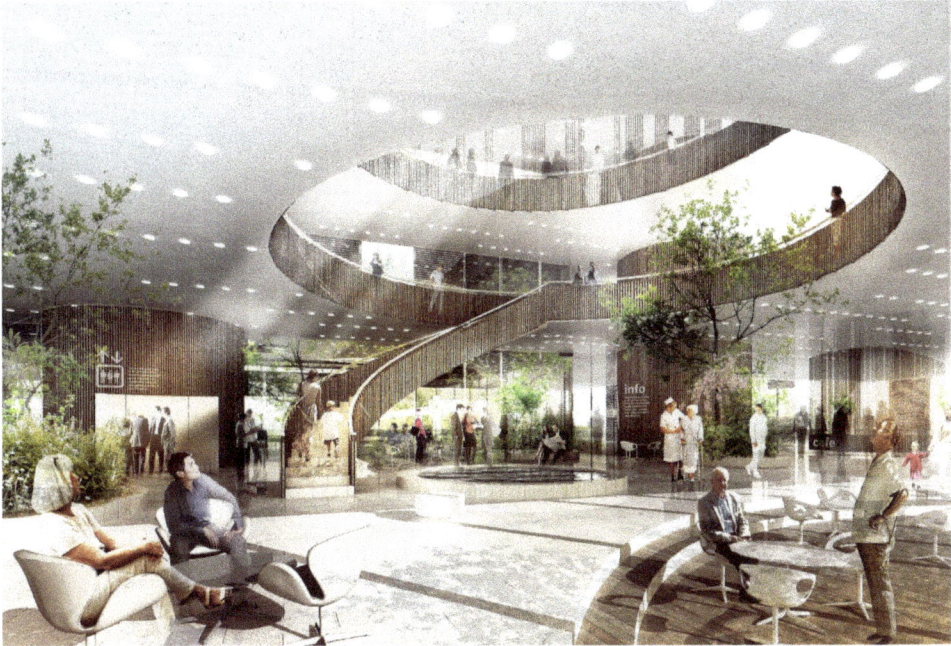

5. *The foyer is the central compartment with clearly marked routes and contact with the green atrium; it is spacious, friendly and welcoming.*

how this issue can become an architectural and professional challenge.

The design group tried to bring ordinary and positive qualities from housing design into the healthcare building. They worked with scale, materials and some of the fundamental architectural virtues of the profession.

They believe that hospital design should encompass functional and sensory aspects, and this idea is comprehensive and essential in architecture for humans. Hospitals are handicrafts on a very large scale. Applied art is characterized by functionality and form/architecture, which are mutually reinforcing and not contradictory. So far, the Central Denmark Region has seen the design group through the competition phase; the next steps are design and execution. The clinical structure and location of the func-

tions are orderly and rational. The building plan is compact and this minimizes walking distances for staff and saves operating and labor costs as well as energy. This was a goal and an important design parameter from the start.

The concept of the hospital is new for the design team. Prior to this competition the design team had gained extensive experience in the design of low building structures such as Skejby Hospital. They were also familiar with high-rise bedward towers such as those of Herlev or Aalborg. In this project the design team did something else.

The hospital's main functions are:
- outpatient clinics
- treatment options
- wards
- laboratories.

Outpatient clinics are located on the

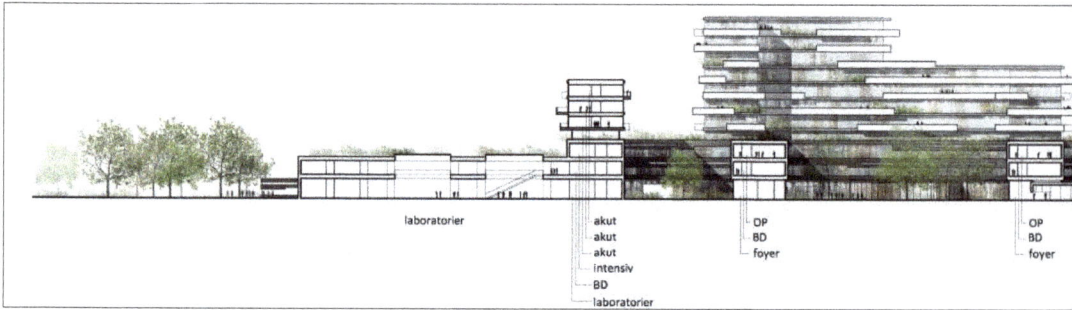

laboratorier

akut
akut
akut
intensiv
BD
laboratorier

OP
BD
foyer

OP
BD
foyer

50   *6. Architecture - overall section.*

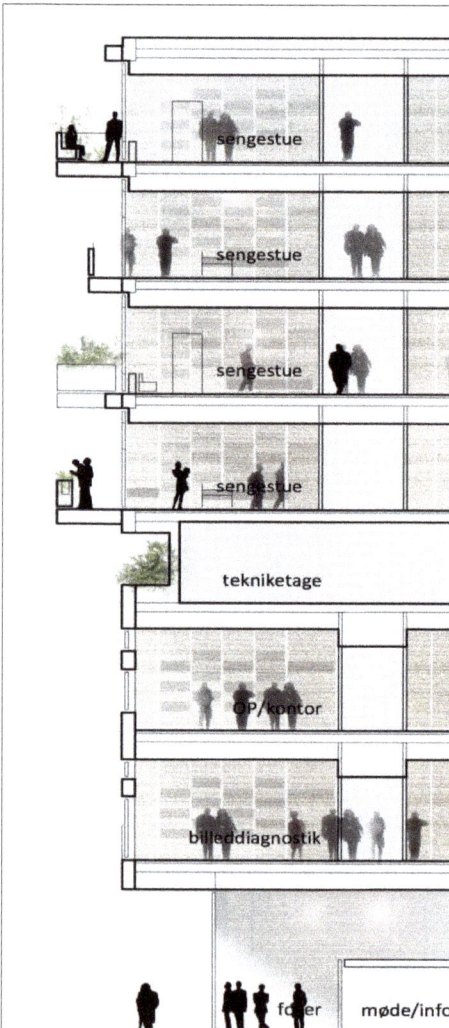

sengestue

sengestue

sengestue

sengestue

tekniketage

OP/kontor

billeddiagnostik

foyer   møde/info

7. Architecture - detail of section.

ground floor, imaging and operating theaters are located above the central foyer, and wards are located upstairs. The central foyer is not a gate, a limitation or a closed façade, but rather a glass envelope open to the natural landscape on both sides, such as a path through a garden. It has many functional and architectural benefits.

The design group sought inspiration from:
- the landscape's vastness and horizontality;
- the ease of the unbroken skyline;
- the living fence and precision directions.

The landscape inspired the design with a simple and straightforward architectural concept.

The hospital has a heavy base where outpatient clinics, imaging and surgery areas are located. The base anchors the hospital to the site and ensures flexibility and elasticity. Wards float as slices above the base. This ensures a very robust concept that can accommodate changes and adaptations over time. The layout is simple and straightforward. The main entrance is on the north side. The desire for a clear layout and to provide clear elective and acute flows has been achieved. Each cluster will have separate building sections.

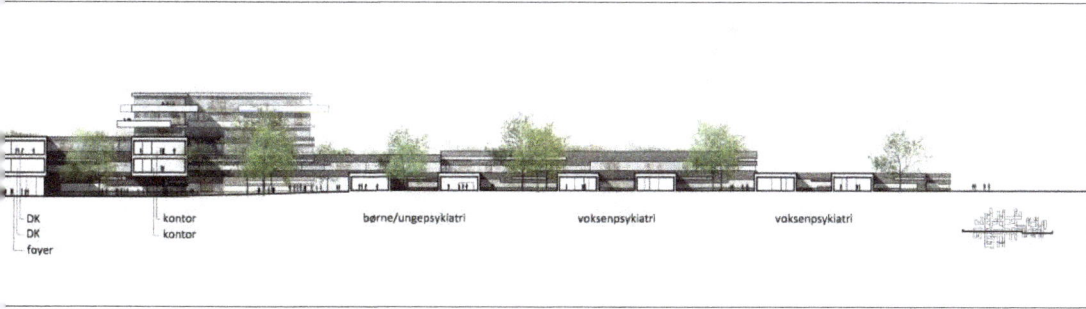

DK
DK
foyer
kontor
kontor
børne/ungepsykiatri
voksenpsykiatri
voksenpsykiatri

51

The base edge is constructed in a north-south direction with respect to the landscape; fingers radiate into the ground and between them the landscape penetrates the foyer in its entirety.

A user-friendly and comfortable feel is created in the environments through the use of partitions in rustic oak, clear signage and wayfinding, and lots of green inside and out.
The foyer is the central compartment with clearly marked routes and contact with the green atrium; it is spacious, friendly and welcoming.

The psychiatry cluster has a clear layout: the wards are located on the ground floor, the outpatient clinics are on the first floor and there is good visibility for staff and various options for shielding.

The architecture has stronger materiality and the transition between the buildings and the landscape is lobed and varied. The base is a brick masonry construction with relief and there are several oak slats that add acoustic variation.
The façade of the bed wards has a layer of terraces and narrow service balconies on the outside of the envelope. The inside is clad respectively and covered with planks of oak.

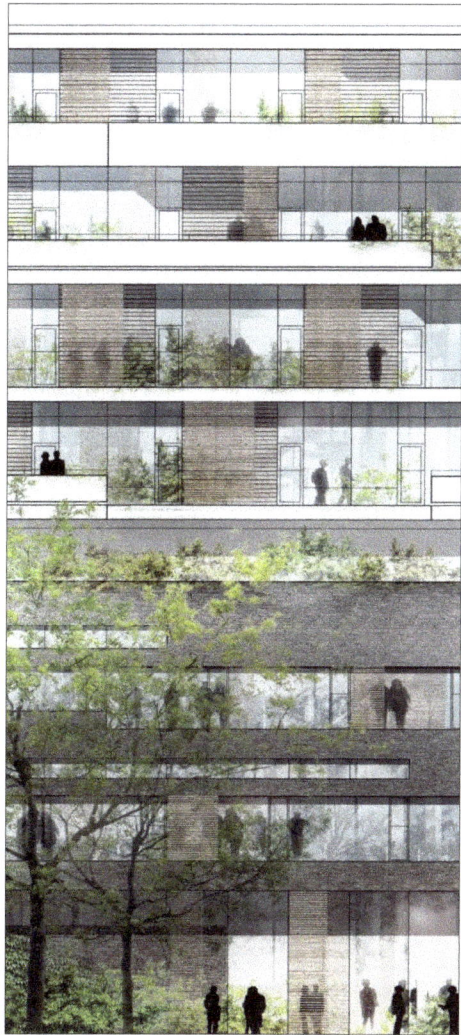

8. Architecture - façades.

TESIS Inter-University Research Centre "Systems and Technologies for Social and Healthcare Facilities"
University of Florence, Italy

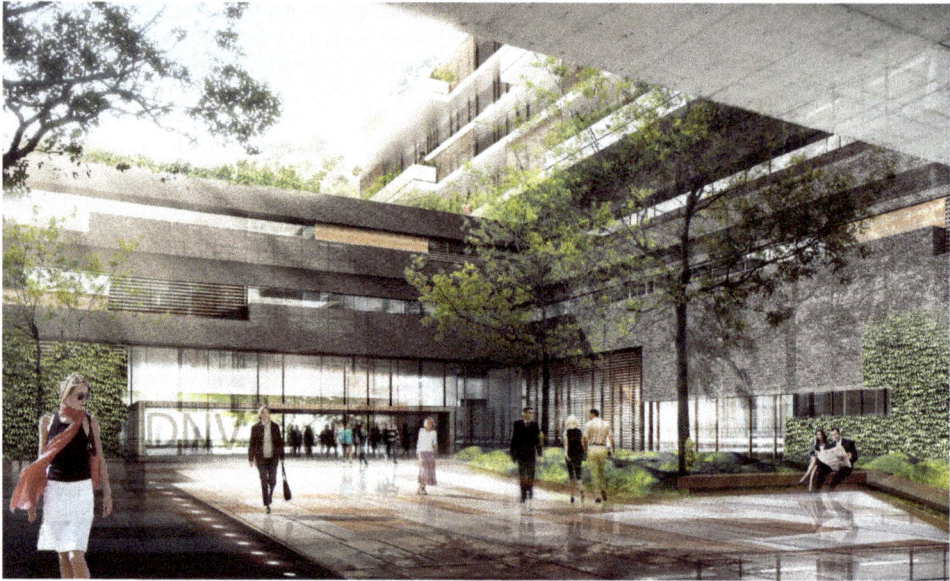

9. The main entrance is scaled down and has a different feel, tactile and sensory.

The main entrance is scaled down and has a different feel, tactile and sensory.

The project includes a wide range of passive and active measures: 2015 Energy Class, compact building body, sun protection, high daylight factor, efficient building envelope, demand-controlled ventilation, smart lighting, etc.

Countryside and hospital

The landscape architecture reinforces the existing forest features and hedgerows through paths and water elements.

Architecture – Façades

Horizontal bands of windows, with varied parapet and skirt heights, depending on the underlying functional distribution, is the recurring motif which is interrupted by a floor with a prevalence of glass at the entrances, seating areas and lobby area.

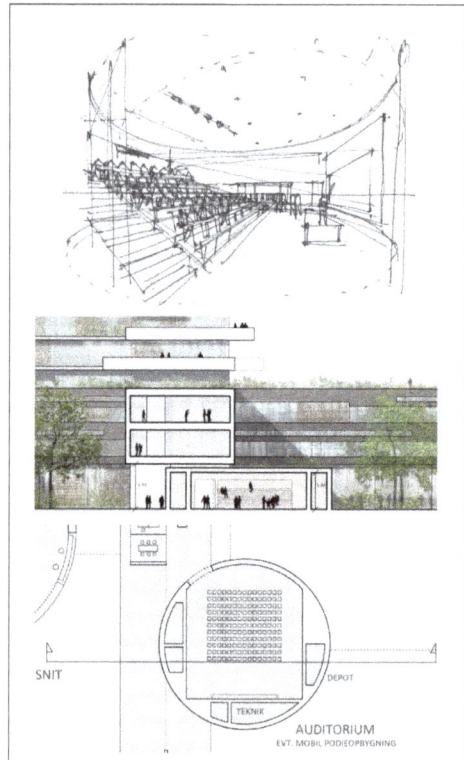

10. Auditorium.

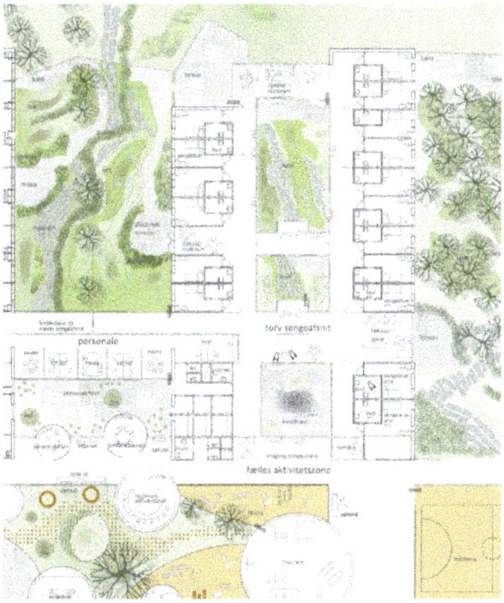

11. *Psychiatry cluster.*

Concept

The project qualities are:
- a compact and functional concept;
- a robust and adaptable project;
- a clear and orderly layout, wayfinding;
- a building that fits into the landscape;
- human architectural expression and quality materials;
- sustainable and energy-optimized solutions.

Arrivals

The new arrivals entrance significantly improves accessibility. Parking has been moved closer to the entrance and is lo-

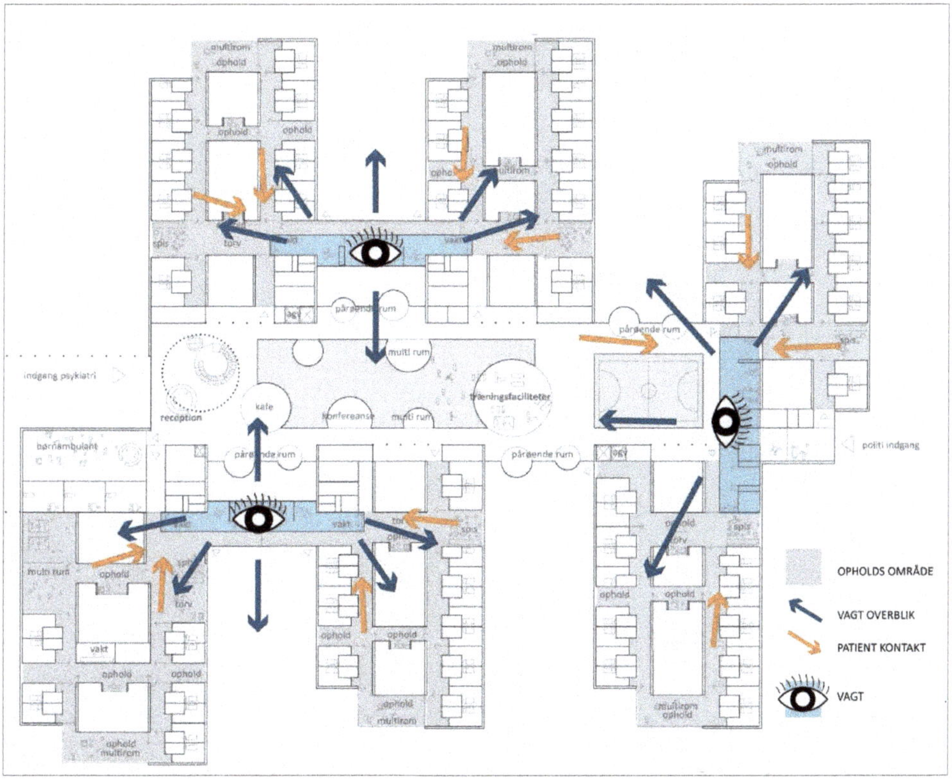

53

12. *The layout of the psychiatry cluster is clear: wards are located on the ground floor, the outpatient clinics are in the first hall, staff have good visibility and there are various options for shielding.*

cated on the arrivals path. Parking is now generally required to be near stations and in convenient locations. At the main entrance, moreover, there is a space for larger vehicles for the disabled.

Transport room

Only outpatients, relatives and personnel use the foyer as a living room area. Patients who must be transported in bed

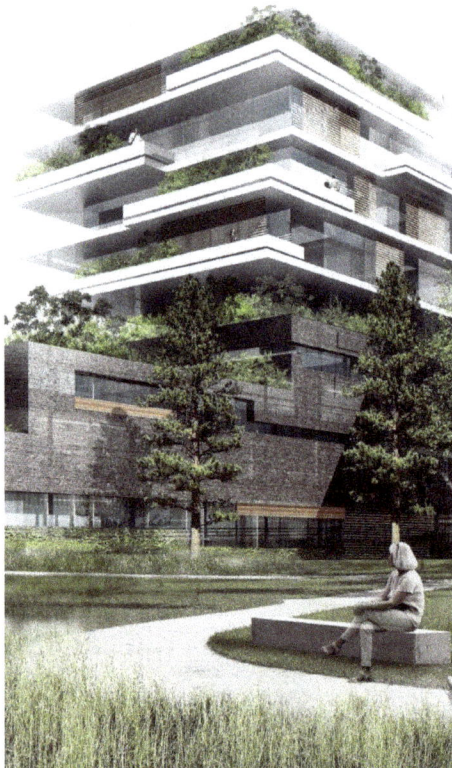

13. The base is a brick masonry construction with relief and there are several oak slats, which add acoustic variation.

from the ward to the outpatient clinics on the first floor are taken in the bed elevator directly from the floors down to the outpatient clinics in the living room area. The vertical flows include separate elevators for beds, people and supplies.

Transport 1

Bedridden patients are transported separately from other patients; bed transportation takes place in "non-public" areas. Bedridden patients arrive at the imaging area from the bed elevator located outside the core department. Here there are temporary waiting places for beds close to the diagnostic study area. Acute bedridden patients and patients from the emergency unit arrive at the imaging area independently from each other.

Patients arrive at the outpatient clinics, sometimes even with relatives, and proceed directly from the foyer up to the respective imaging or day surgery area of the central core.
The transport of bedridden patients for theatre treatment is organized through transport operations and not the Command Center for that operating theatre. Space is set aside next to the Command Center as a temporary waiting area for bedridden patients. Acute patients from the emergency unit on the 1st floor are taken via a separate lift for acute patients into the operating area on the 2nd floor.

Heliport

It has been stated that EH101 type helicopters will be used and the heliport location requires an angular range of more than 180° at which operations are possible. The figure shows a noise charge

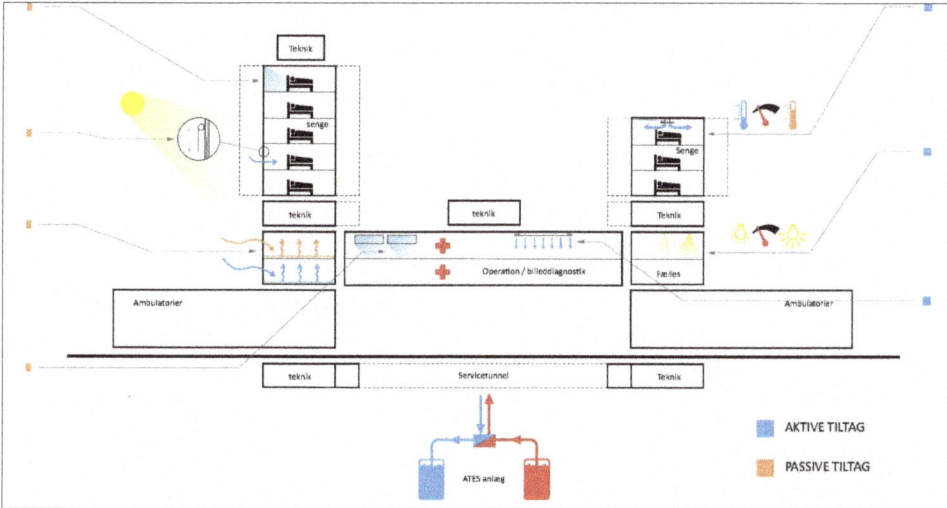

14. *The project includes a wide range of passive and active measures.*

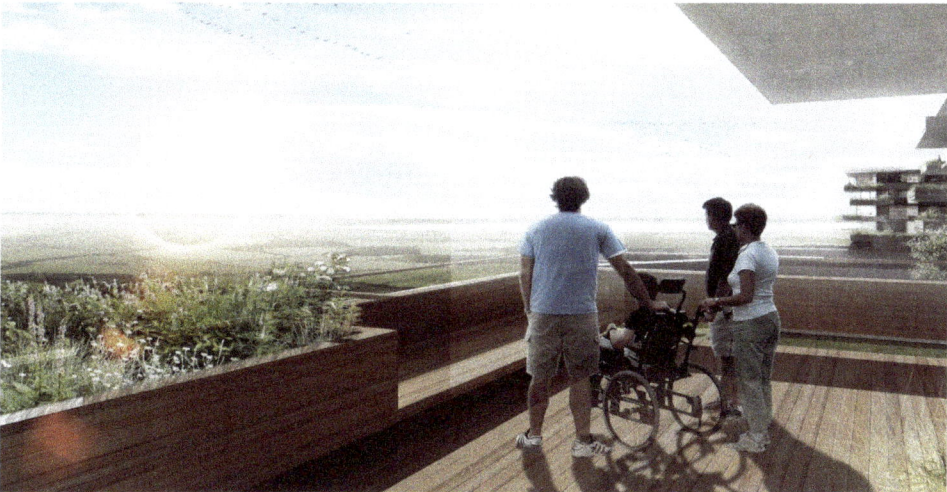

15. *There is a row of terraces and narrow service balconies on the bed wards façade.*

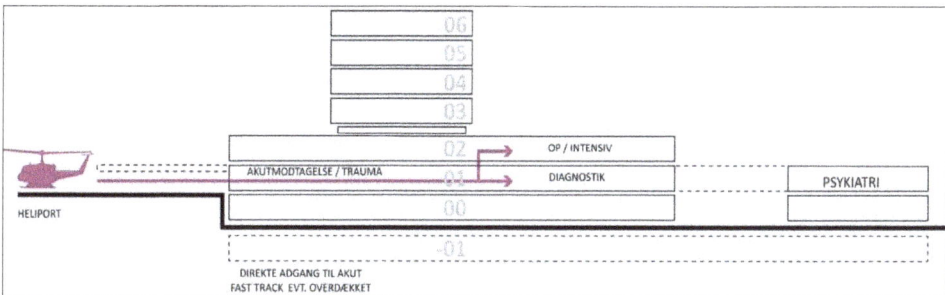

16. *Heliport, section.*

TESIS Inter-University Research Centre "Systems and Technologies for Social and Healthcare Facilities"
University of Florence, Italy

56

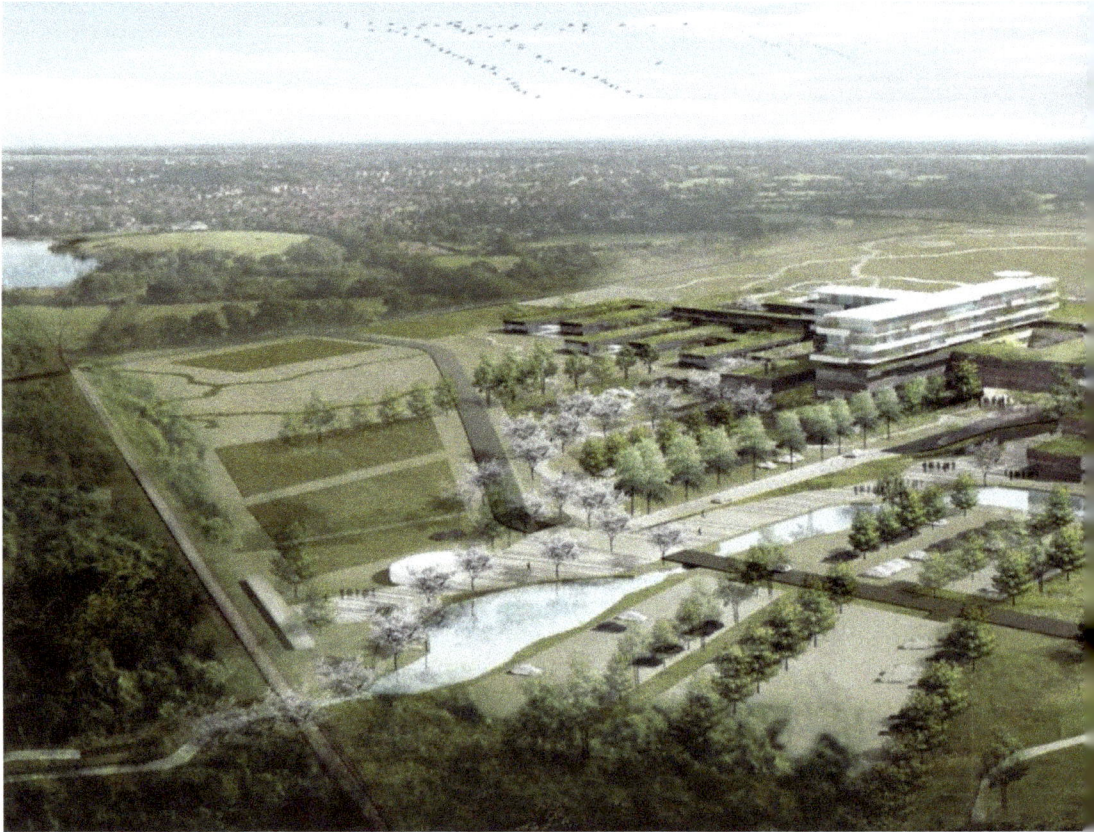

17. The hospital as seen from the northwest.

for one approach at a compass direction of 340°. A helicopter approaching from this direction will pass over Snejbjerg at a height of 300-400 m. The noise level in the Snejbjerg passage will be about 75 dB(A).

The noise contour by starting from the opposite direction towards 160° will be about the same. Helicopters approaching from other directions will pass over open country with only a few farm buildings.

Figures 16 and 18 show the heliport position. The noise level at the hospital building is a high of 80 dB(A) for the

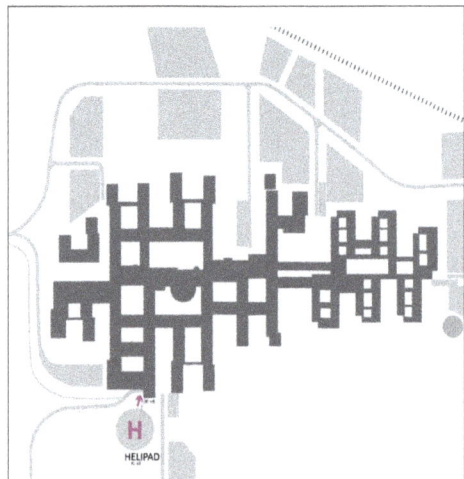

18. Heliport, plant.

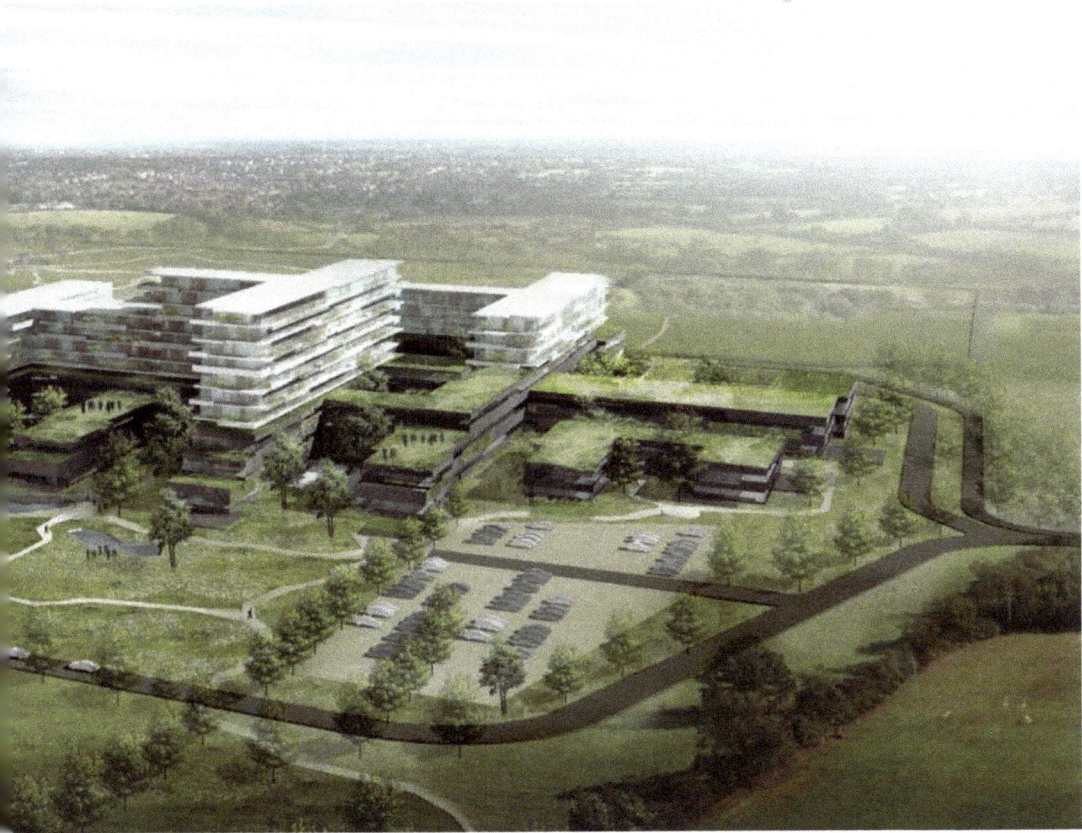

nearest buildings and between 70 and 80 dB(A) in a large area.

The receiving of acute patients has been improved, as has the clarity of the two affected hubs, and there are integrated waiting areas at the lifts.

Psychiatry

In the units and common areas of the psychiatry department, the following points are important:
- the cluster has an active center with a combination of open and private areas for interviews, therapy and activities;
- all wards are located to the east or west and thus have good daylight conditions;
- all wards are located on the ground floor with views of nature;
- outdoor protected areas are defined, many courtyards have different characteristics;
- ability to establish shielded units, 2-4 wards with private seating areas and outdoor area;
- office space for staff between two wards for better flexibility and overview;
- opportunity for staff security in order to delimit the personnel area;
- flexibility between wards if the number of wards required in the future changes.

TESIS Inter-University Research Centre "Systems and Technologies for Social and Healthcare Facilities"
University of Florence, Italy

TESIS

Flexibility

Session introduction

During the session the speakers provided a critical reading of the topic of flexibility in the design and planning of healthcare buildings. The theme was examined from several viewpoints, and each of the speakers expressed their vision on the basis of their different professional skills.

· · · · · · · · · · ·

Peter Sher's talk opened by highlighting how until now studies on flexibility have not been translated into significant improvements in the quality of healthcare environments or the rationalization of construction costs. Facilities built with the aim of being future proof have not been able to accommodate changes so that in certain cases they were even demolished. In view of this, according to the author, future research should shift the focus onto issues such as flexibility, growth and adaptation from a new perspective in which more emphasis is placed on approaching the problem based on an analysis of the real needs rather than addressing it solely from a theoretical standpoint.

Peter Sher
p. 61

Roelof Gortemaker presented the design experiences of his architectural firm, De Jong Gortemaker Algra architects, in which he highlighted the most common configurations of buildings that provide a flexible combination of spaces dedicated to care. If we carefully read the history of some buildings that remained in use for decades, it is clear that some particular architectural solutions are able to ensure the facilities remain flexibile over time. According to the author, in addition to the functional organization, the shapes of buildings in the future may be changed by measures for the reduction of energy consumption.

Roelof Gortemaker p. 73

Jørn A. Limi's presentation focuses on the problems that made the expansion of Akersus University Hospital (Ahus) necessary and on the new construction phases. In the mid-nineties Akersus University Hospital was unable to meet the healthcare demand of the reference catchment area and structural problems occurred in the same period. Following the process of renovating the hospital, it emerged that in the next few years it will be necessary for the buildings to accommodate new training programs and the latest technologies, optimally evaluating the risks and costs of the facilities.

Jørn A. Limi

p. 87

According to Tarald Rohde it is possible to observe how design choices made in the name of flexibility have sometimes resulted in the creation of environments lacking from an aesthetic point of view and in certain cases that remain unused due to rapidly changing needs. Examining the changes made at the Rikshospitalet over the last ten years it is clear that it would be appropriate to analyze the present needs rather than trying to foresee the future and creating inadequate architectural solutions.

Tarald Rohde p. 93

TESIS Inter-University Research Centre "Systems and Technologies for Social and Healthcare Facilities"
University of Florence, Italy

1. 50 years of ideas in healthcare buildings.

	in the 1940s		1950s		1960s
Ideas in medicine	World Health Organisation Antibiotics. Kidney dialysis.	Open heart surgery. Kidney transplant. DNA Structure.	Drug resistant bacteria. Hospital infection. Early ambulation	Progressive Patient Care. Intensive Care Units. Ultrasound.	
Ideas in architecture and building	The modern movement.	Industrial production. Prefabrication. Modular co-ordination.	Design research Nuffield investigation. Physical environment.	R.I.B.A.plan of work. Low rise v high rise. Systems theory.	
Ideas in society and people	Postwar housing, education, health, employment. Welfare state.	"Festival of Britain" New towns. Local health centres. Co-operation.	"The Death and Life of Cities".	Consumer movements. "What's Wrong with Hospitals?"	
Ideas in health care policy and the NHS	Universal access to free healthcare. The NHS national and regional structures.	Friesian's automated hospital design. The D.G.H. The Hospital plan.	Research development Guidance. Greenwich D.G.H. Traffic flows.	Best buy Hospital Harness. Community Hospitals Nucleus.	

Flexibility for Adaptation
Background, Definition and New Guidance

Peter Sher
B.A. (Arch.)
R.I.B.A. Architect-Research-Consultancy, London

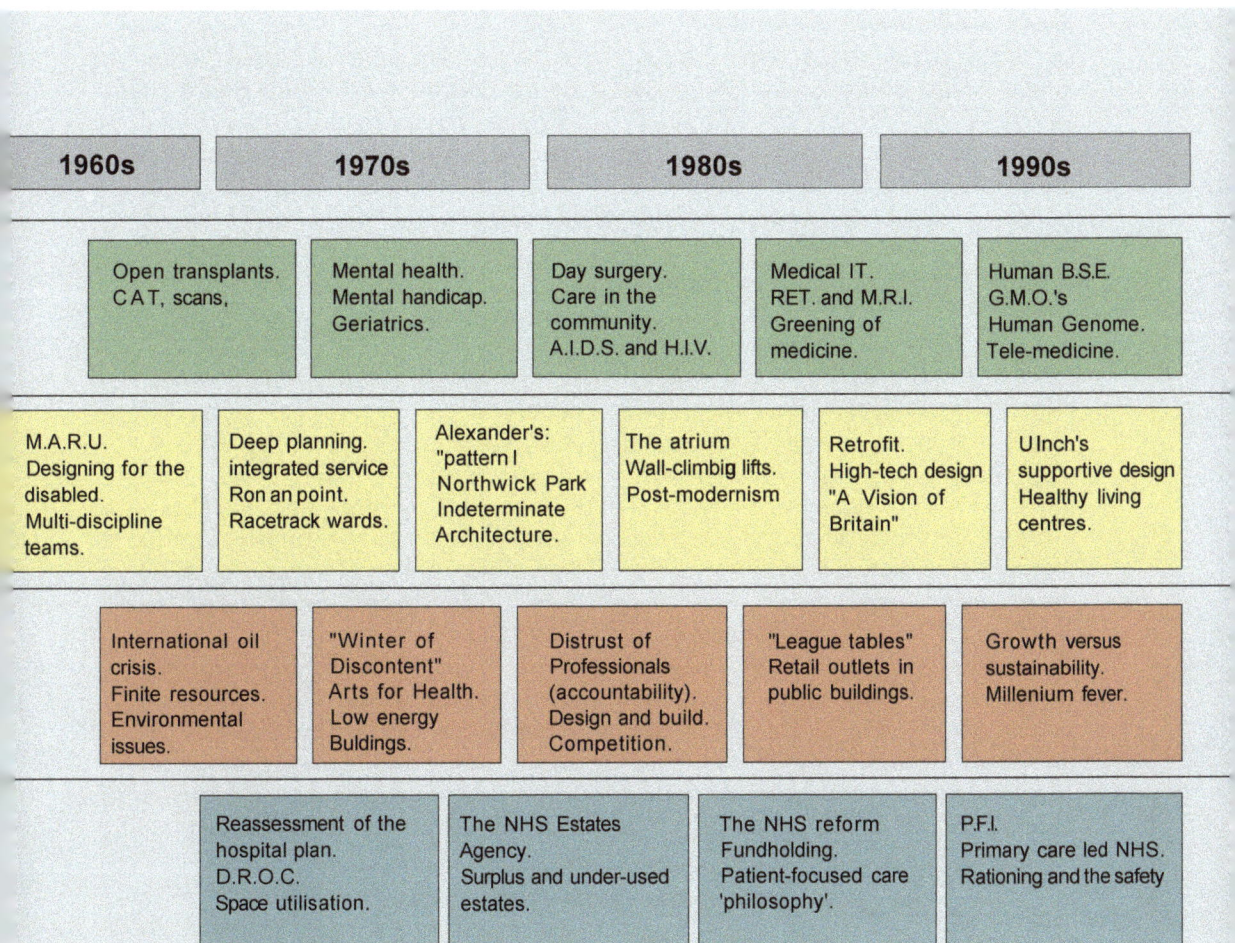

61

1960s	1970s	1980s		1990s
Open transplants. C A T, scans,	Mental health. Mental handicap. Geriatrics.	Day surgery. Care in the community. A.I.D.S. and H.I.V.	Medical IT. RET. and M.R.I. Greening of medicine.	Human B.S.E. G.M.O.'s Human Genome. Tele-medicine.
M.A.R.U. Designing for the disabled. Multi-discipline teams.	Deep planning. integrated service Ron an point. Racetrack wards.	Alexander's: "pattern I Northwick Park Indeterminate Architecture.	The atrium Wall-climbig lifts. Post-modernism	Retrofit. High-tech design "A Vision of Britain"	U Inch's supportive design Healthy living centres.
	International oil crisis. Finite resources. Environmental issues.	"Winter of Discontent" Arts for Health. Low energy Buldings.	Distrust of Professionals (accountability). Design and build. Competition.	"League tables" Retail outlets in public buildings.	Growth versus sustainability. Millenium fever.
	Reassessment of the hospital plan. D.R.O.C. Space utilisation.	The NHS Estates Agency. Surplus and under-used estates.	The NHS reform Fundholding. Patient-focused care 'philosophy'.	P.F.I. Primary care led NHS. Rationing and the safety

Abstract

Since the mid-twentieth century there has been a continuing acceleration of advances in medical science and technology and of radical changes in patterns of disease, society, demography, healthcare organisations and finance. In reaction to the mismatch between the speed of change and the construction time needed to build or to adapt healthcare facilities there has been a demand for healthcare facilities to be designed to be "flexible to adapt to future changes of use."

Attempts to meet this demand include research and development in the growth, change and ageing of hospitals, the combination of interstitial floors for environmental engineering services with demountable partitions within long-span structures and the use of "templates". Despite the claims of designers their effectiveness over the subsequent life of built examples has never been independently examined.

Requiring the design of healthcare facilities to be flexible to adapt to future changes of use has been almost universal for decades. Yet flexibility and adaptation have never been defined and future changes of use are always characterised as "unknown"! By defining adaptation and flexibility a framework can be established to enable project teams, comprising clients/users and design teams, to effect known changes of use.

Working definitions are proposed for Adaptation, Growth and Flexibility. A continuum for Flexibility is proposed as a series of levels, 1, 2, 3, etc. from minimal upwards. The proposed levels apply once an adaptation is decided upon. The levels will be refined through independent testing by means of field observations/surveys of actual adaptations in existing health facilities. This understanding of the background and definitions is offered to project teams involved in healthcare building developments and their use.

Keywords
flexibility, adaptation, growth and change

Introduction

The presentation at the seminar in Florence in 2008 discussed Adaptation and cited a variety of built examples [1], whereas the presentation at the seminar in Buenos Aires in 2009 gave an account of the research project entitled "Adaptability and Innovation in Healthcare Facilities" funded by the Howard Goodman Bursary [2], and offered conclusions about flexibility. This theme is continued below.

Background

In the past healthcare buildings were developed in response to immediate and urgent need and the capability for adaptation or for flexibility was never expressed. It certainly was never mentioned in Florence Nightingale's seminal and influential book Notes on Hospitals (1861)[3]. By the mid-twentieth century most developed countries had acquired over time a large number of widely varying types of healthcare facilities. It was becoming increasingly difficult to accommodate, by adapting these buildings, the rapid acceleration of advances in medical science and technology and

62

the radical changes in patterns of disease, demography, healthcare organisations and finance.

Yet even in 1955 the outstanding Nuffield Studies in the Function and Design of Hospitals devoted only one section, just under a page in length, to Flexibility and Growth [4]. This "critical, fundamental study was focused on practical issues, and . . . conclusions were related to practical possibilities." However, 'Clients' for the design of healthcare facilities, especially those in national or local government health services, reacted to their experiences of rapid change[5] by specifying the absurdly impractical requirement for designs to be "flexible to adapt to future changes of use." Designers and the construction industry responded by developing a number of innovations, e.g. the combination of interstitial floors for environmental engineering services with demountable partitions within long-span structures and the use of templates. The brief but sensible discussion of flexibility and growth in the Nuffield Studies was impressively developed in the 1960s with studies by Professor Peter Cowan[6] and the development by John Weeks of his theory of Growth and Change[7] demonstrated in the design of Northwick Park Hospital in London, opened in 1970. At the same time another new development was the Greenwich Hospital, opened in 1969. It was designed and built embodying innovative ideas for maximum flexibility in the physical planning to accommodate future changes in layout and equipment[8]. Neither of these significant and innovatory projects was independently examined in use and Greenwich Hospital was finally demolished by 2007. However in 1975, in response to an economic crisis and politi-

63

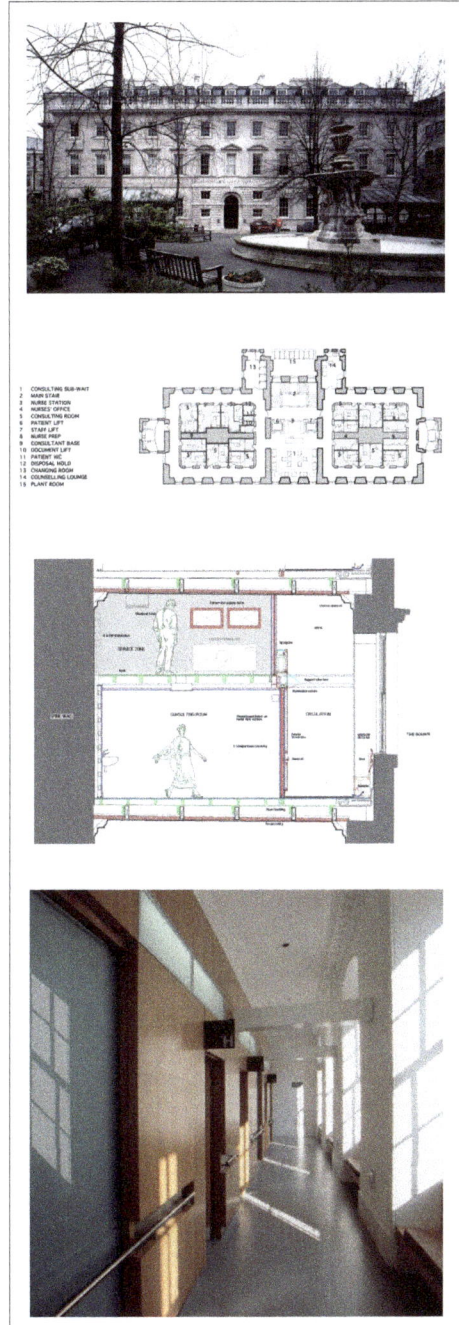

2. Seminar in Florence 2008, Adaptation of 18th-century ward block to 21st-century Cancer Care Centre.

TESIS Inter-University Research Centre "Systems and Technologies for Social and Healthcare Facilities"
University of Florence, Italy

64

The report: "There is a need for more sophisticated research . . . We must understand what 'flexibility and adaptability in the built form' amounts to and how . . . we can recognise 'the potential to accommodate future changing needs'."

3. Seminar in Buenos Aires 2009.

cal imperatives in the UK, the 'Nucleus' system was introduced. Templates combined the capability for growth with flexibility for all basic departmental plans. The Howard Goodman Bursary research project showed that there are serious obstacles even to examining the responses to changes required by government policies, financing and contracting requirements[10].

Another result has been the alarming development of "Futurology". This has been an ongoing industry in academic and policy fields remote from experience in healthcare design and construction, but its glamorous outputs have been of little or no practical use [5, 6]. Nevertheless "Futurology" is still flourishing with extensive academic "research" not adding noticeably to design or construction practice. Its glamorous outputs have been of little or no practical use[10, 11, 12].
The undefined mantra that designs should be flexible to adapt to future

changes of use continues in current briefings, though now absorbed within the wider topic of "Sustainability". The gap of understanding between "futurologists" – both academics and policymakers – and designers and the construction industry needs to be bridged. The gap is born of a lack of clarity in communicating and it is a typical example of the ever-recurring gap between theory and practice[13].

Defining Terms

The term change needs no definition. We know there will always be changes of use but we cannot specify for each building or space – where in the building will need change, when the change will be needed, or what change will be needed. We are asked to make designs flexible to meet future changes of use – unspecified change.
This will ensure the designs are 'Sustainable'!

Working definitions of the terms adaptation and flexibility were proposed and set out in the presentation at the Buenos Aires seminar. So far they have not been challenged and they will be developed further here.

Adapt, adaptation, adaptable, 'adaptability'.

In this field adaptation applies to change in the function of the building, i.e. what users do in the building; it describes a transformation from one use to another, a process.

When it is possible to adapt to a change in any set of circumstances the outcome is adaptation. No conceivable set is adaptable to every conceivable change. The term adaptable should only be applied to each specific set and specific change to it.

(E.g. this nursing unit is adaptable for a change to an outpatient clinic.)
There have been many unique examples of changes of use – adaptations – in every building type as well as hospitals, and from the small to the very large scale. Since all adaptations are specific and unique 'adaptability' is not a quality that can be usefully evaluated. Generalizations about a building design being "adaptable", "more adaptable than" another, "not adaptable" and so on have no useful meaning.

But when the term 'adaptability' is used, to many it implies a variable quality because it resembles terms like permeability or visibility which are defined variables to which numerical values are assigned. Unlike these 'adaptability' has not been narrowly defined and its use should be avoided.

Level of Flexibility	Define Duration	User Considerations Notes
	Time needed *in situ* from end-date of existing use to start-date of changed use	Disruption to clinical function. Procedures and approvals Staff changes and training Commissioning All costs including administrative
1	Very short Overnight or weekend	Minimal, informal approvals. Very limited areas affected No changes to 'whole' systems
2	Up to 2 weeks	Significant minor works Large areas and some 'whole' systems may be modified
3	Up to 3 months	Capital project affects clinical services Large areas and some whole systems modified
4	Up to 6 months	Similar to level 3
5	Up to 1 year	Similar to level 3 Some expenditure may fall within two 'financial years'
N/A Not flexible	Over 1 year	Similar to level 3 Total expenditure over more than one 'financial year'

4. Levels of Flexibility – Table 1: User considerations.

TESIS Inter-University Research Centre "Systems and Technologies for Social and Healthcare Facilities" University of Florence, Italy

65

Level of Flexibility	Define Duration	Clinical function (Adaptation)		Building Elements (Flexibility)		
	Time needed *in situ* from end-date of existing use to start-date of changed use	Operational	Technical services and equipment Infection control	All building elements and loose furniture	Mechanical, Electrical and Sanitary engineering	I.T. Telecoms Security Safety P.A.
1	**Very short Overnight or weekend**	**Own staff including specialists +visiting specialists for equipment procedures**		**Own staff including specialists+ visiting specialists in all elements**		
2	**Up to 2 weeks**	**Own staff including specialists +visiting specialists for equipment procedures**		**Own staff including specialists+ visiting specialists in all elements**		
3	**Up to 3 months**	**Own staff including specialists +visiting specialists for equipment procedures + Professional Project Management required**		**In-house or outside contract and professional Project Management required**		
4, 5	**Up to 6 months Up to 1year**	**Similar to level 3**		**Similar to level 3**		

5. Levels of Flexibility – Table 2: Clinical functions and building elements.

Flexible, future changes of use, flexibility

We can design buildings using building elements that are flexible in that they may be more or less independently and readily reconfigured. Future changes will always remain unknown.

Claiming that a design is 'flexible to adapt to future changes of use' that cannot be identified with any certainty makes no sense.

Flexibility applies to the building/built environment; it may be defined as a variable quality of the process required for adaptation.

It is possible to speculate about the future but very few predictions are fulfilled accurately. [To quote the "futurologist" Alvin Toffler, "The future always comes too fast and in the wrong order."] De-signs cannot be "futureproofed" because the future political, economic, social, medical or technological environment at any specific future date cannot be predicted.

Levels of Flexibility

It has been proposed that flexibility should be defined as a variable quality of the process required for an adaptation. We may assign values to assess flexibility in different ways. For example an adaptation will have a measurable cost, take a measurable length of time to be implemented, effect a measurable saving in energy usage, effect a measurable change in operational efficiency, and so on. Differing proposals to adapt to a specific change may be compared on the basis of one of these single measures. For example, using the one variable of cost, a rule was adopted for public buildings in need of substantial change that if adapting the building were estimated to cost 75% or more of the estimated construction cost of demolishing and replacing it with a new building then the adaptation was defined as 'uneconomic' and a new building was justified.

The cost of the physical process by itself however is only one aspect of an adaptation. We assign values to these measures in option appraisals but a single combined value cannot be expressed for an adaptation.

The value of each specific measure (cost, energy use, etc.) may represent a level of flexibility for the adaptation. As the extent of a change becomes more elaborate the other factors – operational, energy use, staffing, etc. – may also become increasingly significant. Differing proposals to adapt to a specific change may readily be compared on the basis of any one of these single assessments.

Measuring flexibility using time or duration as the key variable is proposed. This is because the duration of the adaptation process is of prime importance to every stakeholder. For obvious reasons the time from end-date of existing use to start-date of changed use affects all users of the building, the operational managers, the design teams and the construction and specialist contractors.

The adaptation, for example of an existing outpatients unit as an emergency centre, would be planned in advance and include all the hospital operational consequences and all the changes to the building and services. All temporary and permanent construction work, hospital staff changes and operational system changes, and all costs, would have to be established. Together with this material

67

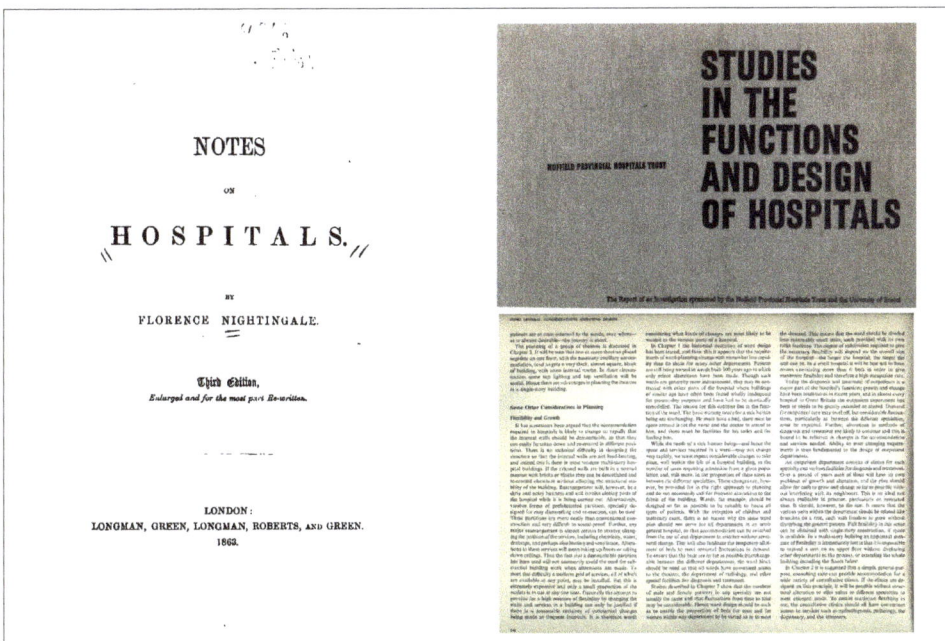

6. Nightingale (1863) to Nuffield (p. 146 Flexibility and Growth, 1955).

TESIS Inter-University Research Centre "Systems and Technologies for Social and Healthcare Facilities"
University of Florence, Italy

68

the duration between the end-date of use as an outpatients department and the start-date of use as an emergency centre would be worked out. The duration will determine the Level of Flexibility.

In using space in a building the minimal change is to rearrange the furniture for a change in use. The maximal change is to abandon the space or building and replace it with a different one for a change in use. Between minimum and maximum there is a continuum through which changing the built space becomes a more and more elaborate process. The suggested continuum is a series of Levels of Flexibility, 1, 2, 3, etc. and these are outlined in Tables 1 and 2. For each Level of Flexibility a maximum duration is set and Table 1 notes some of the key User Considerations at each level. Table 2 outlines requirements to implement Flexibility in the Building Elements and for the Adaptation of the Clinical Function. By ensuring that the adaptation of the Clinical Function is fully worked out by the healthcare client and that the flexible changes to the Building Elements are fully worked out by the contractor(s) the full duration and Level of Flexibility is established. These levels need independent testing by means of field observations/surveys of actual adaptations in existing health facilities to refine and expand the definitions.

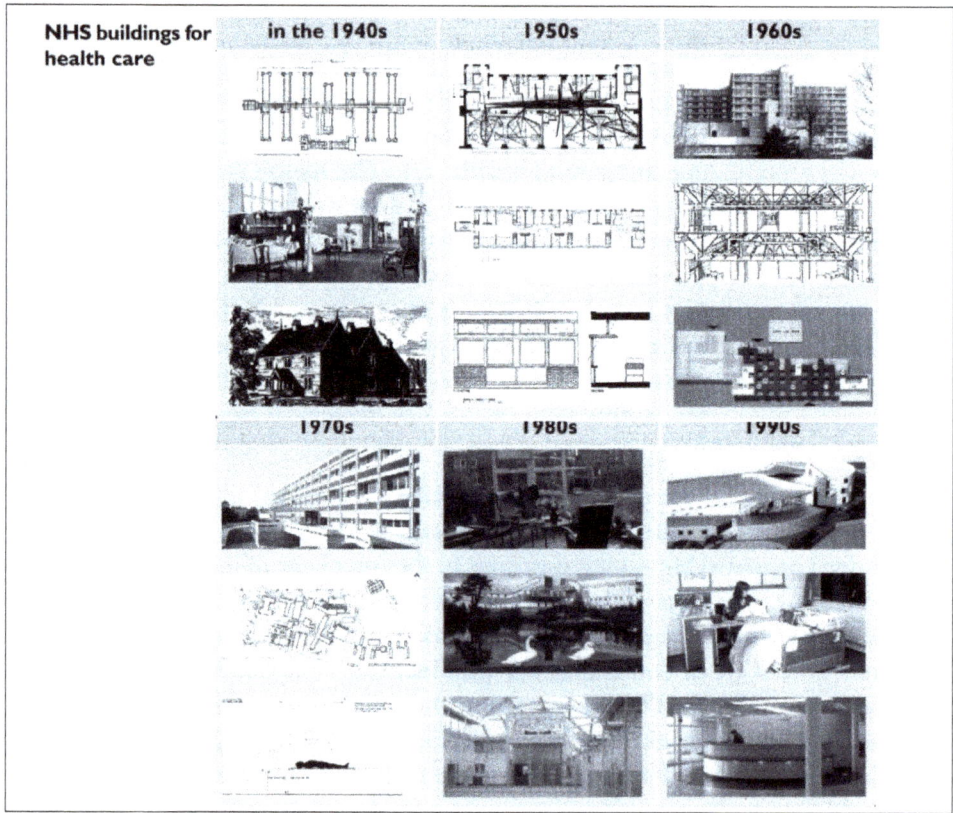

7. *Accelerating Change – from c. 1950.*

Discussion

So far a pragmatic response has been given to the sterile academic speculations about "future healthcare" and "the hospital of the future".

When the desired change is known and specified it is possible to get to work to make the change. But it is also certain that the future will bring unpredictable dramatic changes (consider the disasters of the last ten years), above all in the global population growth and in global climate change.

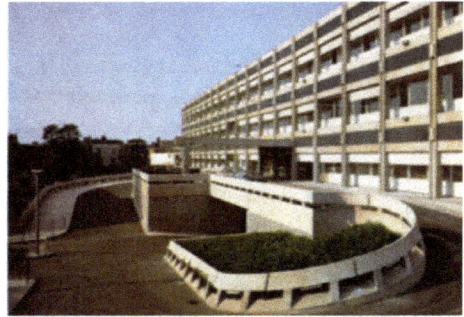

8. *Greenwich Hospital 1969.*

The time-honoured formula for designs to be flexible to adapt to future changes is now part of Sustainability.

In the British NHS "Sustainability" means "Future-proofing investment" and "Robust and flexible planning for change – Whole life investment, expansion/contraction"[14]. This was required before the unpredictable dissolution of the NHS now taking place. (British politicians predict that the NHS will soon be "unsustainable".)

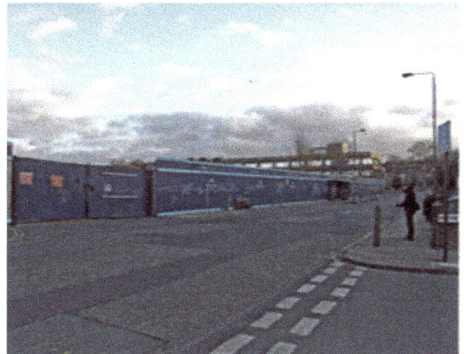

9. *Greenwich Hospital 2007.*

"Expansion" or "Growth" is usually included with flexibility as they are both consequences of change. But the capacity for physical growth is a function of site availability although it is profoundly affected by the way the existing facilities have been designed.

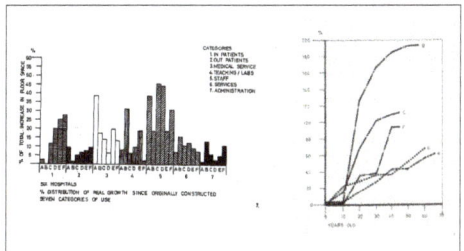

10. *1965 Growth and Change studies, Cowan.*

There have been some valuable studies of planning for growth[15] and, of course, innumerable built examples, successful and unsuccessful, worldwide. This should not be confused with flexibility within existing facilities.

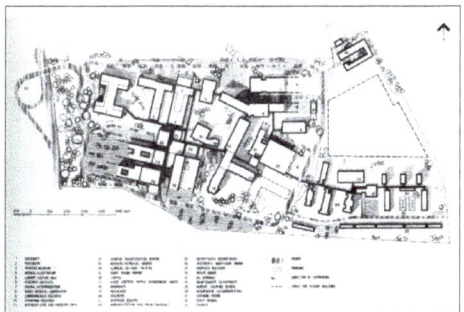

11. *1970 Northwick Park Hospital, Weeks.*

69

70

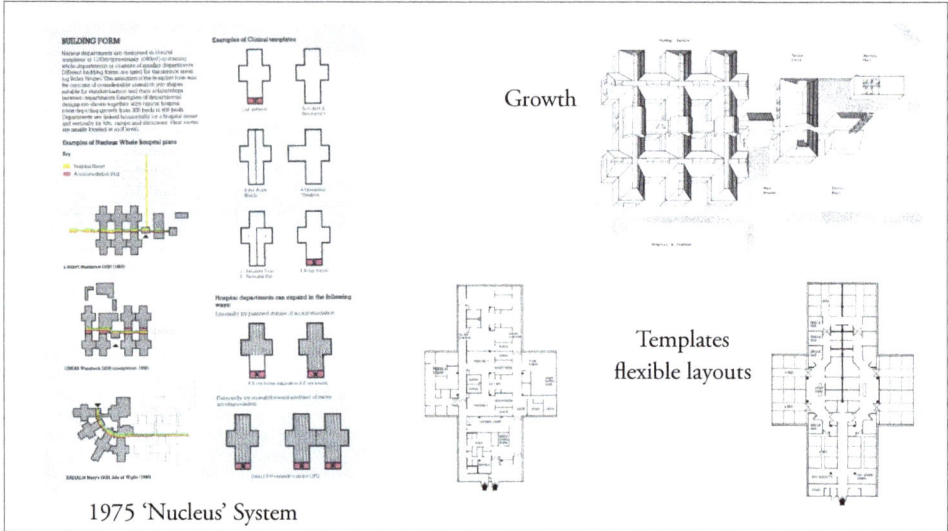

Growth

Templates
flexible layouts

1975 'Nucleus' System

12. Growth and Change and Flexible Layouts.

To sum up, an attempt has been made to clarify some of the exceedingly unclear habits found in the use of important key terms in professional practice and in academic work. These terms must have different and distinct meanings if we are to make sense in communicating with our communities, not to say with each other.

Once more, they are:
flexibility, adaptation, growth, change, sustainability.
It would also be an idea to do without the following terms of high-grade humbug:
future change, future-proofing, hospital of the future.

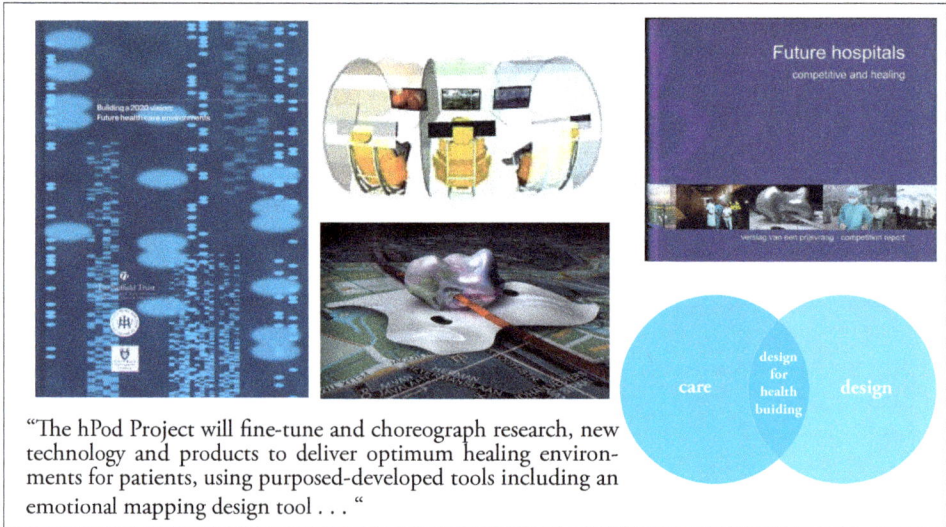

"The hPod Project will fine-tune and choreograph research, new technology and products to deliver optimum healing environments for patients, using purposed-developed tools including an emotional mapping design tool . . . "

13. Futurology.

References

1 Scher, P. 'Lessons in Humanising Future Health Care Architecture'. *The Culture for the Future of Healthcare Architecture. Proceedings of the 28th International Public Health Seminar.* Florence, Alinea editrice s.r.l. 2009.

2 Barlow, J. Köberle-Gaiser, M. et al. *Adaptability and innovation in healthcare facilities.* London, HaCIRIC, Imperial College, 2009.

3 Nightingale, F. *Notes on Hospitals.* London, Longman, Green, Longman, Roberts and Green, 3rd edition, 1863.

4 Davies, R.L. and Weeks, J. *Studies in the Function and Design of Hospitals.* London: Nuffield Provincial Hospitals Trust, O.U.P. 1955.

5 Francis, S, Glanville, R, Noble, A and Scher, P. *50 Years of Ideas in Health care Buildings.* London. The Nuffield Trust. 1999.

6 Cowan, P. and Nicholson, J. 'Growth and Change in Hospitals' *Transactions of the Bartlett Society, Volume 3 1964-1965* London 1965. Bartlett School of Architecture, University College London.

7 Weeks, J. 'Hospitals for the 1970s' *R.I.B.A. Journal,* London, December 1964, pp. 507-516.

8 Goodman, H. 'Greenwich District Hospital. An exercise in logistics.' *Hospital Management, Planning and Equipment,* London, October 1966 pp. 574-577.

9 Barlow, J. Köberle-Gaiser, M. et al, *op. cit.*

10 Francis, S. and Glanville, R. *Building a 2020 vision: Future health care environments.* London, The Stationery Office, 2001.

11 *Future hospitals, competitive and healing.* Utrecht, Netherlands Board for Hospital Facilities, 2005.

12 Mazuch, R. 'A sense of place', *World Health Design,* April 2008, p. 29.

13 Scher, P. 'Bridging the Gap'. *Building,* 17 November 1972, pp. 123-127.

14 Department of Health. *NHS Design Review Panel Guidance,* London, Department of Health, 2007.

15 Carthey, J. and Chow, V. 'Flexible and Adaptable Hospitals - Australian Case Studies'. Proceedings of HaCIRIC International Conference, London, Imperial College, 2009.

71

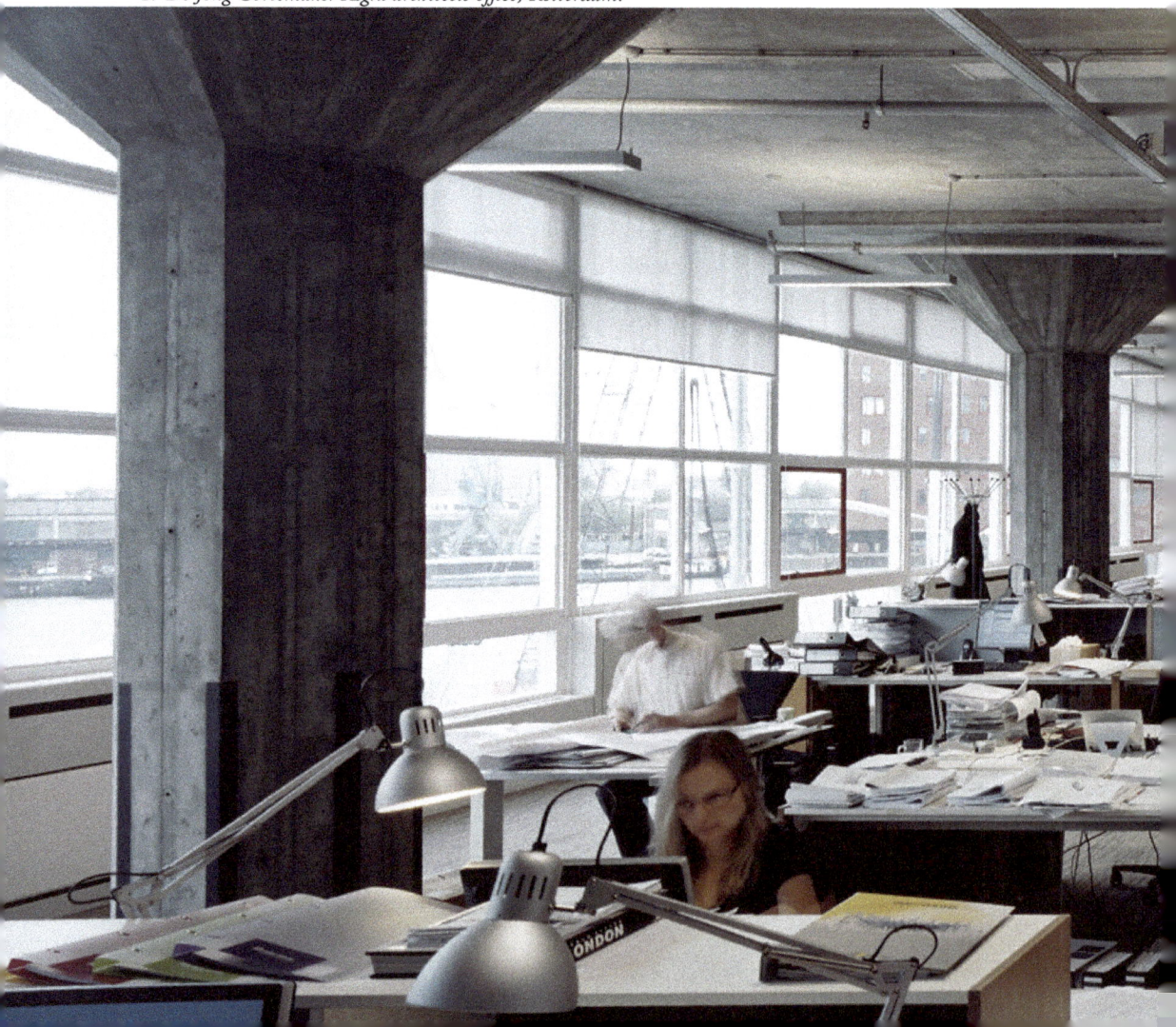

1. *De Jong Gortemaker Algra architects office, Rotterdam.*

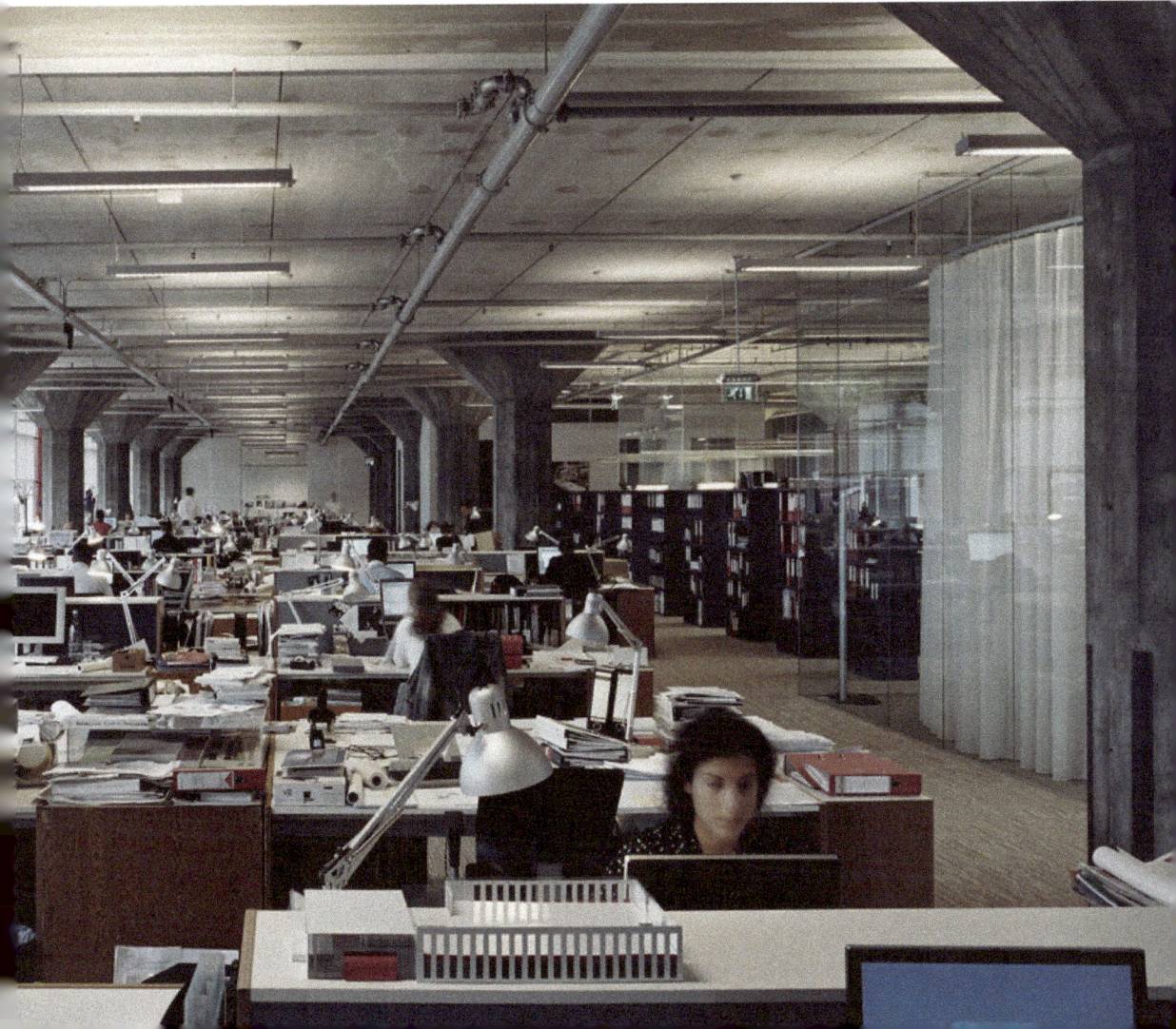

Flexibility and Robustness - 3 Strategies

Roelof Gortemaker
De Jong Gortemaker Algra Architects, Rotterdam, The Netherlands

73

Introduction

The office of De Jong Gortemaker Algra architects is located in a 50-year-old building. Originally built as a warehouse for a ship company, over the years it has been used as an exhibition hall, a dance hall and an outlet shop. Today it is an office building. Despite its age and the original design, the building is flexible and sustainable.

Hospitals compared to airport buildings

To achieve flexibility and robustness in buildings three main strategies can be followed: the grid, pavilions and the hall (pavilions under a big roof). To explain

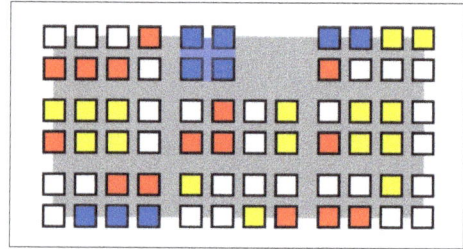

2. *Organizational model: matrix.*

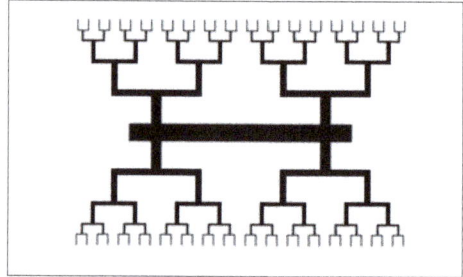

3. *Organizational model: tree.*

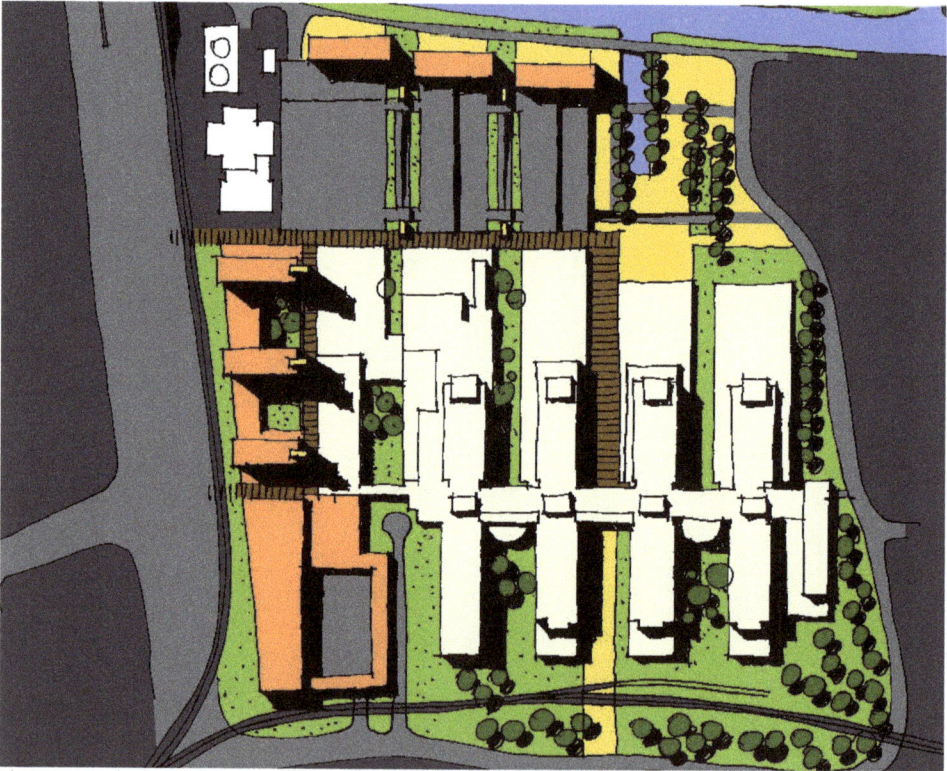

4. *Saint Anthony Hospital Nieuwegein: tree structure.*

74

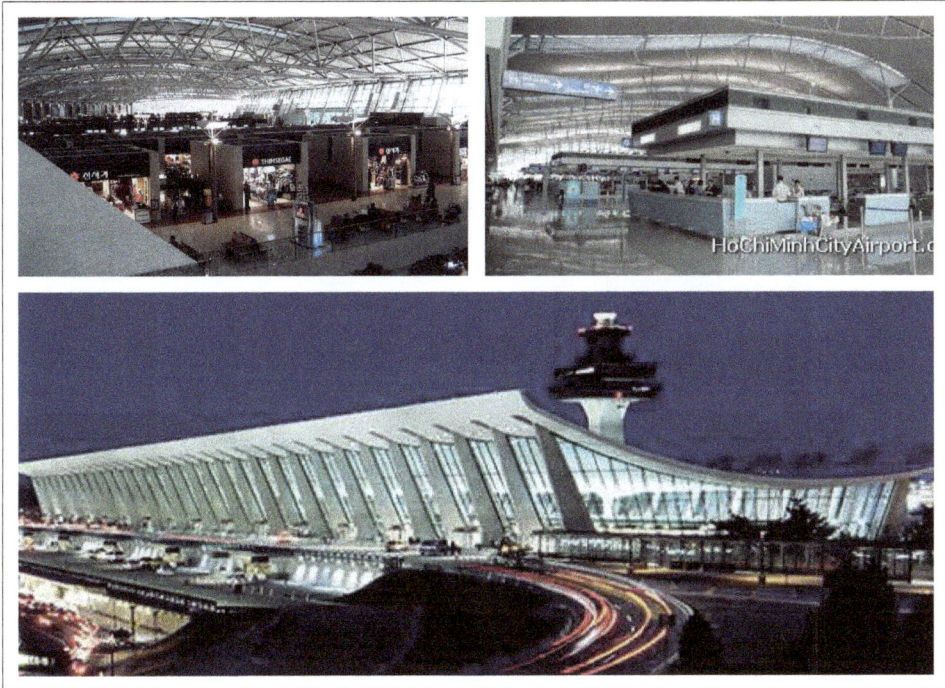

75

5. Airport buildings: matrix structure.

these strategies it is first important to determine two different kinds of organisation: the matrix organisation and the tree organisation.

Most hospitals have a tree structure. We recognize a main axis, namely a street with building parts connected to it. There is only one way to walk from A

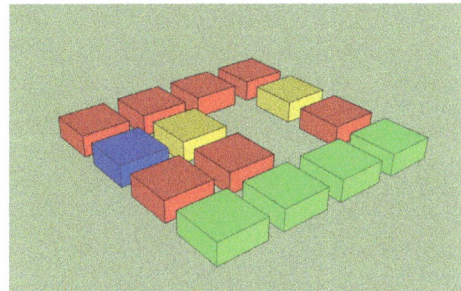

7. Strategy 2: simple pavilions can easily be replaced.

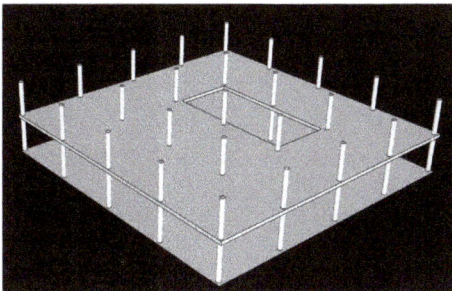

6. Strategy 1: a grid structure for all possible functions.

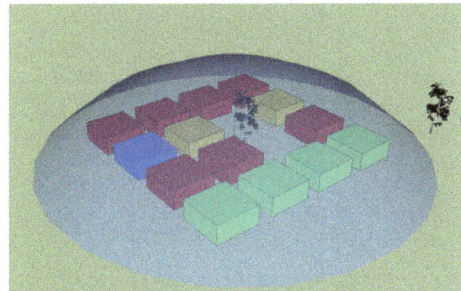

8. Strategy 3: sustainability with one big roof.

TESIS Inter-University Research Centre "Systems and Technologies for Social and Healthcare Facilities"
University of Florence, Italy

76

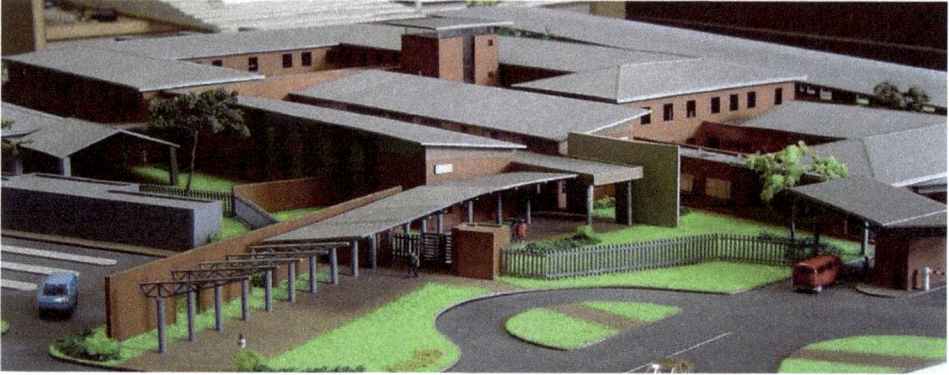

9. *Tembisa Hospital South Africa.*

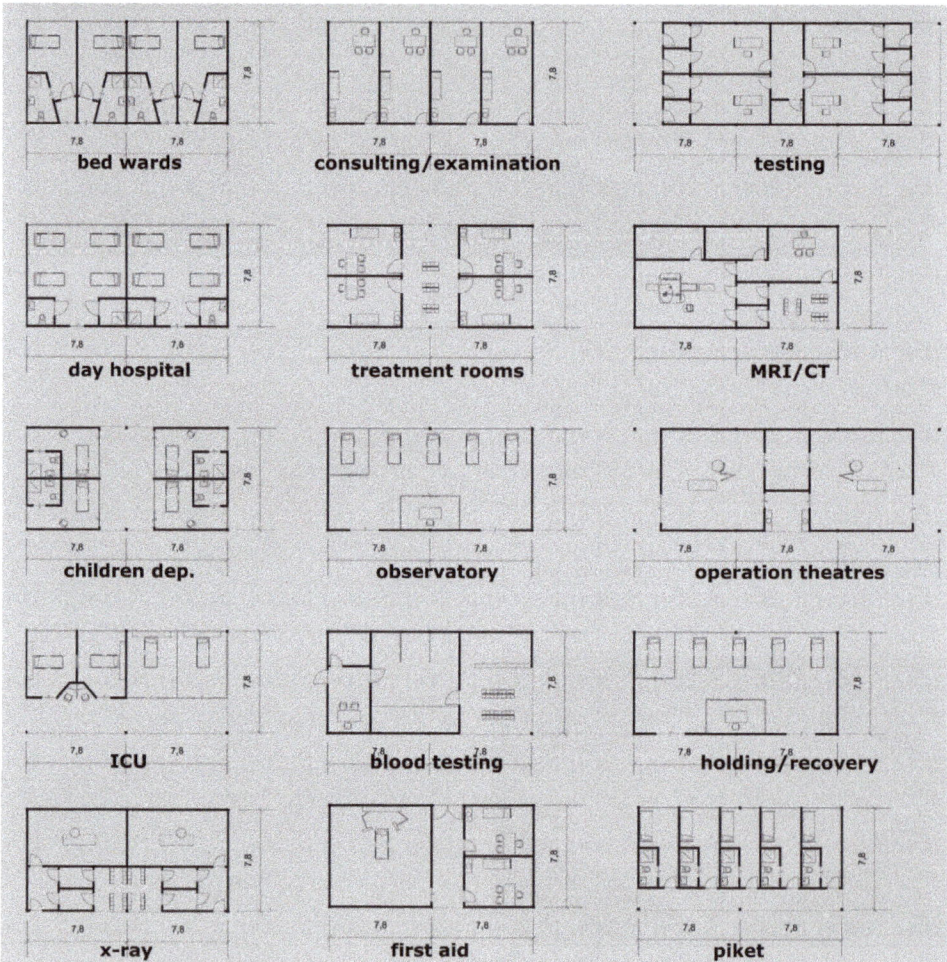

bed wards

consulting/examination

testing

day hospital

treatment rooms

MRI/CT

children dep.

observatory

operation theatres

ICU

blood testing

holding/recovery

x-ray

first aid

piket

10. *One size fits all: 7.8 x 7.8 m grid.*

to B. When the hospital organisation changes its procedures or specialties it is difficult to adapt the building to the new situation.

This is quite different in other large public buildings such as shopping malls, exhibition halls or airports. These buildings often have large halls with glass roofs and little pavilions within them. Some examples are John Foster Dulles Airport, HoChiMinh City Airport and Incheon International Airport in Korea. In airport buildings one large expensive structure can be made with small, cheap pavilions placed inside.

In a matrix organisation there are alternative routes compared to a tree structure.
When the hospital organisation changes its procedures or specialties it is relatively simple to adapt. With a matrix structure hospitals can achieve flexibility.

77

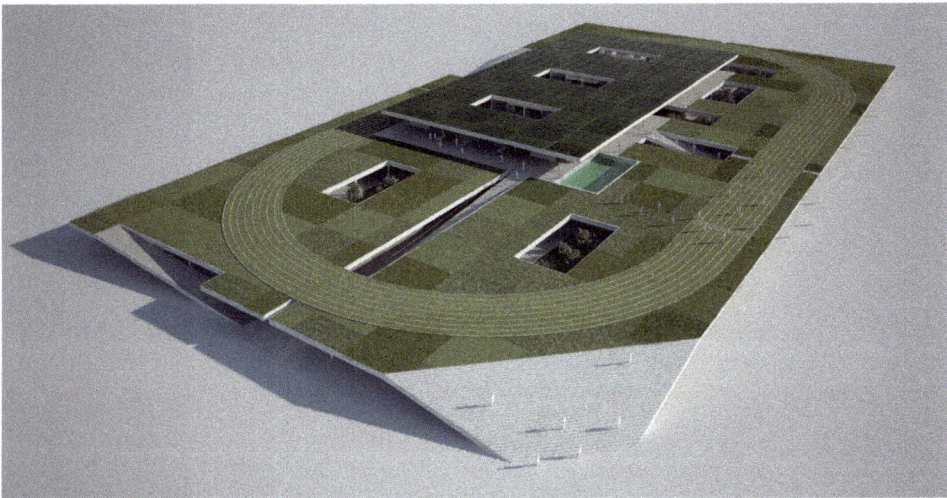

11. *Small Hospital Big Idea competition, California 2011, view of the green roof.*

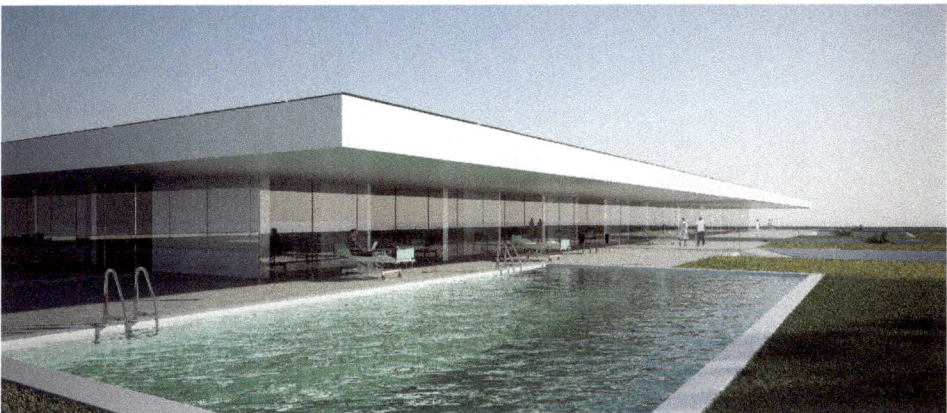

12. *Small Hospital Big Idea competition, California 2011, the swimming pool.*

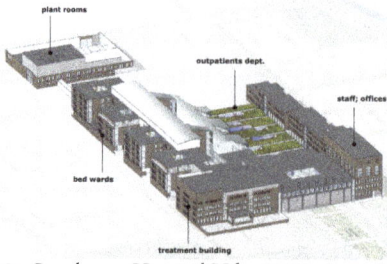

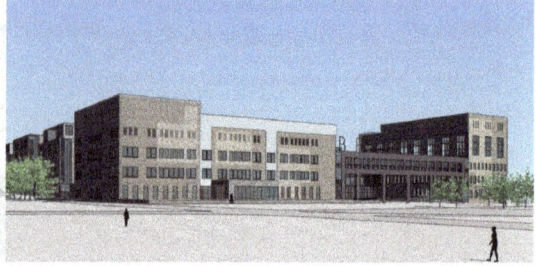

13. *Bernhoven Hospital Uden 2011.*

78

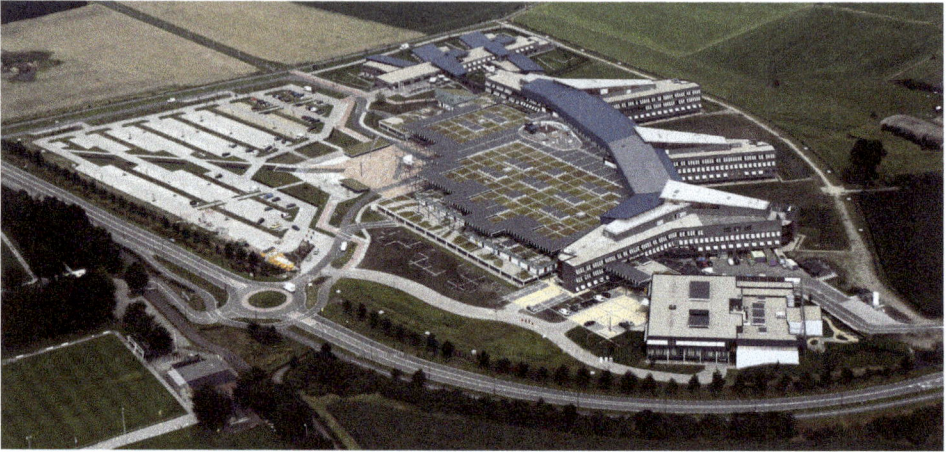

14. *Deventer Hospital 2008, aerial view.*

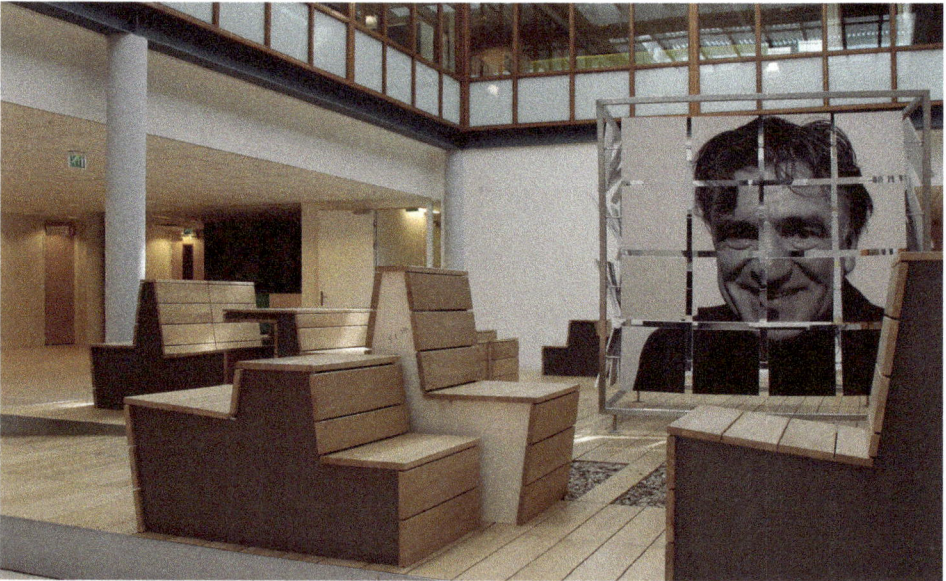

15. *Deventer Hospital 2008: hall.*

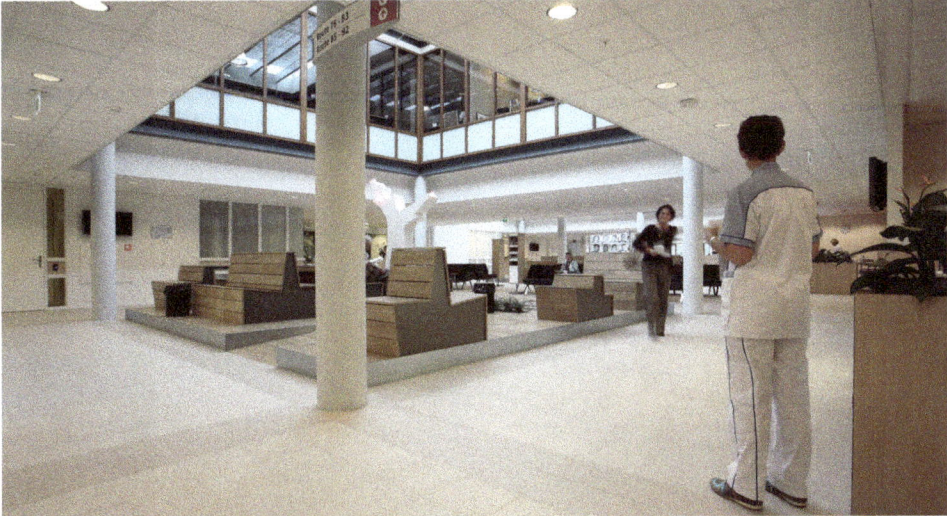

16. *Deventer Hospital 2008: hall.*

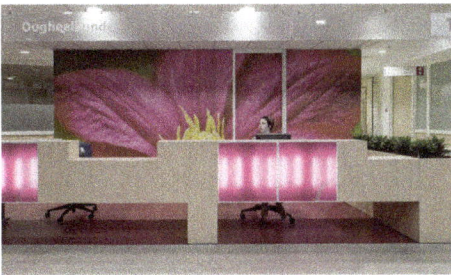

17. *Deventer Hospital 2008: reception.*

Design strategies

The first strategy is the grid with over-dimensioned columns and floors. The column distance, floor-to-ceiling height and floor type should be chosen carefully. For a new hospital in Zeeland a 7.8 x 7.8 meter grid was developed, one size fits all. It ensures the possibility of accommodating all possible functions.

The second strategy is the use of pavilions, which can easily be replaced as they are cheap and functional.

The third strategy is the hall: one big hall with a simple pavilion structure inside it. Sustainability is easily achieved here.

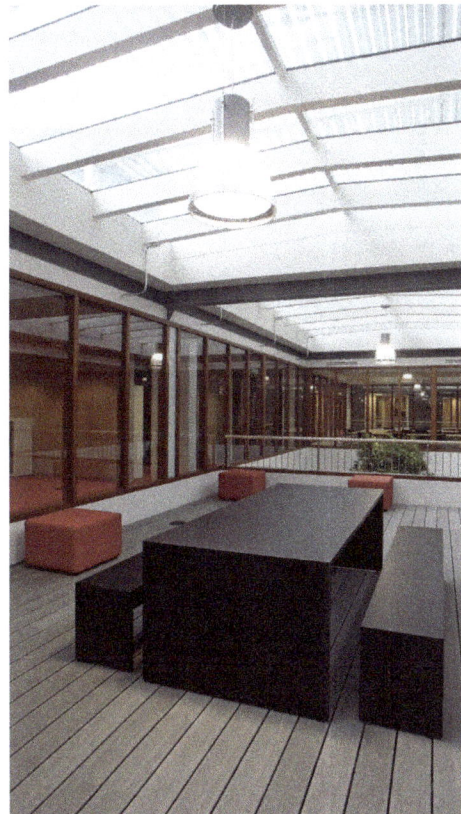

18. *Deventer Hospital 2008: staff relaxation area.*

TESIS Inter-University Research Centre "Systems and Technologies for Social and Healthcare Facilities"
University of Florence, Italy

Grid

The grid strategy was used in the design competition Small Hospitals, Big Idea (California, 2011): the design proposal was a small hospital combined with facilities around. All functions fit into a 30 x 30 foot grid. Daylight patios are situated in the middle of the building and can be placed in different positions on the floor. The bed wards, with single beds, are at the level of the outdoor sports facilities. Beds can be moved to the terraces outside.

Pavilions

The pavilion strategy works well in countries with a good climate and functions that are not particularly complex.

19. *Knokke Hospital competition 2009, form determined by energy efficiency.*

20. *Cruise ship and hospital: same layering of functions.*

21. *Knokke Hospital competition 2009, aerial view of the project.*

Tembisa Hospital in South Africa was designed using this strategy. For a big hospital or a hospital in a cold climate this is not the most appropriate strategy. Hospital Bernhoven in Uden (The Netherlands) is a good example. Every function has its own building. When a building is not needed anymore it can be sold or let to another company.

Hall

For the Dutch climate the hall strategy is more appropriate: pavilions under a big roof like the matrix structure of

an airport. Deventer hospital is an excellent example of this strategy. In the project many measures were taken to improve sustainability: 98% of the permanent measures and 85% of the variable measures from the national package for sustainable building. As a result, the Deventer hospital is a demonstration project for sustainable decision-making. In the field of energy, it is a European demonstration project of the European Commission. Thanks to this approach, the energy consumption of the hospital is 40% lower than that of a comparable hospital.

81

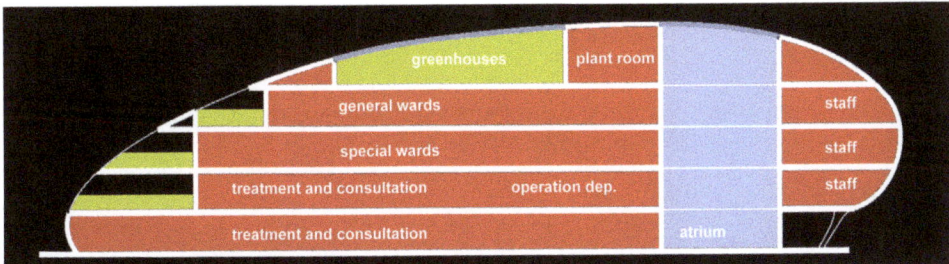

22. *Knokke Hospital competition 2009, teardrop form.*

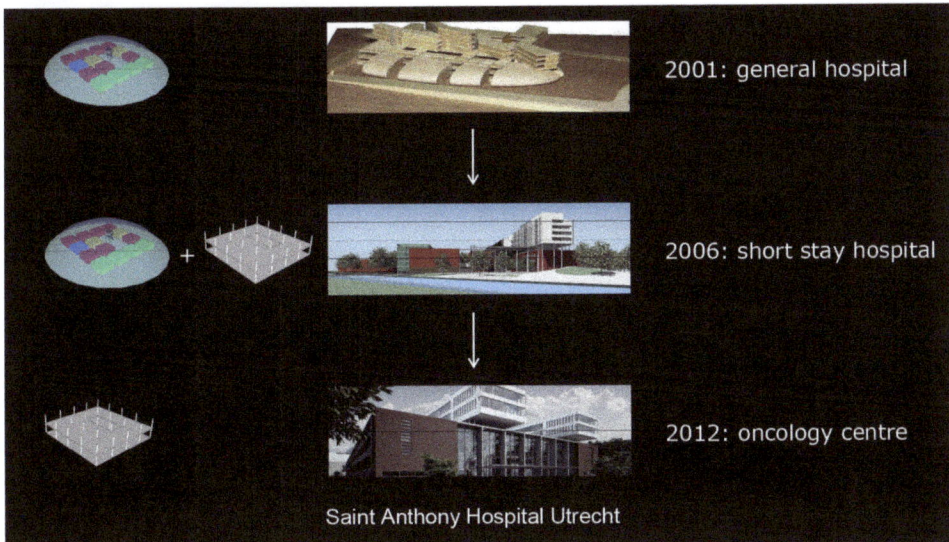

23. *Evolution of design in 10 years.*

TESIS Inter-University Research Centre "Systems and Technologies for Social and Healthcare Facilities"
University of Florence, Italy

TESIS

Oostkust health centre in Knokke (Belgium) was the project presented in collaboration with UNStudio for a design competition.

The hall is influenced by the orientation of the building to achieve maximum energy efficiency. The hospital has a compact structure which allows for good orientation and short walking routes. The teardrop form also has certain technical advantages such as reduced wind influence, improved direct sunlight and improved energy yield.

Case study: Saint Anthony Hospital, Utrecht

The design of the Saint Anthony Hospital in Utrecht has adopted different strategies over the last 10 years. Due to

82

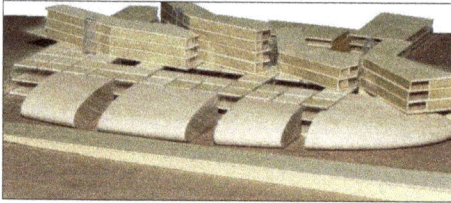

24. *Saint Anthony Hospital Utrecht 2001: hall structure with bed wards on top.*

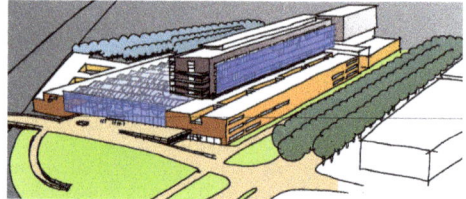

25. *Saint Anthony Hospital Utrecht 2003: big hall in the middle of the grid.*

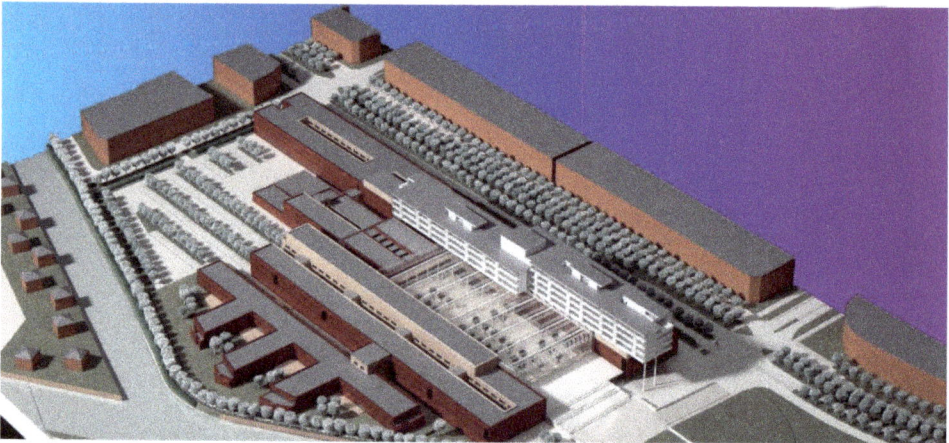

26. *Saint Anthony Hospital Utrecht 2004: maquette.*

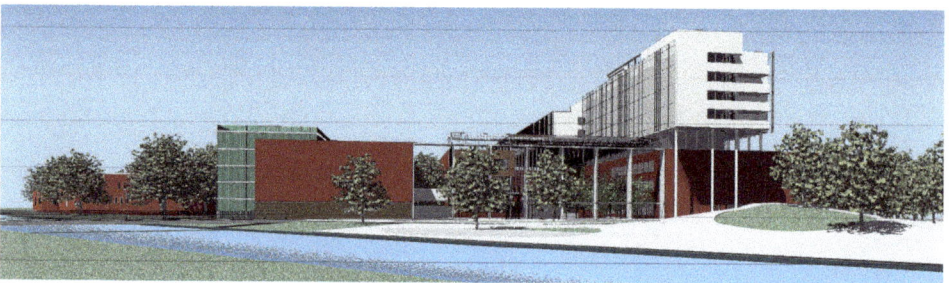

27. *Saint Anthony Hospital Utrecht 2005: external view.*

a change of location and a change in function all strategies were considered. In 2001 a general hospital was planned. The hall strategy with one big roof was applied.

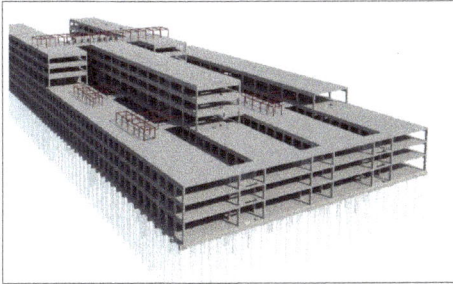

28. *Saint Anthony Hospital Utrecht 2008: simple concrete grid 7.2m x 7.2 m, daylight patios and corridors in two directions in a matrix structure*

In 2006 the plans changed from a general hospital to a short-stay hospital. In line with this change the design strategy also changed to a combination of the hall strategy with a grid. The function of the hospital has now changed to an oncology centre, and a starting point for the design strategy was the grid.

Building costs and renewal costs

83

The grid accounts for 33% of the building costs. This is a high rate due to the over-dimensioning of columns and floors (cost index = 120). Regarding the application of the design strategy of pavilions, after a renewal process nothing

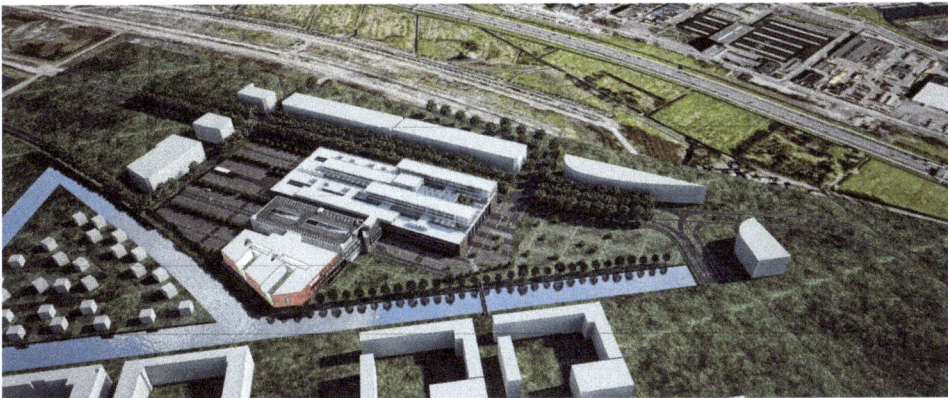

29. *Saint Anthony Hospital Utrecht 2011: aerial view of the project.*

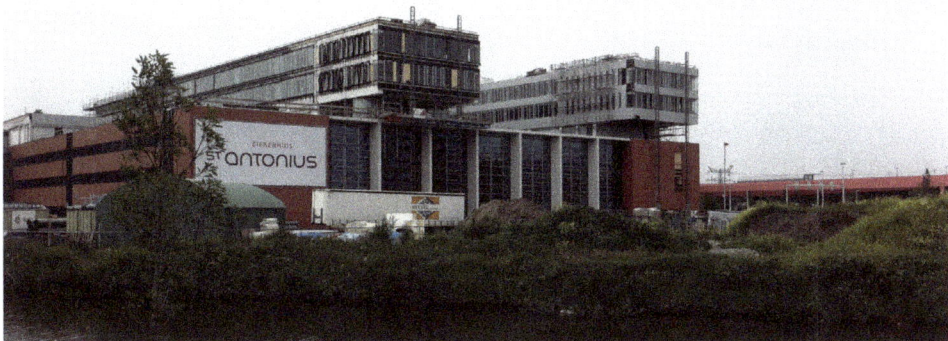

30. *Saint Anthony Hospital Utrecht 2012: after 10 years of design the building is under construction.*

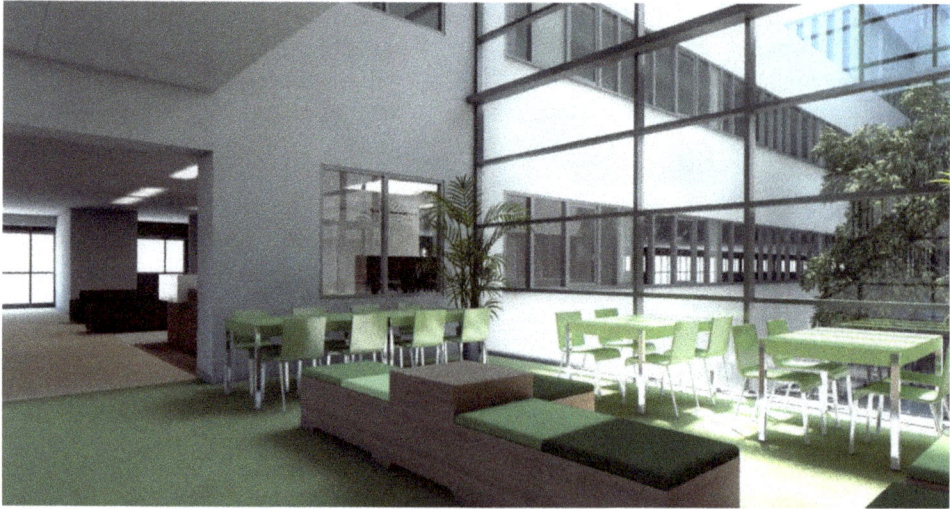

31. Saint Anthony Hospital Utrecht 2011: winter garden.

remains and pavilions are cheap buildings (cost index = 100). The sustainable hall is very expensive (cost index = 150) but it remains even if there is a process of renewal; pavilions are cheap and easy removable.

Conclusion

Change in hospital organisations affects the use of facilities. Flexibility is required to fit these changing functions. Three main design strategies – grid, pavilions and hall – can be applied to obtain flexibility, sustainability and robustness. A combination of these strategies can work together.

We started by comparing hospitals with airports. The comparison ends with hospitals and cruise ships. Big cruise ships and ferries have the same functionality and type of organisation as a hospital: the parking and logistics are situated below, the kitchens come next, above them are public spaces with restaurants, and the rooms are on top.

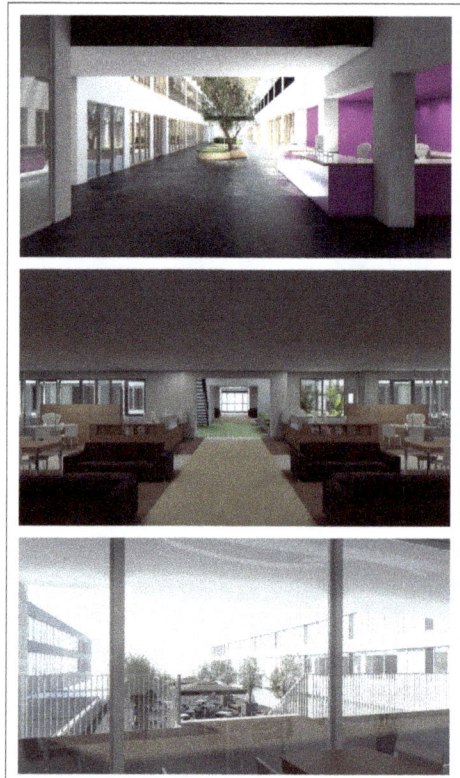

32. Saint Anthony Hospital Utrecht 2011: interiors.

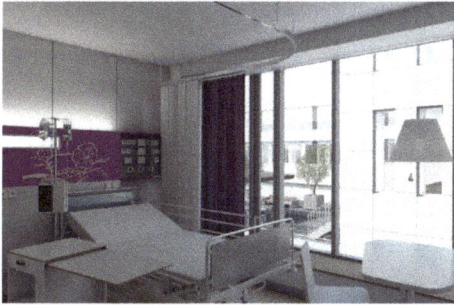

33. *Saint Anthony Hospital Utrecht 2011: ward.*

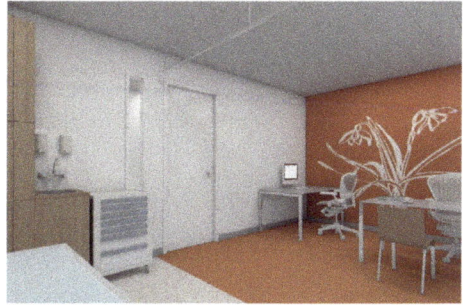

34. *Saint Anthony Hospital Utrecht 2011: examination room.*

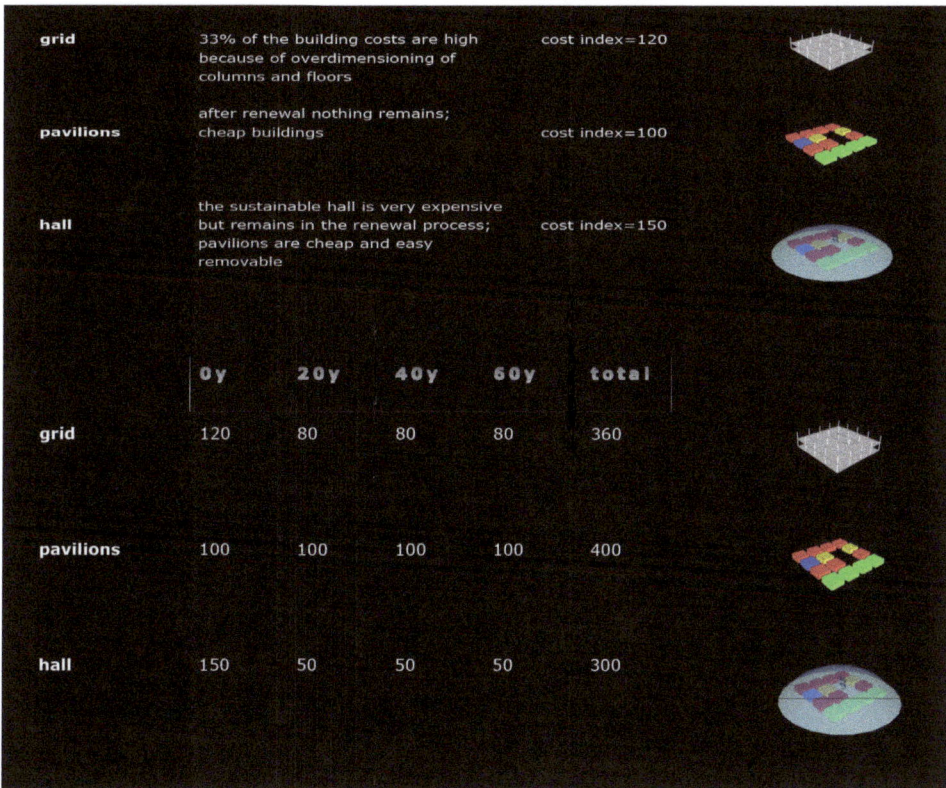

85

grid	33% of the building costs are high because of overdimensioning of columns and floors	cost index=120	
pavilions	after renewal nothing remains; cheap buildings	cost index=100	
hall	the sustainable hall is very expensive but remains in the renewal process; pavilions are cheap and easy removable	cost index=150	

	0y	20y	40y	60y	total	
grid	120	80	80	80	360	
pavilions	100	100	100	100	400	
hall	150	50	50	50	300	

35. *Cost comparison: buildings costs and renewal cost.*

Yet the form is quite different from a hospital because the form of a ship is strongly influenced by its function of sailing.

The form of a modern sustainable hospital should be entirely determined by climate, ventilation and energy savings.

Hospitals, airports and cruise ships have all the same layers of functionality, but different forms.

TESIS Inter-University Research Centre "Systems and Technologies for Social and Healthcare Facilities"
University of Florence, Italy

1. *Akershus University Hospital, Oslo, Norway.*

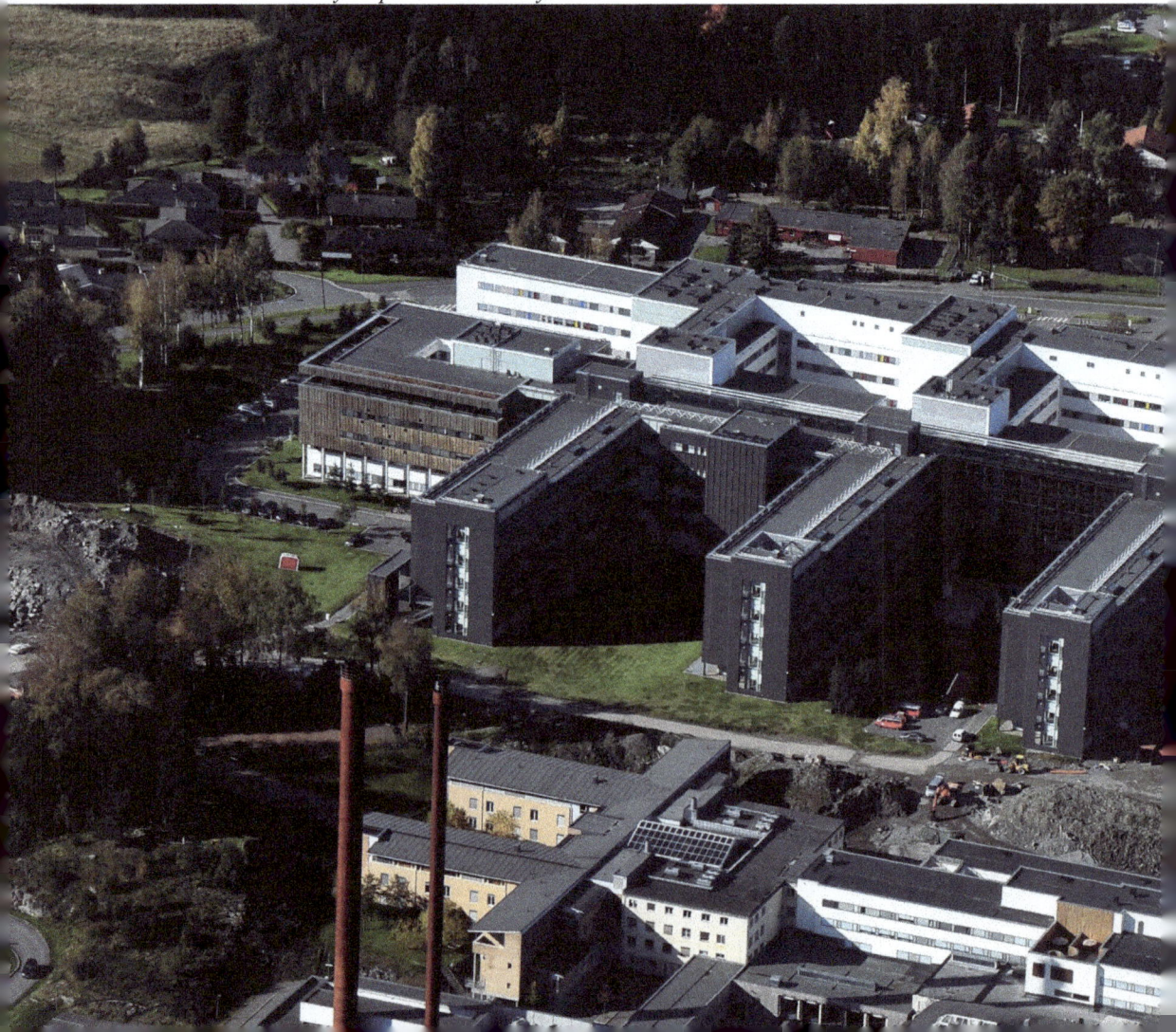

How Has Our Hospital Coped With New Demands?

Jørn A. Limi
CFO Akershus University Hospital

87

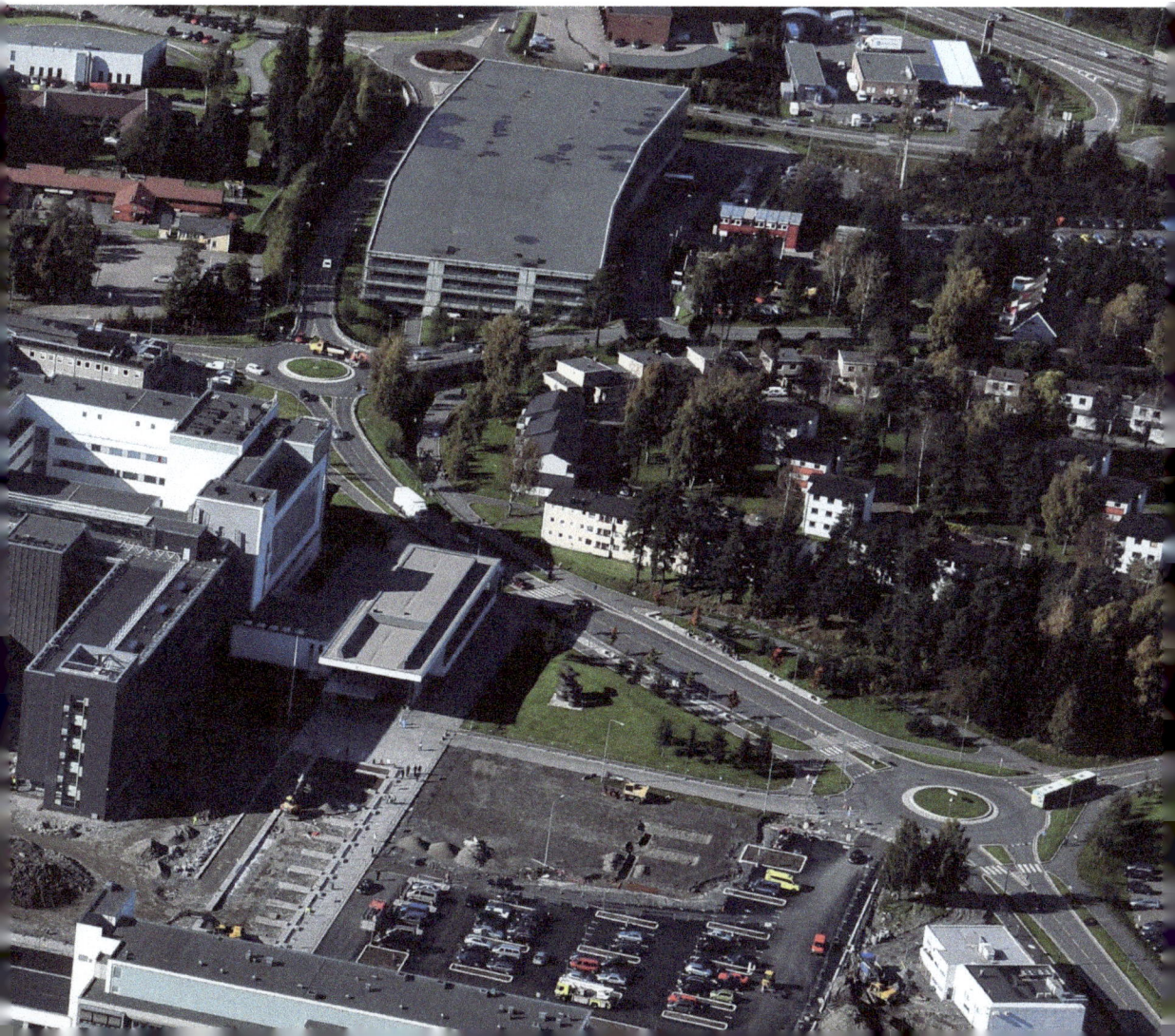

About Akershus University Hospital

The diverse and interesting catchment area of Akershus' main hospital

Akershus University Hospital (Ahus) covers a diverse, challenging and interesting catchment area encompassing a mixture of suburban districts, rural districts and neighborhoods in Oslo.

Ahus is a complete urban hospital whose catchment area comprises a large share of the immigrant population. It is a full-service hospital offering emergency and planned assistance, and serves all inhabitants of the catchment area in all age ranges, from newborns to geriatrics.

Ahus is Norway's largest and most modern emergency assistance provider as well as being a university hospital with fruitful research and development activities.

Why was the new hospital built?

Background

The old Akershus University Hospital had become too small by the mid-1990s (population 270,000) due to population increase and a demographic shift (growth in the number of elderly people).

Structural problems were encountered because the oldest parts of the buildings were built with bad concrete and there was an intense management situation (patients residing in the corridors presented a safety risk). Furthermore at that time a large property for development had been acquired.

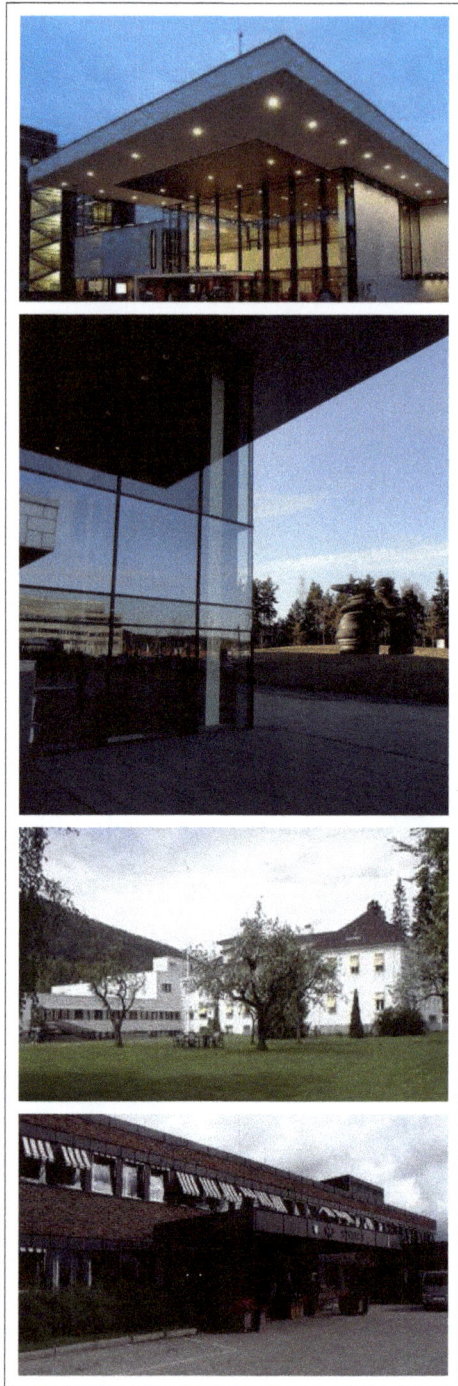

2. Akershus' main hospital.

88

Planning and building process

Planning started in 1995 with an in-house general plan, and several plans and documents were submitted for an architectural competition in 1999. The final plan was chosen in 2002 but the government declared the project too expensive. Therefore re-planning was necessary and the new final plan was presented in May 2003. The board gave its approval on 18 December 2003 and the building process started on 1 March 2004.

The new hospital was officially opened on 1 October 2008. Phase II started on 1 January 2011 and was finished in spring 2012.

The new hospital has the following capacities: 22 operating theatres (8 used for day surgery); 570 beds (in the new building); 73 beds in the patient hotel; 90 day-patient places; 108 outpatient rooms; 23 rooms for diagnostic imaging. The basic structure is comprised of a technical centre, a psychiatric unit, bed cluster wards, a pediatric clinic, emergency rooms, treatment wings, a chapel, a main entrance, a car park, a glass promenade, university/administration and a patient hotel.

Project planning goals (for 2015) provide for: 40,400 patients, 25,200 daytime consultations, 186,500 outpatient consultations and a population of 340,000.

89

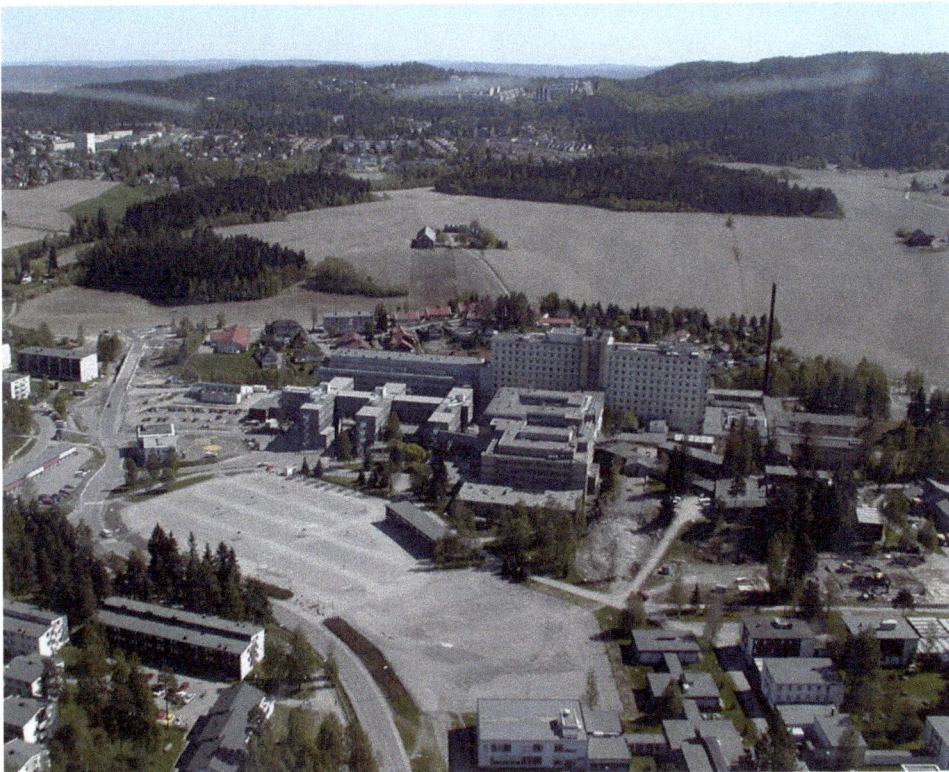

3. *Aerial view of Akershus hospital.*

TESIS Inter-University Research Centre "Systems and Technologies for Social and Healthcare Facilities"
University of Florence, Italy

TESIS

90

The final plan, dated 28 May 2003, provided for a total area of 137,000 m2, more effective performance such as 240 days per year and 10 hours per day, outpatient clinics, day care patients and day surgery, diagnostic radiography, elective surgery, 11 hours per day of postoperative care, a change of 20% from overnight patients to outpatients and an investment of NOK 6.9 billion (2003)/ NOK 8.6 billion (2011).

In order to achieve these objectives special architectural solutions were implemented such as a compact hospital design which reduces distances; separating day patients who enter through the main entrance from emergency patients who enter via the ambulance entrance; emergency rooms (ER) on the 2nd floor and a gate to the emergency unit; the day surgery separated from other surgical activities; and office areas between bed and treatment areas.

By observing the current needs it is possible to identify some solutions for the future such as automatic solutions and the use of robots in the laboratory centre; up-to-date image diagnosis equipment; smart cards for doors and IT. Modern logistical solutions may deliver goods and dispose of waste: AGVs/pneumatic tube system, automatic waste tube and laundry distribution system. Up-to-date standardized storage processes and systems may be applied in a regional warehouse and the use of bar codes may be implemented.

Major changes decided from 2008

Changes to the hospital structure in the Oslo area and in particular to Oslo University Hospital were decided in 2011 due to the growth of Ahus' catchment area, which increased to 450,000 inhabitants. In 2012 further sequence changes were decided in line with the Coordination Reform: increased resources aimed at limiting and preventing disease; length of stay expected to be reduced in 2012; primary care services financed to increase capacity within 4 years (nonsurgery patients).

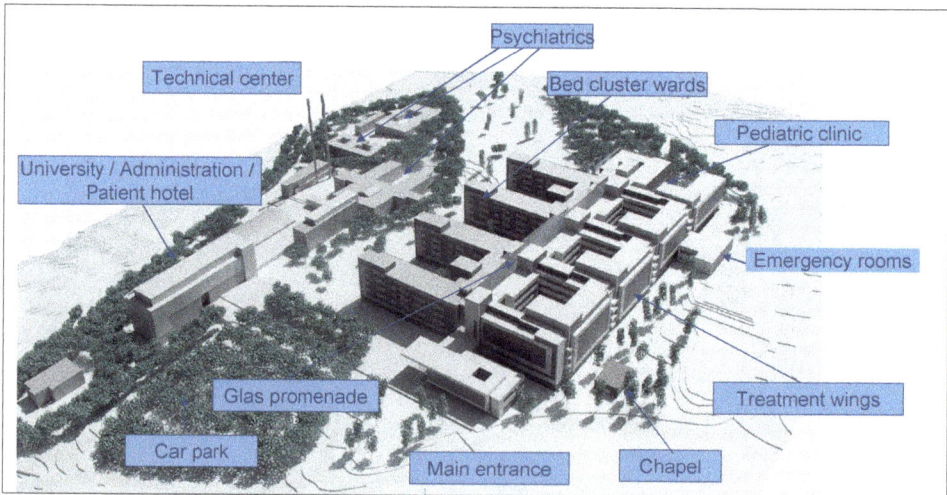

4. Basic structure.

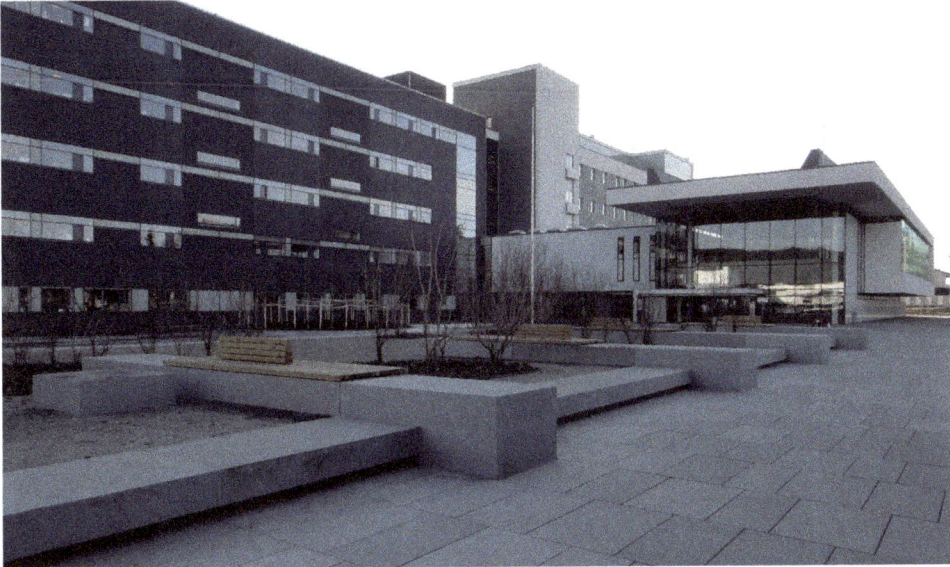

5. Main entrance.

A comparison between patient activity in 2011 and the 2015 goals reveals the following: 53,536 patients (+33%); 41,171 daytime consultations (+63%); 208,245 outpatient consultations (+12%); a population of 455,000 (+34%).

Some additional investments are needed for patient care at two additional locations, which were originally due to be closed, mainly designed for outpatient and day care consultations (plus a day surgery). Furthermore there is a need for minor rebuilding works at the new hospital to convert office space to outpatient and day care areas, an emergency unit (2012), and space for new MR and CT equipment. There is a need for new buildings for offices and some other functions.

Experiences

Moving from a traditional labor-intensive hospital to a new high-tech build-ing implies a number of changes and involves a training program, some start-up issues (too much new technology at once), fundamental risk change (systems run 24/7/365), and a change in the cost structure. The Ahus culture also shifted: most of the employees stayed and new management challenges include taking into account financial and risk challenges and culture change.

Changes bring future costs…

Original investments were cut and the 2002 investment cut reduced support functions, storage areas, offices, etc. Additional investments will be required in a few years. The regional trust wanted to use the hospital's capacity from day one: bed capacity is already full, with some patients in corridors (85% capacity is planned for 2015) and new investments are needed for expected population growth (+25% by 2025).

TESIS Inter-University Research Centre "Systems and Technologies for Social and Healthcare Facilities"
University of Florence, Italy

1. *Rikshospitalet, National Hospital of Oslo.*

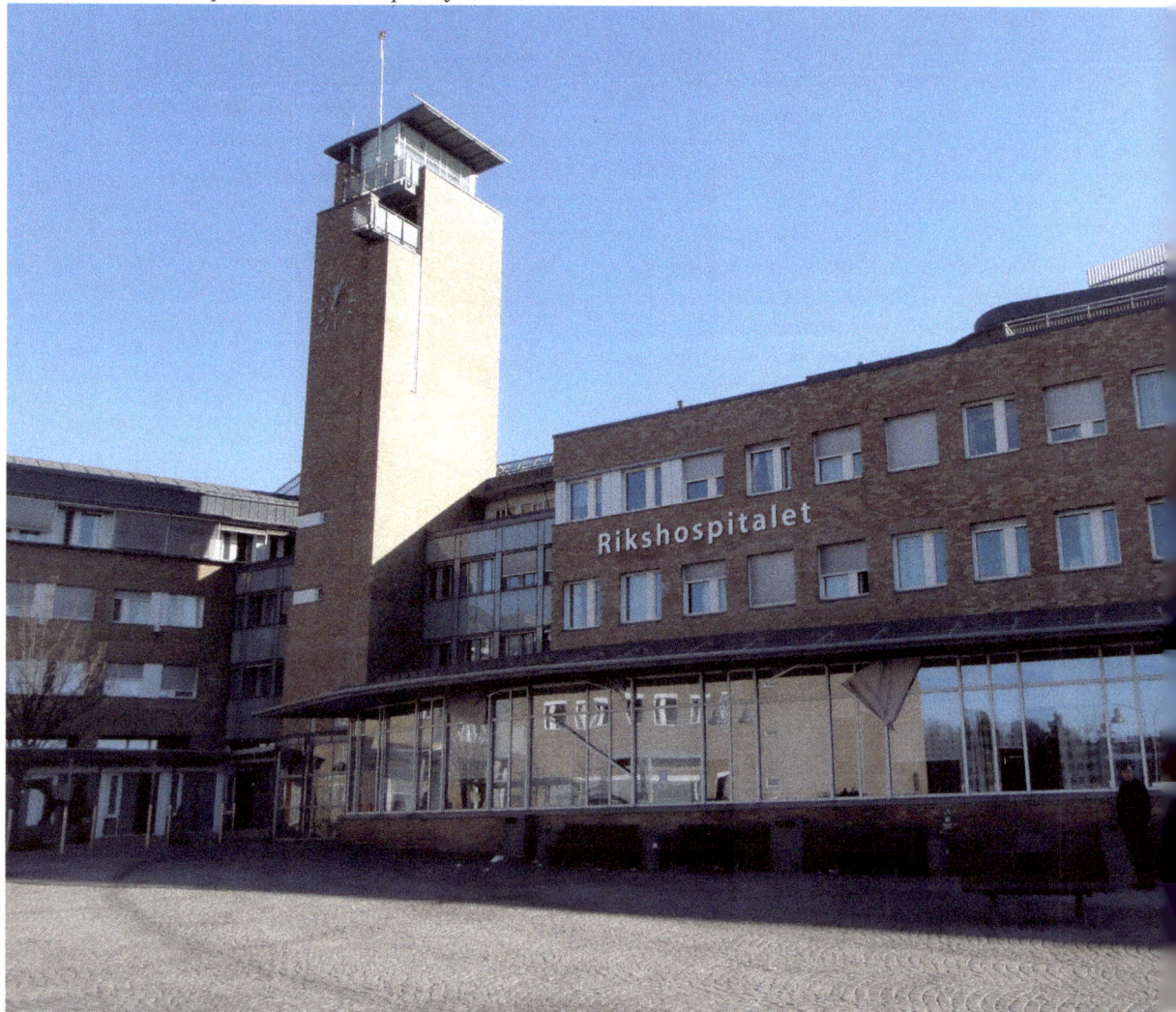

Building Changes in the National Hospital of Oslo 10 years later

Tarald Rhode
Senior Advisor SINTEF Health Research

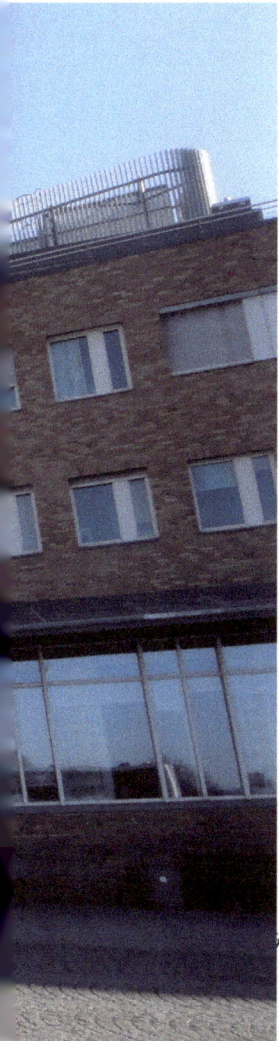

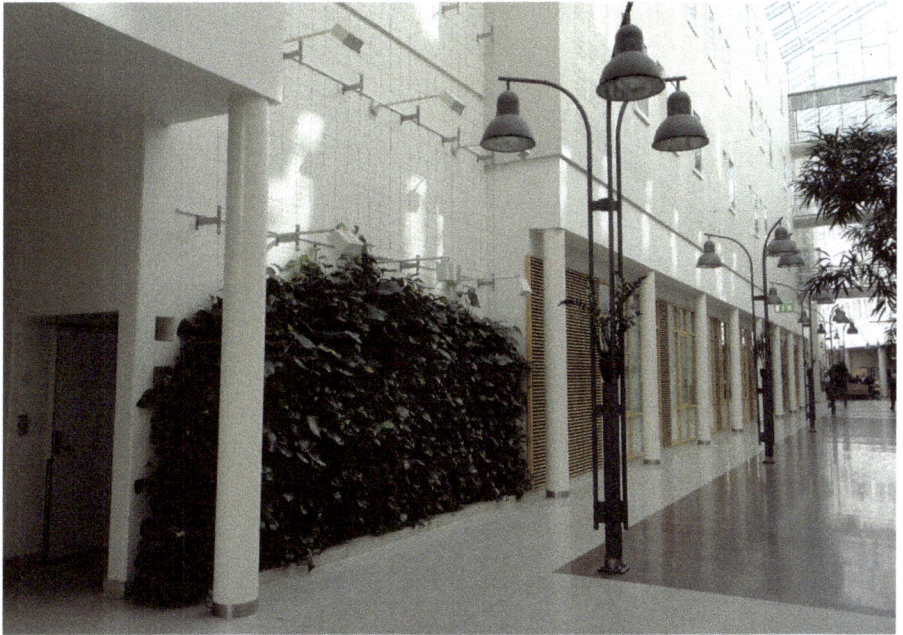

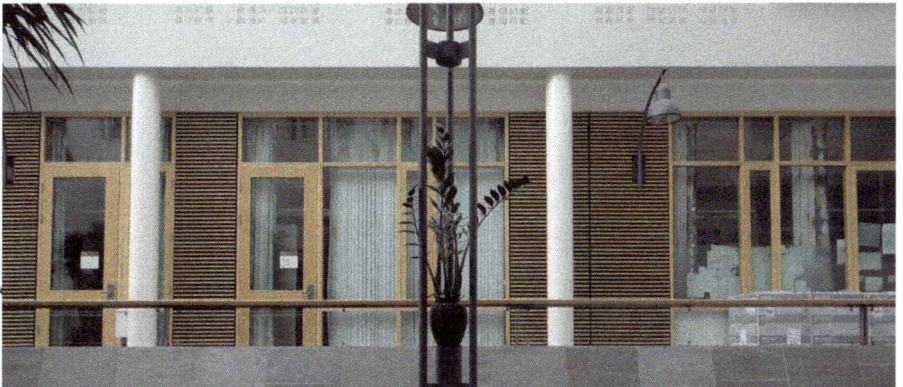

93

Flexibility is often the mantra when planning hospitals. But what really changes and how well is it possible to prepare for changes to come. This short presentation starts with the New National Hospital in Oslo, Norway. It was finished in 2001 and has therefore been operating for 10 years. What kind of changes has this hospital undergone in 10 years?

Our forefathers had already had second thoughts about what would happen in the future, so let this quotation set the tone for what is to follow.

According to Old Norse wisdom poetry, entitled Håvamål, "You should not know your destiny in advance, that makes you only grieve." From this point of view we must ask ourselves if flexibility is a mantra to escape the present?

It is easy to talk about what may happen and forget the task at hand. In some

94

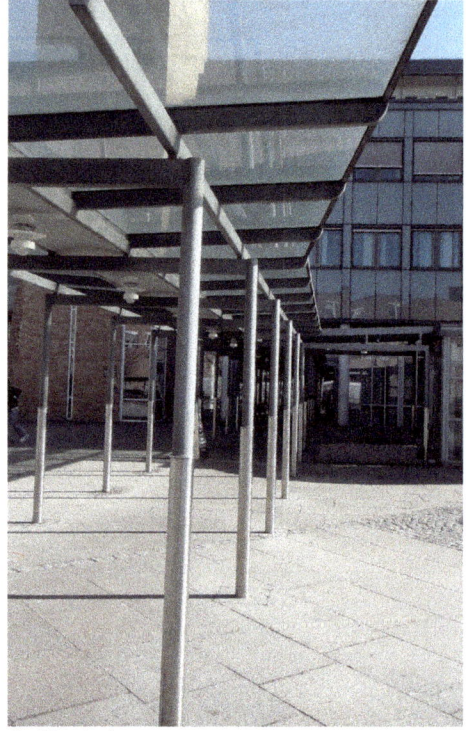

2. Hospital entrance.

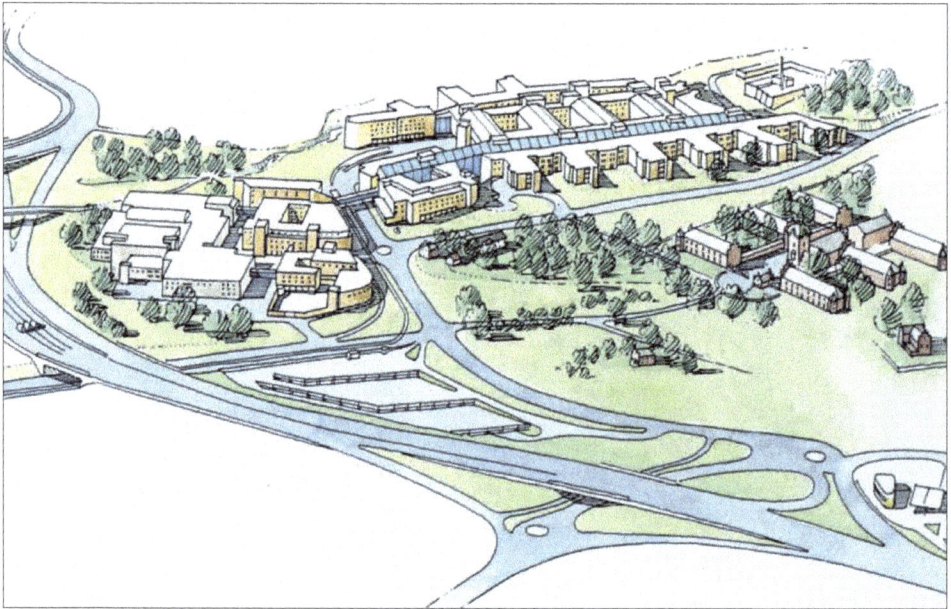

3. A project sketch of Rikshospitalet.

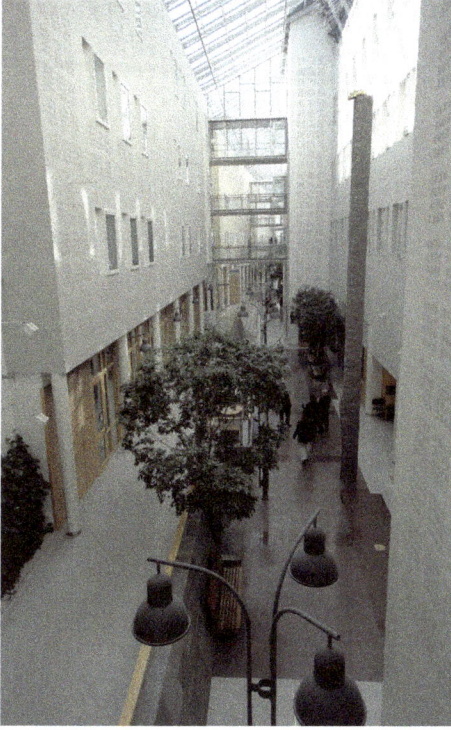

4. *View of the connective tissue.*

cases the possible outcome of a "flexible" hospital may be areas that nobody likes or expensive technical solutions because the building has to be prepared for the most demanding situations. The most probable result of planning for the future: the future turns out to be different.

The story of the construction of the National Bank of Norway is an example of knowing what will happen. At that time Oslo municipality was planning what they called the baseline street through Oslo: a motorway that was supposed to pass by where the bank was to be built. It was planned that this motorway would pass through a tunnel under the building. Up until 1985 no firm decision had been made on whether to proceed with this plan. The Norwegian Bank reached an agreement with the municipality whereby they would refund the bank for some of the expenses incurred for the

95

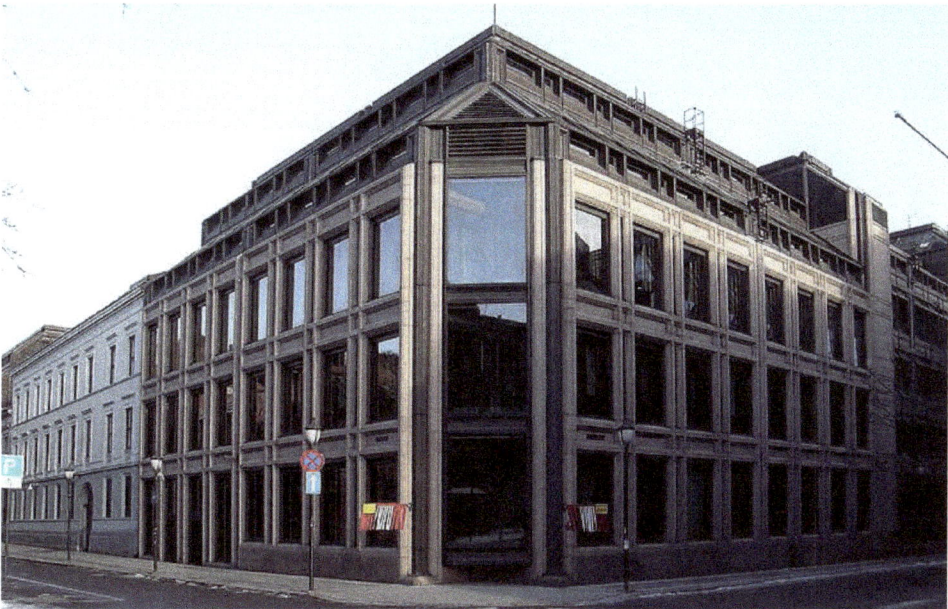

5. *The National Bank, a motorway in the basement.*

TESIS Inter-University Research Centre "Systems and Technologies for Social and Healthcare Facilities"
University of Florence, Italy

work necessary to prepare for this motorway. The work was carried out, but in 1985 the plan changed. Today this stretch of a motorway is a parking lot.

While building the New National Hospital preparations were made for a PET scanner and a positron scanner. This was a few years before PACS was a reality, so the radiology archive was placed where the positron scanner was supposed to go.

When the positron actually arrived it was much more expensive to find another location for it in this part of the building, so instead it was placed in a separate building on the north side of the hospital.

Image 6 places the map of the small Norwegian town Røros above the New National Hospital. It is the same size. This is to underline that a hospital is not one building but rather a town, so when talking about flexibility it would be wise to think of town planning.

In Norway most hospitals have now categorized all their built areas into functions. This was already done for the National Hospital when it was built. The pie chart in image 6 shows how much of the area has changed its name/function in 11 years.

Most changes relate to extensions, and include the PET scanner and the positron. Interior changes only account for 2% of the total area.

Of course there have been other changes too. The technical division has brought in more equipment over the years, resulting in problems obtaining enough electricity and challenging the ventilation capacity.

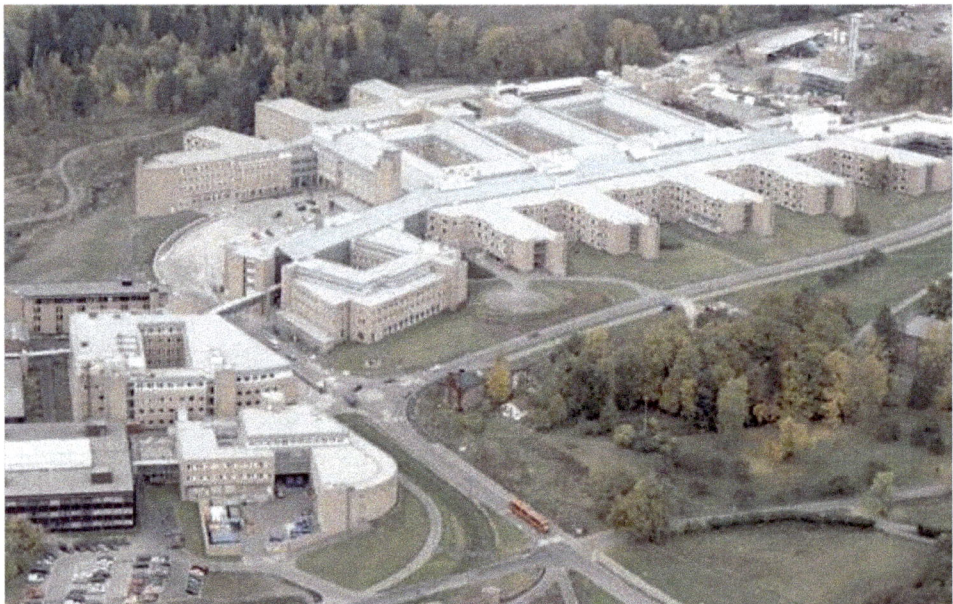

6. Rikshospitalet: the size of a small Norwegian town.

However, there have been relatively few real changes in functions. Looking at the 2% that has changed, the pie chart in image 7 shows what the new functions are: 4% extensions, 2% new functions, and 94% no change.

The following changes have been made to the areas in 10 years: 3% offices to 5% bedrooms; 20% more energy demand; 5% less complicated rooms and 46% offices. Offices are the winners.

Thus it is possible to conclude with another old saying by Confucius, "Make studies of the past if you want to predict the future." Do not fantasize too much about the future before you have a good grasp of the past and the present. Be serious in understanding what the demands of the present are and make good solutions for the present, which will give you the best flexible solutions for the future.

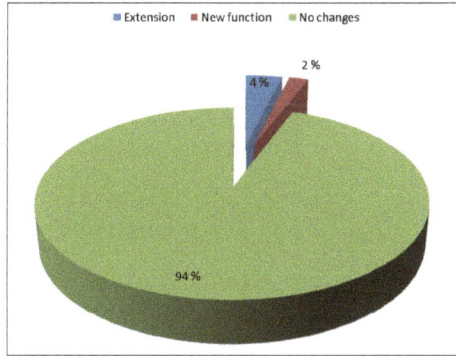

7. *The net area of the National Hospital, changes made since 2001.*

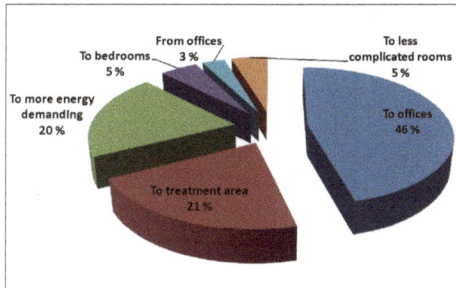

8. *What kind of changes have been made to the areas in 10 years?*

97

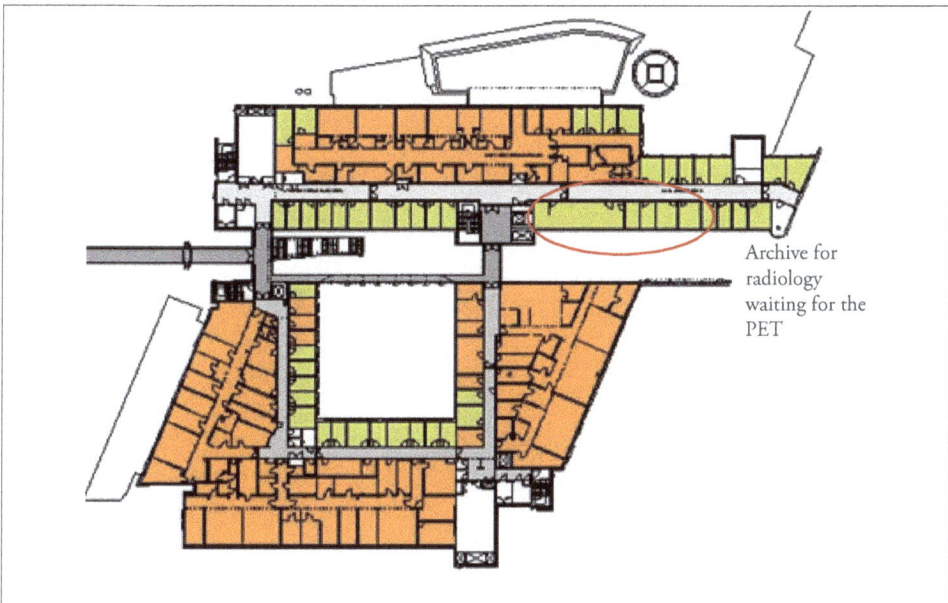

Archive for radiology waiting for the PET

9. *Waiting for the positron and the PET scanner.*

TESIS Inter-University Research Centre "Systems and Technologies for Social and Healthcare Facilities"
University of Florence, Italy

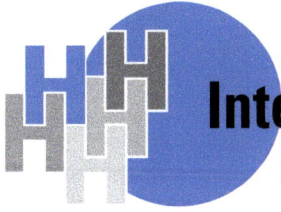

International Hospital Projects

Session introduction

The three case studies presented in the session highlight some design topics with similar features even though they describe works in different parts of the world. Each of the three experiences provides an opportunity to reflect on a particular issue of healthcare design: the relationship between the healthcare complex, pre-existing buildings and the context, the role and tasks of the designers according to the instructions from the public client, and the necessary interaction between the professionals involved in the collaborative project.

The paper by Romano Del Nord describes the experience of designing the portal entrance to the University Campus at Careggi in Florence. This case provided an opportunity to reflect on the relationship that the healthcare complex should have with the cultural and urban context of reference. This intervention avoided closing down the historic university campus and instead a plan for the regeneration and redevelopment of the existing structures was implemented. The design challenge was met by reinterpreting the typological historical models existing in Florence and by adopting innovative construction techniques.

Romano Del Nord p. 101

Warren and Rhonda Kerr's presentation provides an overview of the Australian healthcare system and the methods of planning and designing healthcare facilities. This particular scenario highlighted the topics of the conference, such as the development of technology, flexibility, cost, energy efficiency and patient safety. In the case of the Fiona Stanley Hospital in Perth the designers, as well as following the indications outlined in the Australian Health Design Guidelines, attempted to meet the new needs related to healthcare by applying evidence-based design and a patient-centered approach.

Warren Kerr and Rhonda Kerr p. 113

An important factor that contributes to raise the level of complexity of healthcare building projects is the presence of several professionals who work together in the design and execution phases. The academic exercise presented by George Mann enabled students to understand the issues of the collaborative project firsthand. Students from three different universities and professional experts involved in the project for the Eye Hospital of Pyang in China simulated, through the design exercise, what happens in the real world of professional practice where different professionals and parties involved in the construction process collaborate remotely via web tools.

George Mann and Xi Qiu Huang p. 121

TESIS Inter-University Research Centre "Systems and Technologies for Social and Healthcare Facilities" University of Florence, Italy

1. *Careggi healthcare campus, Florence.*

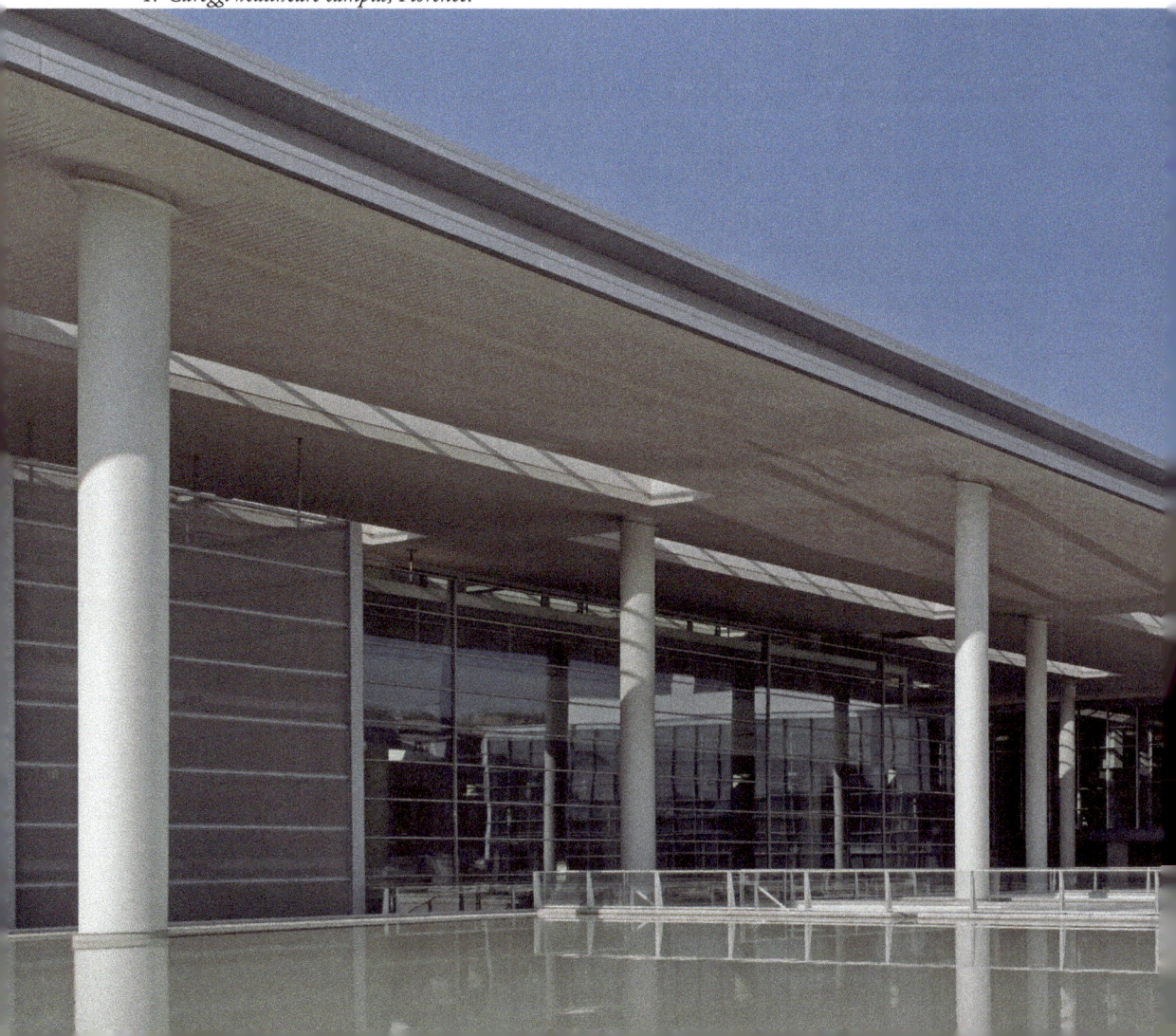

The Teaching and Research Hospital: An Integrated Design Experience

Romano Del Nord
Professor University of Florence
Director of TESIS Inter-University Research Centre

101

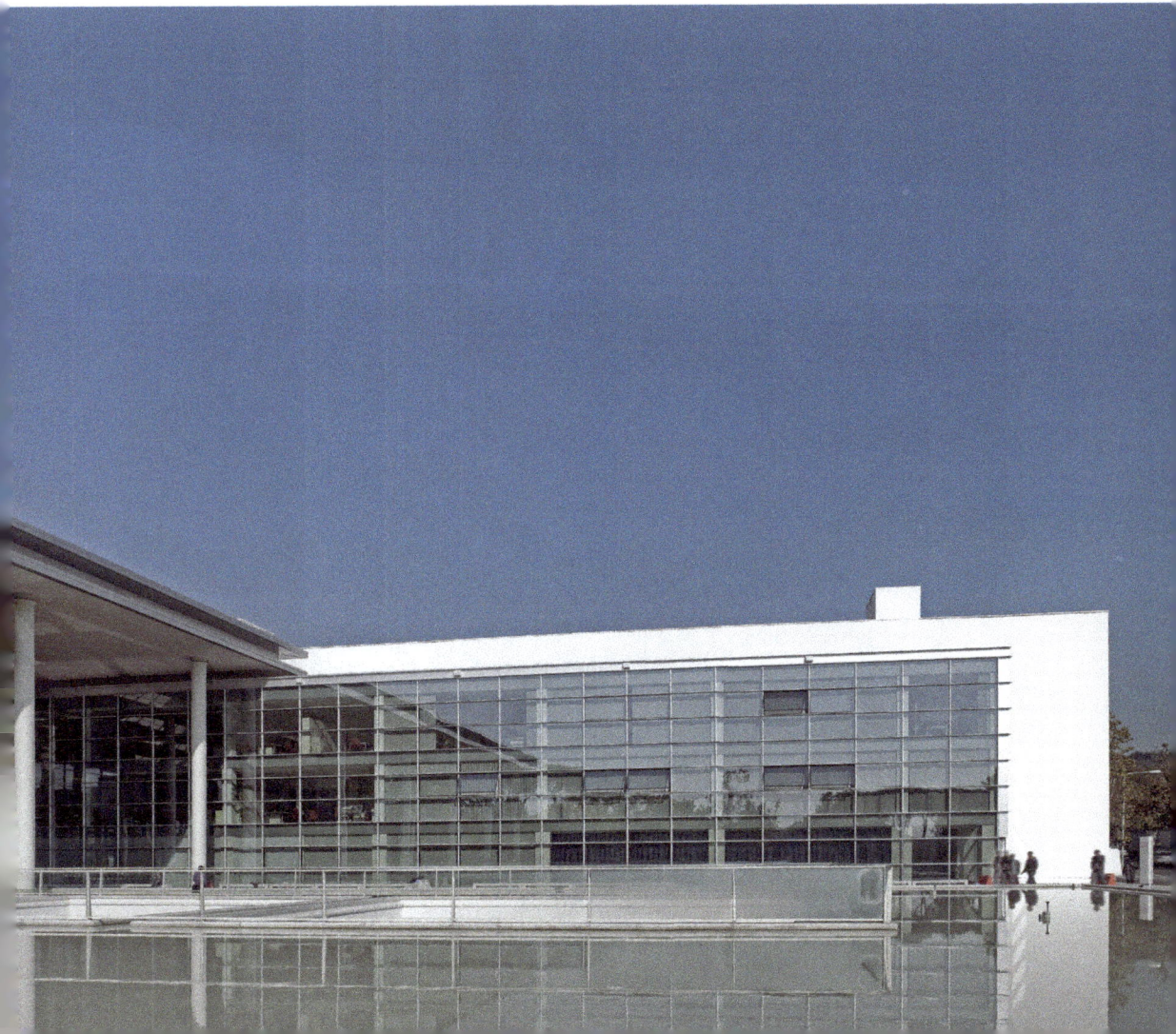

The presentation is about the design experience of a recently opened complex in the Careggi healthcare campus, north of Florence in Italy. The new building is conceived as 'one piece' of a larger mosaic of developments within a master plan that started about ten years ago and has already completed the demolition and reconstruction of 6 major buildings.

102

The significant 'functional core' plays a strategic role in the implementation of the whole reorganization program of the Hospital System in Florence. It is called "an integrated design experience" because its design has provided the opportunity to address three related planning issues:

a. the first is the connection between the 'urban' city and the 'healthcare' city;

b. the second is the creation of a hub where it is possible to manage and develop teaching, research and care activities;

c. the third is the testing of innovative technology and sustainable devices and procedures.

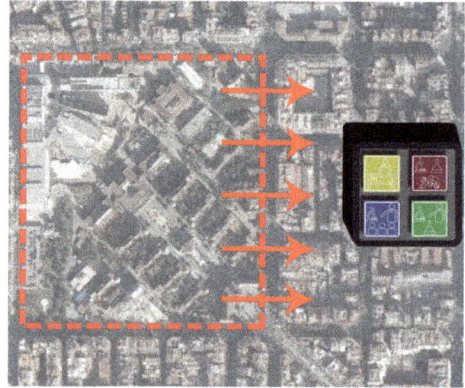

2. Plan strategy: delocalize.

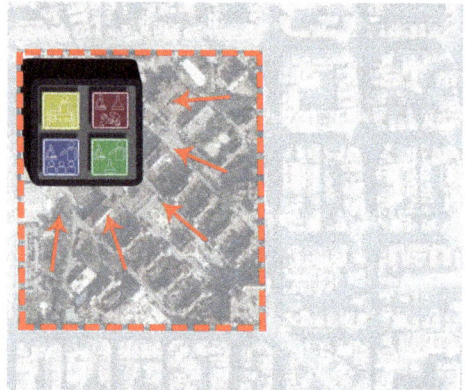

3. Plan strategy: adapt.

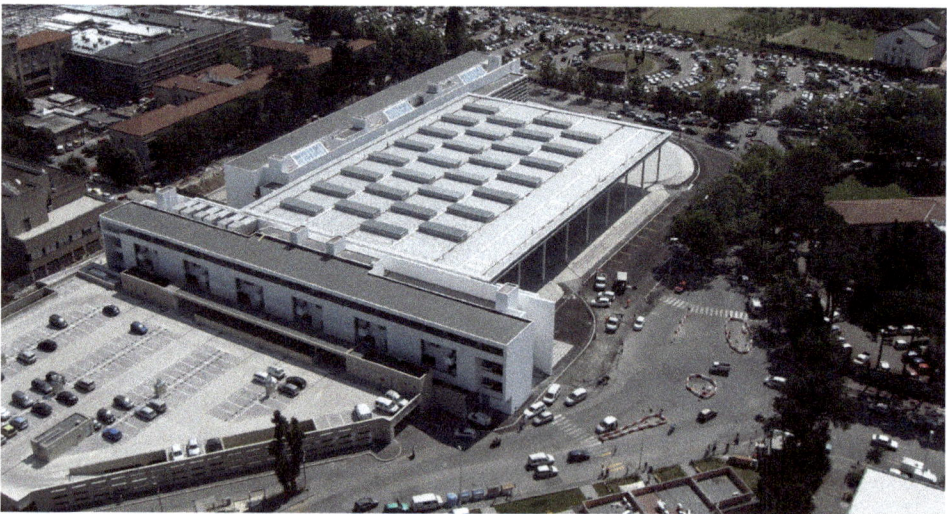

4. Careggi healthcare campus, from 2000 to the future.

The new building must be framed within the decade-long program of the functional reorganization of a hospital campus that started its life in the early Nineties and developed according to the logic of single-discipline pavilions.

In the nineties, for the first time, the Regional Government addressed the updating of the whole campus and commissioned Centro Studi Progettazione Edilizia CSPE to do a Feasibility Study to evaluate the two options: "delocalize" or "adapt". The question was whether it would prove more effective in the long run to move the campus to another area or to start a progressive 'restore and revive' programme up to the 'demolition and rebuilding' of the existing pavilions, without stopping their services.

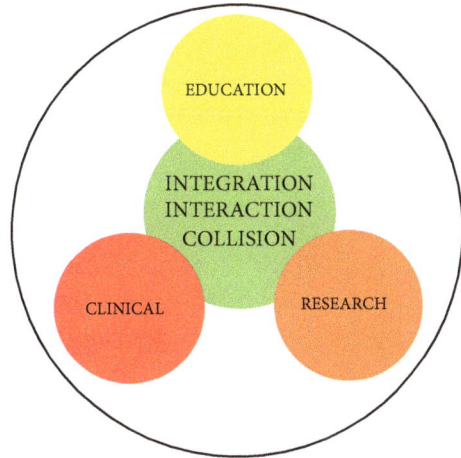

103

5. A new model of care and a new type of integration between care, teaching and research.

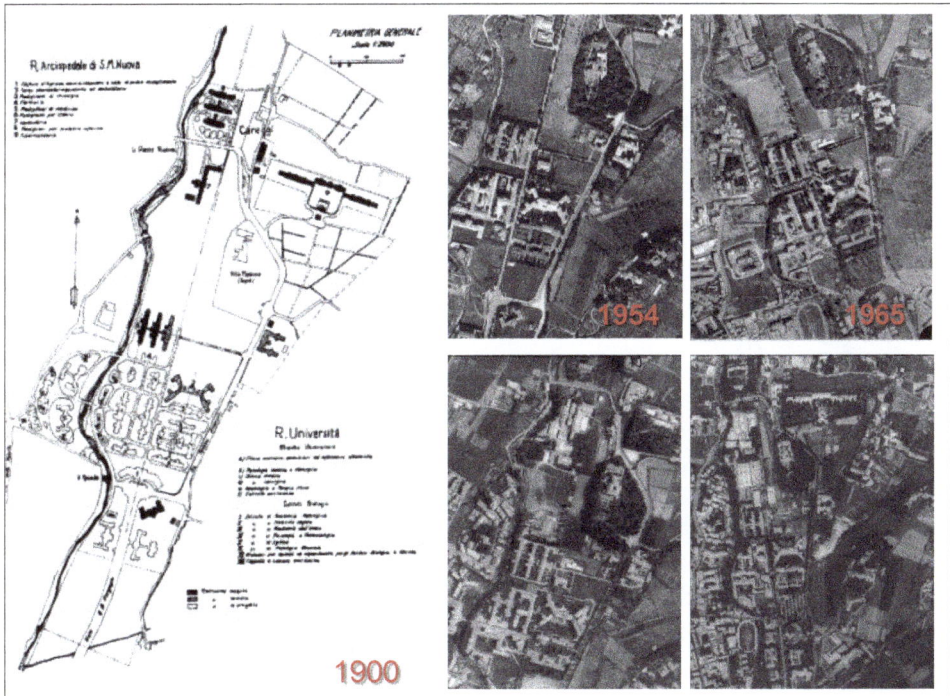

6. Careggi healthcare campus: historical development.

TESIS Inter-University Research Centre "Systems and Technologies for Social and Healthcare Facilities"
University of Florence, Italy

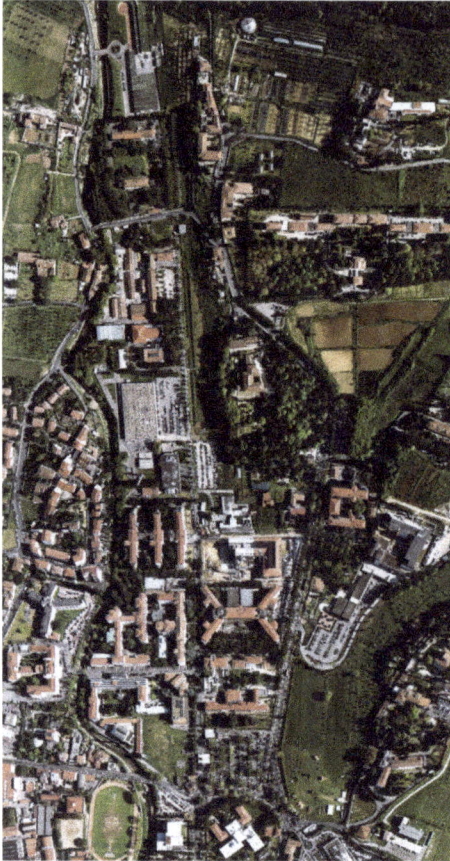

7. Careggi healthcare campus, 2000.

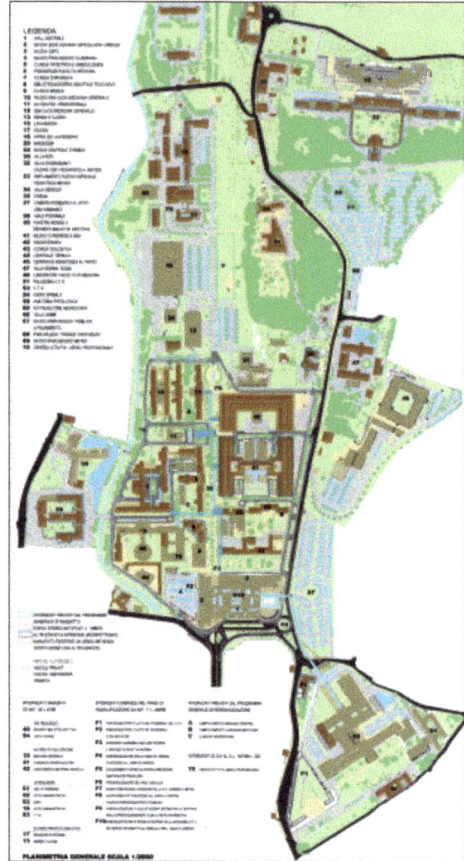

8. The new Careggi plan.

The winning option was to regenerate the whole hospital campus.

The two key factors the new master plan was asked to address were the definitions of:

- a new model of care;
- a new type of integration between care, teaching and research activities.

For the first point, relating to the definition of a model of care fit for the future, the proposal was to centralize all the emergency and trauma care into a single core that would act as the centre of gravity of a satellite ring where all the long-term medical services and care would be concentrated.

For the second point, relating to the functional integration of teaching, research and care activities, CSPE together with the hospital administration decided not only to spread these activities throughout the campus but also to concentrate them into specialized centres.

The aim was to achieve two types of integration. The first conceives of integration as the sharing of objectives among the three functions. The main consequences of this meaning relate to the organizational and management structures of the aforementioned functions.

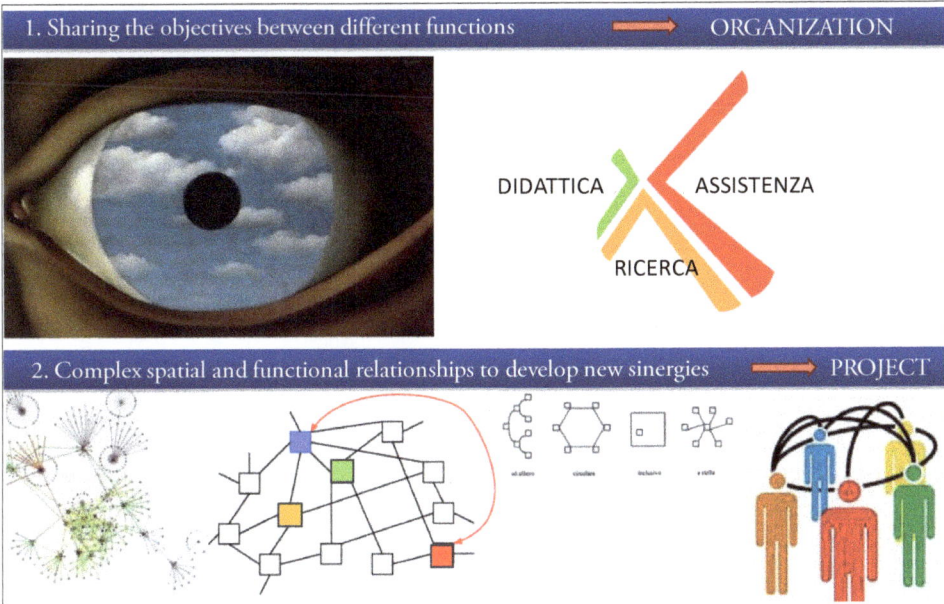

9. Two types of integration.

The second conceives of integration as complex spatial relationships or functional links that support the development of synergy among care, training and research activities. The main consequences are the physical scale and the design of the teaching hospital complex. The proximity of care, teaching and research is vital and can be managed in different ways:
– fully decentralized;
– partly decentralized;
– partly centralized (as is the case at Careggi);
– fully centralized.
In this case the "partly centralized" model was adopted. It means "proximity at macro level" (campus scale) and "proximity at micro level" (in each individual building).
In order to achieve these objectives, the first stage was to design and build the new Trauma and Emergency Depart-

ment at the heart of the intensive and acute area situated inside the inner ring. The second stage was to find a "control cabin" for the integration facilities located inside the new "Gateway Building", which is symbolically at the entrance of the campus.
Teaching, research and care activities required a physical place that would stress the importance of the integration between these three vital functions that are at the centre of innovation.
The new Integrated Centre is a multidisciplinary building used as a hub for cultural exchange and the dissemination of biomedical research, as well as for managing the integration of research, teaching, training and care.
The typological matrix that generated the new architecture is fully rooted in Florentine urban buildings. Most notably, Brunelleschi's Ospedale degli Innocenti right in the historical centre of

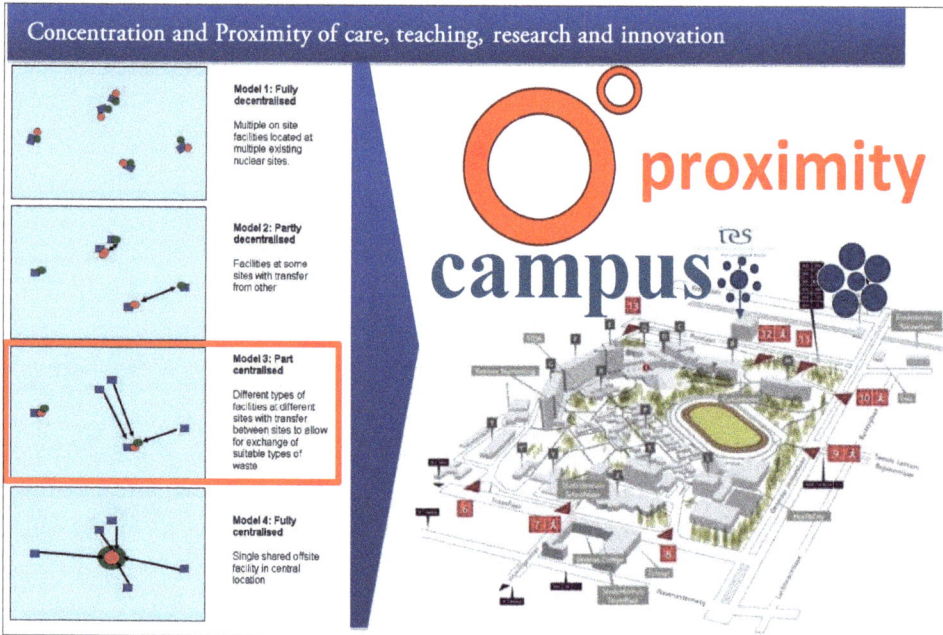

10. Teaching hospital: a concentration of teaching, care, research and innovation.

Florence shows how piazzas and porticos have been traditionally intertwined since the 15th century.

Renaissance Florence shows that "architecture and urbanism", the "private and public realm", and "interior and exterior space" are traditionally connected as part of the same entity.

The team of architects led by CSPE therefore gave a modern interpretation to historical urban spaces in Florence. The design aim of the new Integrated Centre was to update traditional morphologies with modern materials and techniques. This is also highly symbolic of an updated and forward-looking new model of care.

The openness and accessibility between the city and the hospital is reinforced by the new intermodal transport network which uses the New Integrated Centre as a point of reference.

In addition to public transport, which comes right up to the new entrance, there is an adjacent multi-storey car park and public car parks all around the ring road bordering the campus.

To highlight the importance of ongoing exchange between care and biomedical research, CSPE has also designed a bridge that directly connects the new Integrated Centre with the main acute care complex.

Again the purpose is to stress its importance in order to keep the cultural flow alive between researchers and clinicians. Site plan. The new building is composed of three volumes and contains spaces for university teaching and research as well as offices, an information entrance, a reception area and commercial activity. It is linked to a multi-storey car park and cut through by a covered urban street that acts as a direct link between the city

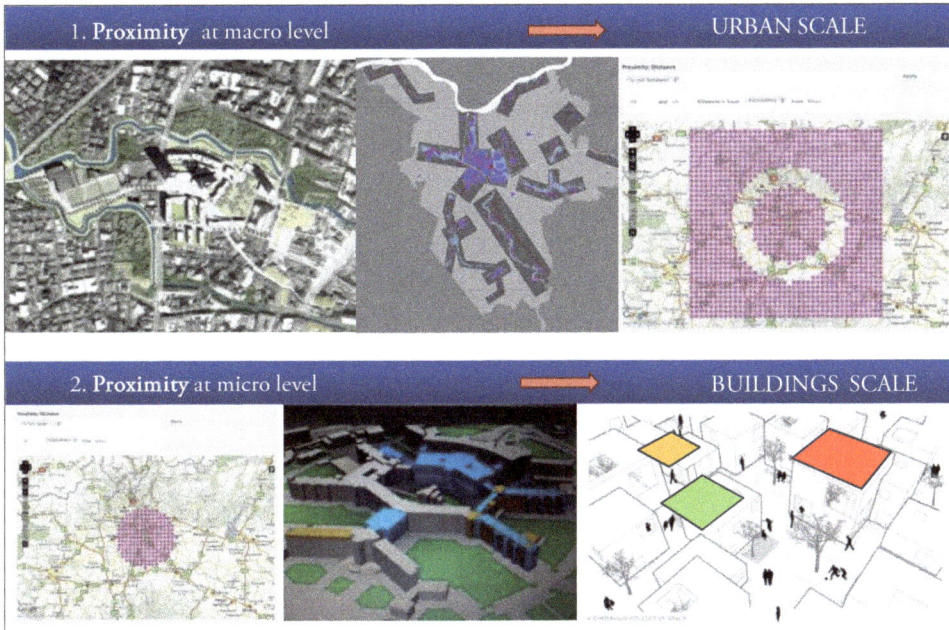

11. *Teaching hospital: proximity at macro and micro level.*

and the campus. The result is complete integration between the public realm and the healthcare city. Overall its total internal area covers 20,000 square meters.

The basement floor is connected with the car park. It contains the more urban activities such as food chains, shops, cafeterias, newspaper kiosks, chemists and restaurants. This is a clear way of integrating the hospital with the city, breaking the assumption that the hospital is a closed-in fortress.

The ground floor is raised above street level by steps that define new boundaries and, most of all, create a new sense of place. The ground floor contains a parking area, laboratories and a research area, classrooms and an auditorium for the Faculty of Medicine and Surgery, as well as the information and reception area.

The upper floors are organized in three

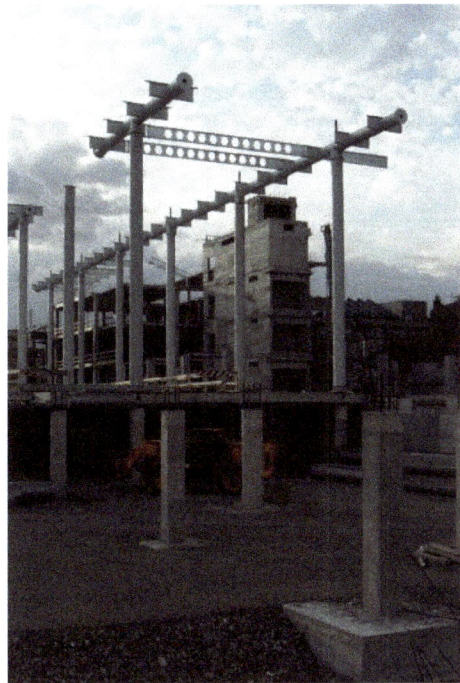

12. *The site during the elevation of the steel pillars.*

TESIS Inter-University Research Centre "Systems and Technologies for Social and Healthcare Facilities"
University of Florence, Italy

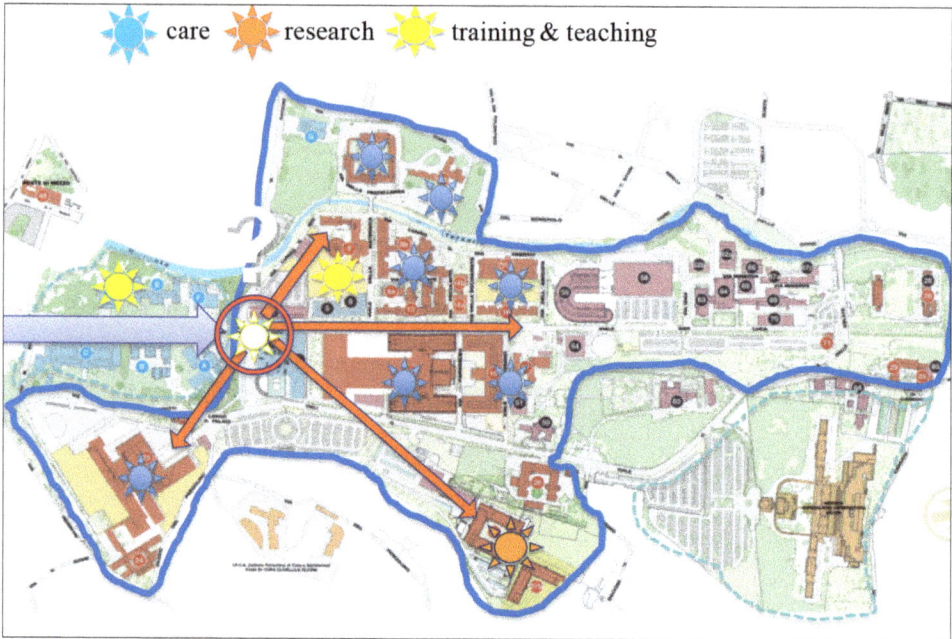

13. *Careggi campus: flows.*

interconnected blocks with research and teaching spaces.

Last but not least, the third aspect to mention is the use of innovative technology based on prefabrication and dry construction systems with wide span trusses. Although widely used abroad, the Italian way of building is still accustomed to in-situ techniques with the large-scale use of reinforced concrete. This type of construction is partly due to the humid Italian climate with hot summers and cold winters that require high thermal masses, lobbying on the part of manufactures, and finally strict seismic rules and regulations. Naturally, beyond experimenting, the aim of this construction is to speed up construction which is an issue that needs to be addressed in hospital building.

The design is characterized by a large roof, supported by slender columns, which projects over the individual buildings giving them a sense of unity. The roof and the large glazed façades create the feeling of being under a covered piazza where people and activities merge in a unique hub. Furthermore, the extensive roof is also a shading device to protect the fully glazed façades and outdoor areas, especially during the hot summer months.

Because of its position on the northern edge of the campus the new centre is also perceived as a gateway, although its particular design components have turned the notion of a "door" into one of piazza and porticos, typical of the Florentine tradition.

The double-height entrance conveys an urban presence capable of relating to the city scale.

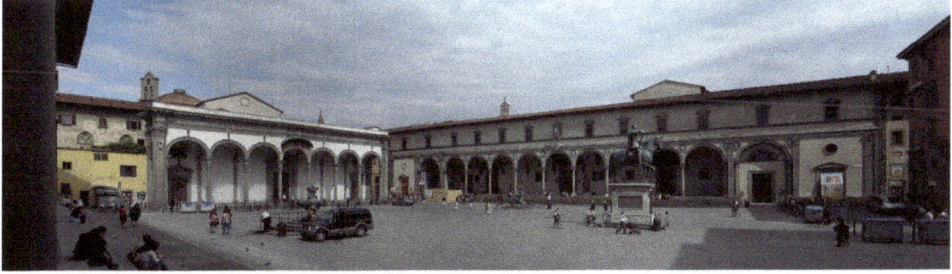

14. Ospedale degli Innocenti, Piazza SS. Annunziata, Firenze.

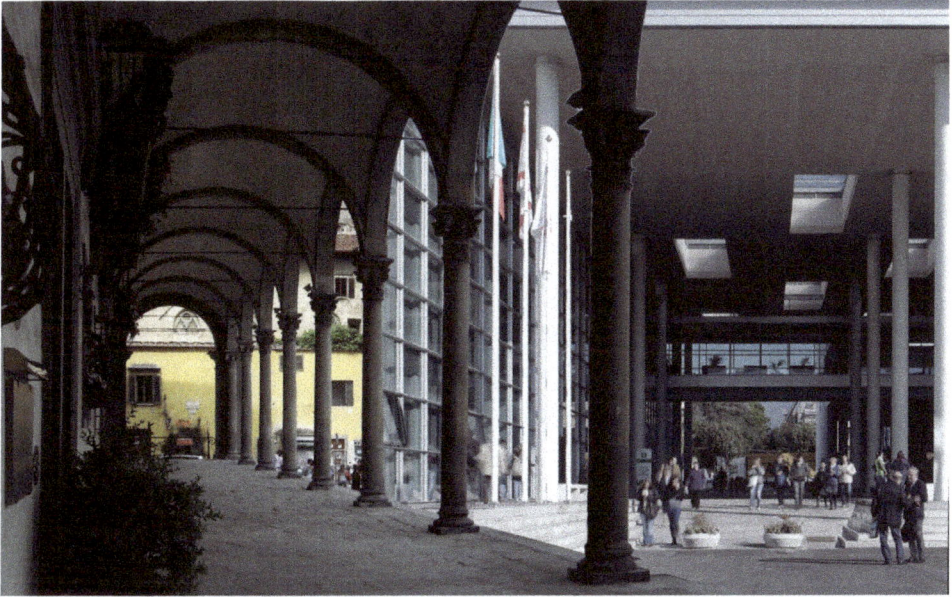

15. Arcades and piazzas identify our public realm.

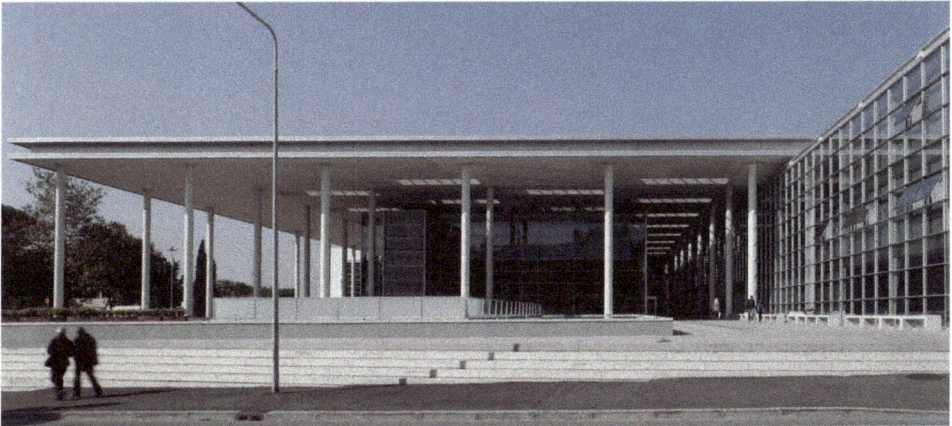

16. Classical modernity.

110

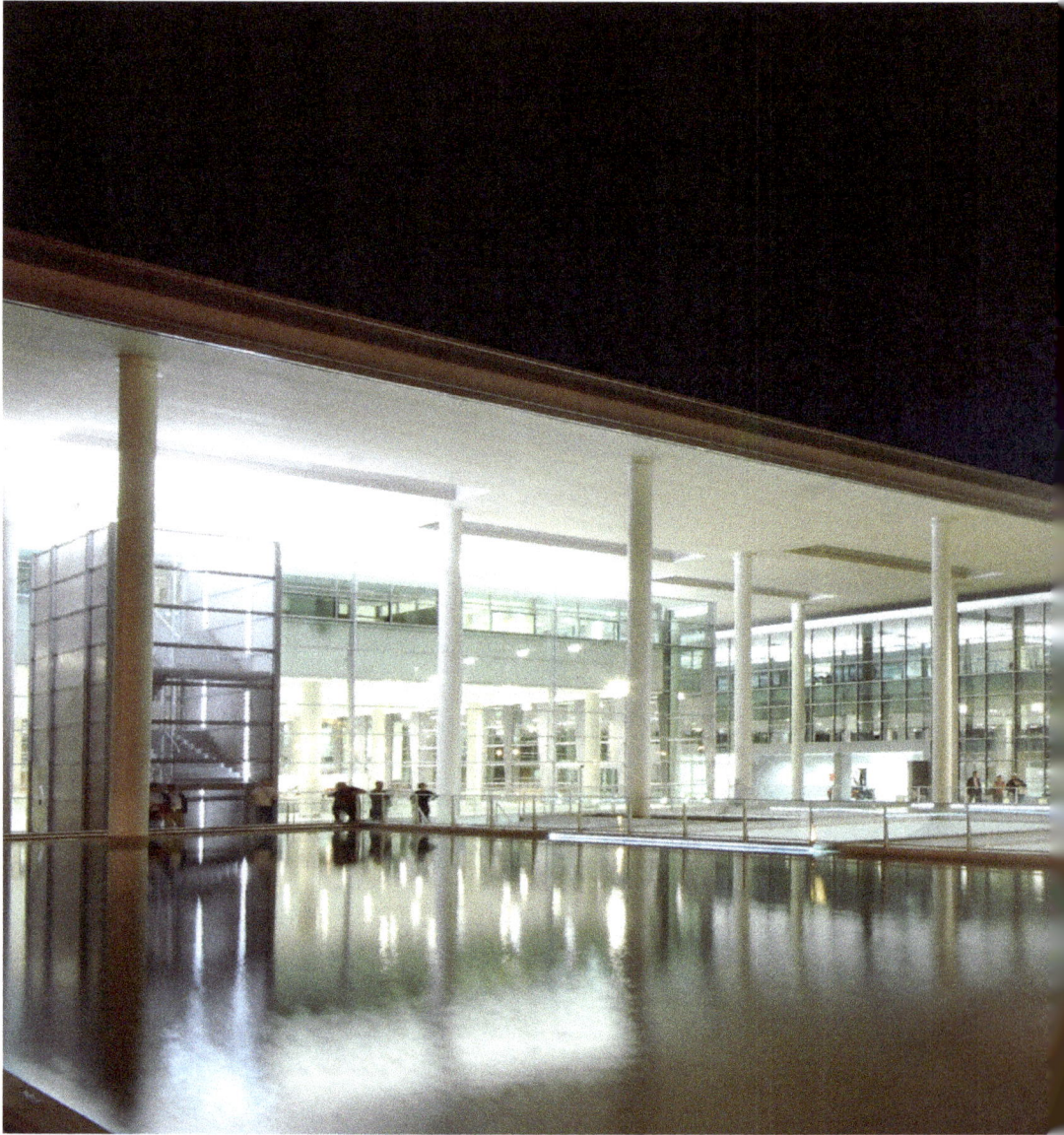

17. A beacon at night.

The extensive use of glass helps to provide an intuitive understanding of the functions and wayfinding. Upper levels are connected by airy bridges suspended on columns.

Materials and details have been chosen to give a sense of openness, and at the same time the strong visual dynamics communicate a vibrant environment with a high level of involvement and exchange.

The view of nature is always present with

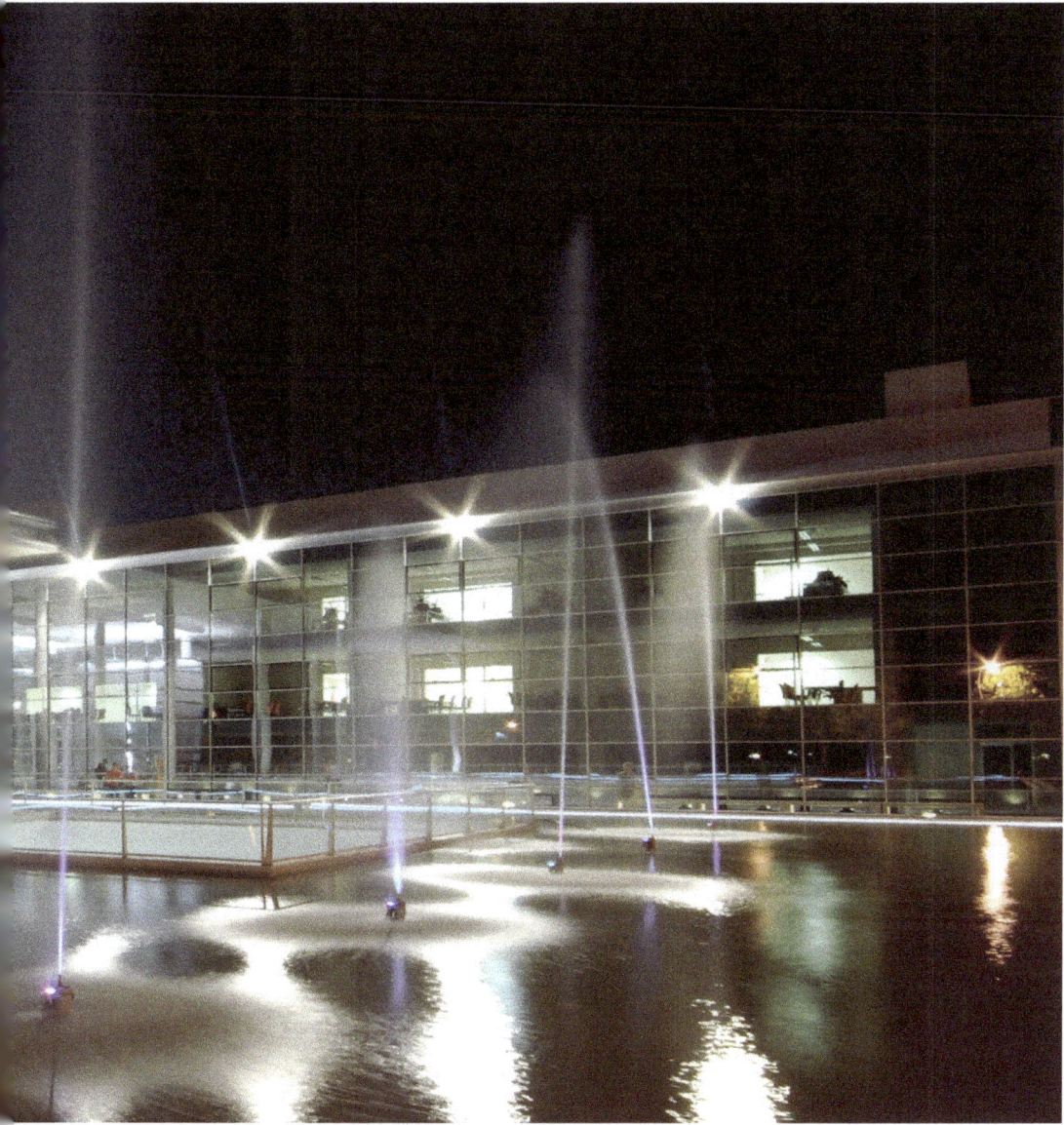

its soothing effect on passers-by and end users.

Inside and outside merge thanks to the dematerialized external walls and open plan interiors.

On the whole this architecture could be defined as classical modernity that will perhaps have a timeless future.

At night the building fills with light and turns into a beacon that attracts attention and reminds us of the importance of this unique place.

TESIS Inter-University Research Centre "Systems and Technologies for Social and Healthcare Facilities"
University of Florence, Italy

1. *Fiona Stanley Hospital, Perth Western Australia. Construction Status, 2012.*

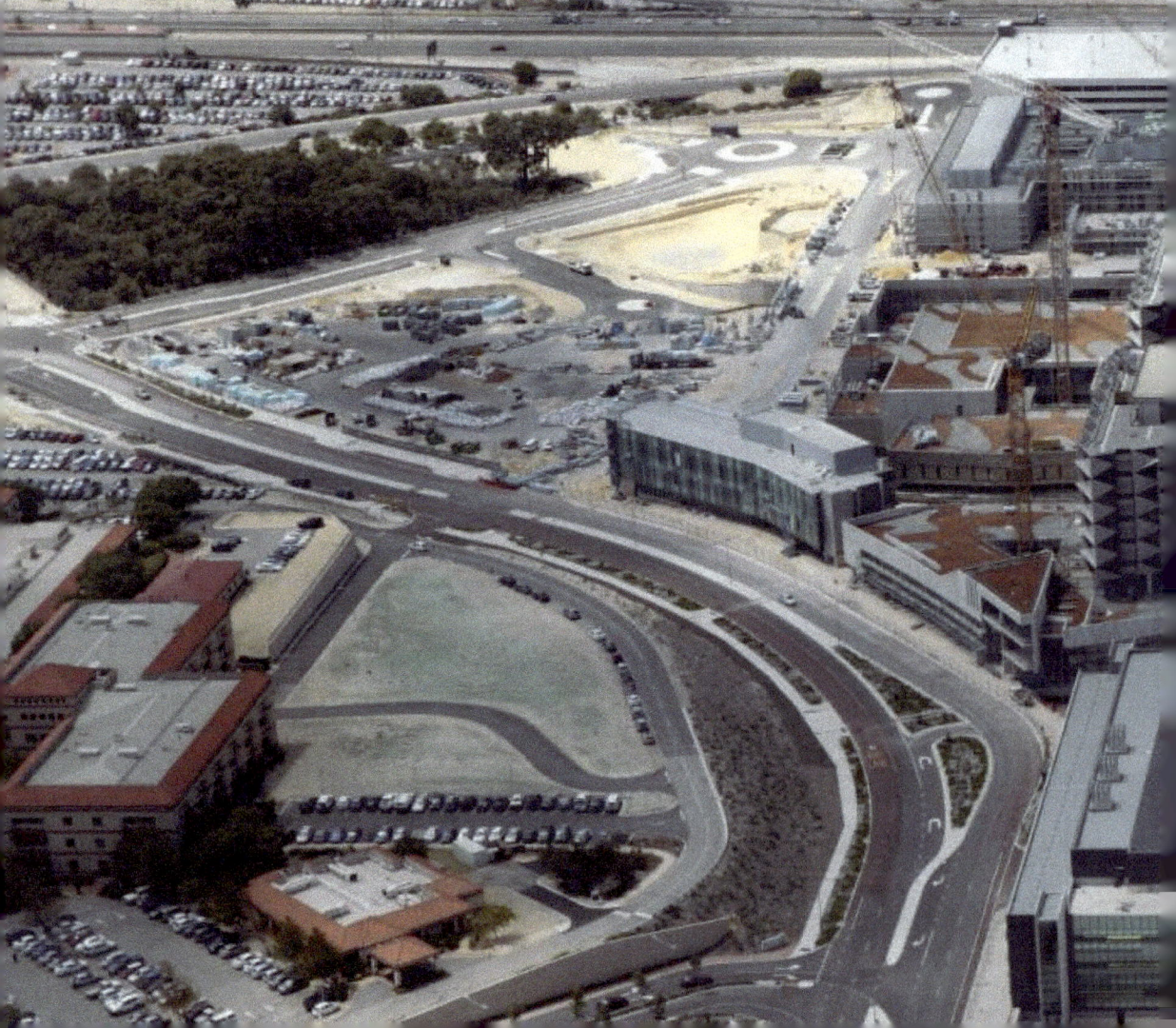

Recent Developments in Health Facility Planning and Design in Australia

Warren Kerr
National Director Hames Sharley

Rhonda Kerr
Principal Health Planner for Hames Sharley

113

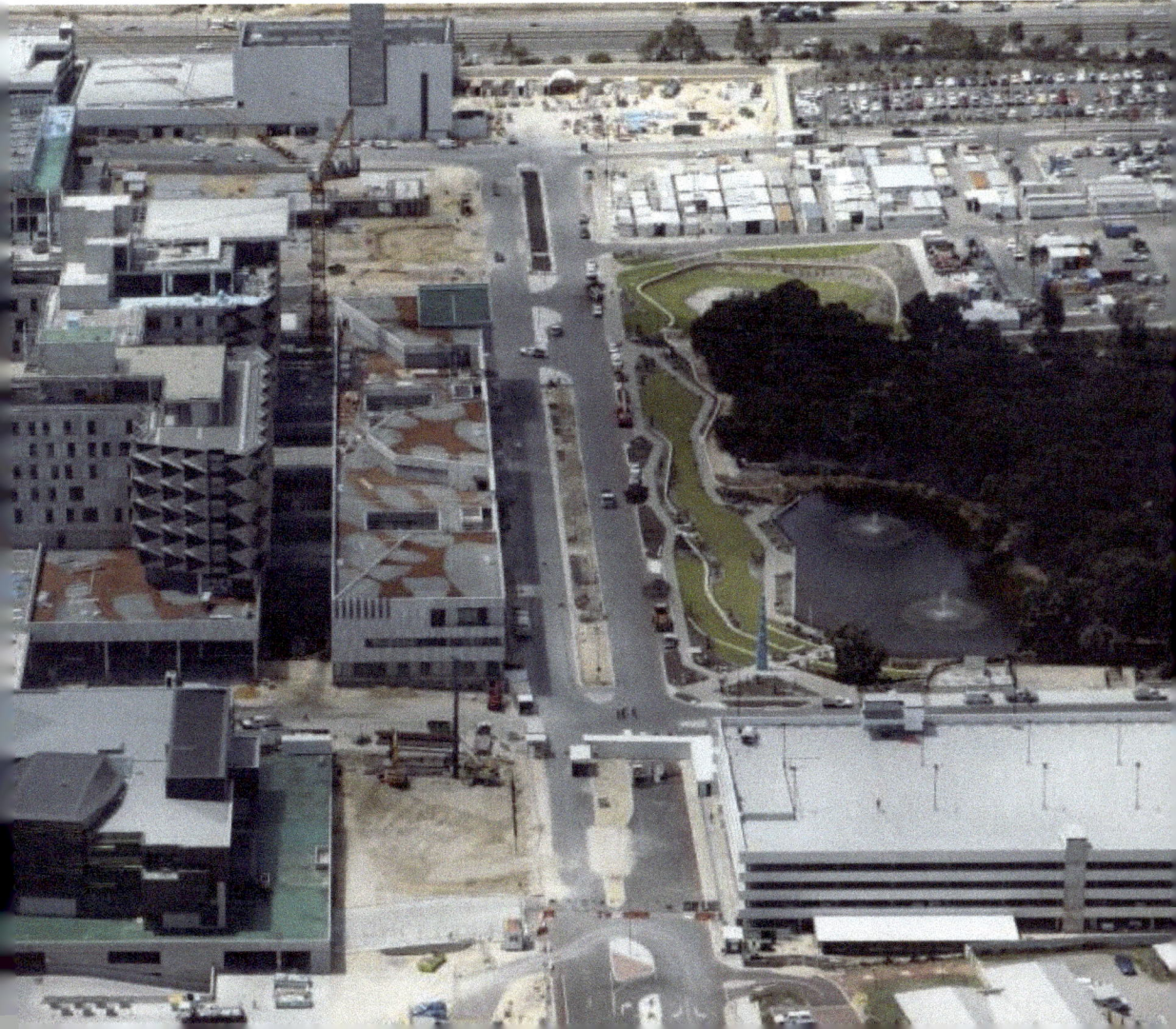

Abstract

This paper provides an overview of the Australian healthcare system and then focuses on the arrangements for health-facility planning and design in Australia as they pertain to the themes of the seminar:
- acute services and the impact on the hospital;
- technology development and its impact on hospitals;
- flexibility in hospital design;
- whether cost is more important than quality in hospital planning and building;
- energy efficient hospitals of the future;
- patient safety in hospital buildings.
The presentation provided details of the roles and responsibilities for healthcare provision by the different levels of government in Australia at Federal, State and local levels, and then addressed how this impacts on the provision of health-care facilities.
This paper provides an outline of the arrangements commonly made in Australia for the delivery, operation and maintenance of major health facility projects including the mix of public and private sector roles normally used in these processes. It covers trends in Australia to provide more energy efficient and sustainable buildings and for the built environment to contribute to the promotion of wellness and good health.
The emphasis is on providing an overview of the changes in the Australian healthcare system as the context for the innovations now being observed in the provision of health facilities. The increasing use of public private partnerships is noted as well as the impact of overseas trends on the planning and de-sign of Australian health facilities.
Hames Sharley have just finished their input into the planning and design of a new $2 billion acute tertiary hospital in Perth Western Australia and examples from this project are used to address the themes of the seminar in technology development, flexibility, cost, energy efficiency and patient safety.

Background

The authors' views are derived from their roles as practitioners based on 30 years of experience in hospital planning and design. Current project responsibilities include a number of hospital projects and leading the Hames Sharley team in a joint venture (with Silver Thomas Hanley and Hassell) for the $2.0 billion Fiona Stanley Hospital project in Perth, Western Australia.

They try to combine work as practitioners, researchers, teachers and advocates for improved processes. Their main research interest is the health outcomes and operational cost implications of planning and design decisions.

An Overview of Australia

The population of Australia is 22.8 million people. Its population comprises a nation of migrants. Even the aboriginal people were immigrants arriving 51,000 years ago. Successive waves of immigrants arrived in 1788, the 1860s, 1890 & the 1950s to form the culture and society that now comprise modern Australia.

Australia became a Federation in 1901 and States retain responsibility for many major issues such as health. The original inhabitants were Australian Aborigines and they account for approximately 2.4% of the population. The land area is 7.7 million sq kms (3 million sq miles). Based on a population of 22.8 million, this results in a density of 2.5 persons per square kilometre.

Australia is the world's 13th largest economy with the 5th highest per capital income, the 3rd longest female life expectancy and the 4th longest male life expectancy. There is low employment in Australia due to a major mining and resources boom.

The Australian Healthcare System

In Australia, health is primarily a State's responsibility. State Governments develop, own and operate hospitals and are also responsible for acute, mental and community health services.

In 1975, the Federal (Commonwealth) Government established the first national health insurance system for Australia and in 1984 this evolved into the current Medicare health insurance system which provides free health services to all Australian citizens. The Federal Government also reimburses General Practitioners and subsidises pharmaceuticals needed for medical purposes. Because the States are responsible for healthcare, there are 9 separate health systems in Australia (one for each of the six States and two Territories plus a separate healthcare system for Aborigines).

There are approximately 1,326 public and private hospitals in Australia (753 public, 280 private and 293 day-only). Approximately 9.4% of Australia's GPD is spent on healthcare (up from 7.6% in 1975).

115

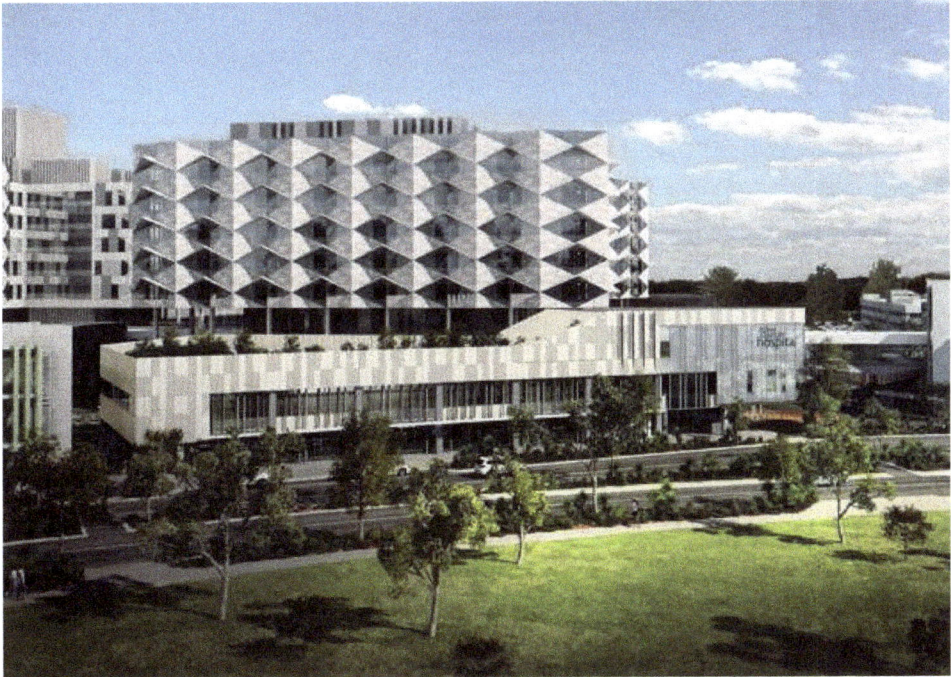

2. *Fiona Stanley Hospital FSH - View from Barry Marshall Drive.*

TESIS Inter-University Research Centre "Systems and Technologies for Social and Healthcare Facilities"
University of Florence, Italy

116

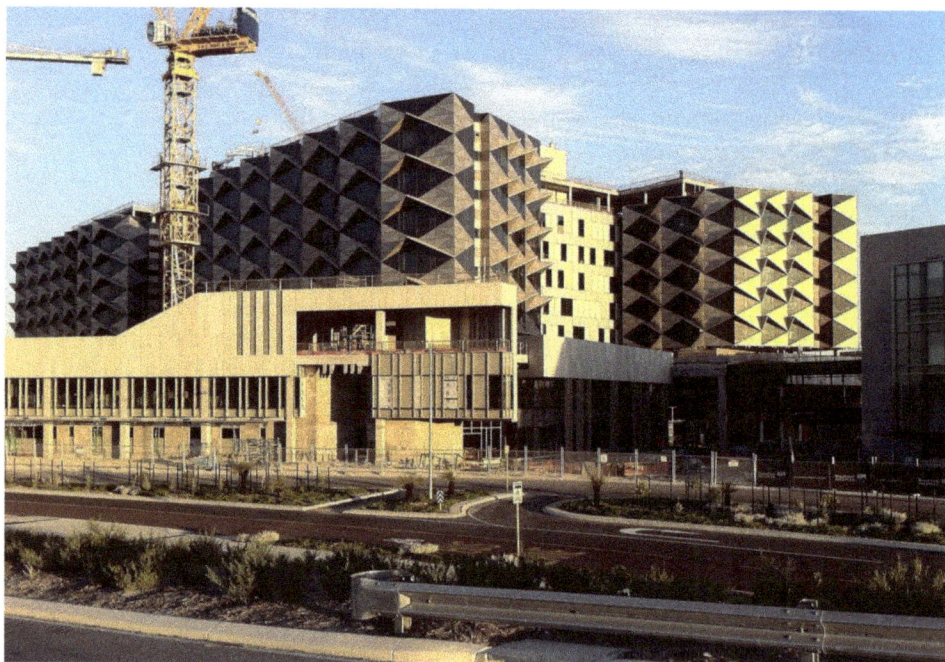

3. FSH - View from Barry Marshall Drive.

Health Facility Planning and Design

The planning, design and construction of public health facilities is a State responsibility. Because Australia is a young country, most hospitals were built after WWII. In many cases they were designed by State Public Works Departments.

However in the 1980s-90s, this work was outsourced to the private sector although traditional procurement methods were still used up to 2000. Since then a variety of procurement methods have been used (including PPPs). However, because each State undertakes its own program of health facilities there is still little sharing of information between the States and no national research centre to facilitate how health facility design can be improved.

Context - Western Australia and Perth

Western Australia is 2.5 million sq kms (1 million sq miles) with a total population of 2.4 million (less than 1 person/ sq km). However, 1.8 million of these residents are located in the capital city, Perth.

The State has huge deposits of mineral wealth with iron ore, nickel, gold, diamonds, etc. Workers required in the mining areas are normally employed on a Fly-in Fly-out (FIFO) basis with most of the workers living in Perth.

All the major tertiary and specialist hospitals are located in Perth. There are three main public tertiary hospitals and the new Fiona Stanley Hospital is currently being constructed on a green-field site to serve the southern half of Perth.

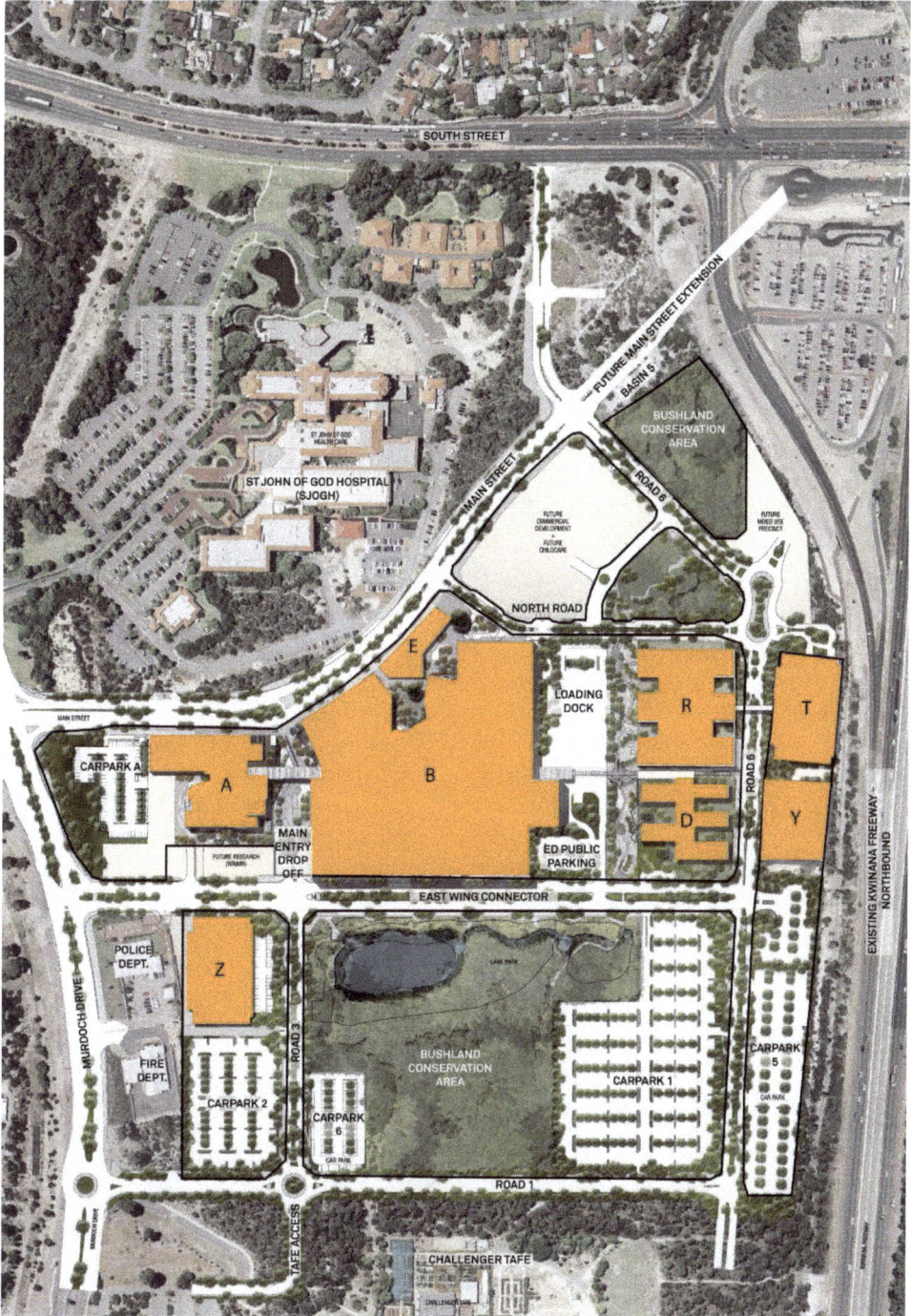

4. FSH Master Plan.

TESIS Inter-University Research Centre "Systems and Technologies for Social and Healthcare Facilities"
University of Florence, Italy

Fiona Stanley Hospital project

The architectural team for the new hospital is the Fiona Stanley Hospital Design Collaboration, which comprises three firms: Hames Sharley, Silver Thomas Hanley and Hassell.

The directors of the Fiona Stanley Hospital Design Collaboration are: Warren Kerr from Hames Sharley, George Raffa from Silver Thomas Hanley and Jeff Menkens from Hassell.

Background - Fiona Stanley Hospital

Fiona Stanley Hospital is a $1.76 billion tertiary hospital, plus $255.7m for the State rehabilitation service. It is the largest single infrastructure project ever undertaken by WA State Government.

Fiona Stanley Hospital - Timeframe

The Government's intention to proceed with FSH was announced in March 2004 and the Project Direction consultants were appointed in 2005. The consultant design team was appointed in June 2007 and the schematic design completed in August 2008. The building contractor (Brookfield Multiplex) was appointed in March 2009. Construction commenced in July 2009 and Stage 2 of this contract was awarded in September 2010.

Completion of construction is scheduled for December 2013 with the opening scheduled for May 2014.

Scope of this Facility:

- 643 acute hospital beds;
- 140 rehabilitation beds;
- 6,300 rooms in the acute hospital;
- 83 per cent single-patient rooms in the acute hospital;
- 161,000 square metres total area;
- 3,600 car bays (600 undercover and 1,450 decked);
- 16 wards (of 24 beds each) in the acute hospital;
- 29 imaging rooms;
- 16 operating theatres + 1 operating theatre in Obstetrics.

Key services to be provided

A full range of acute medical and surgical services will be provided:
- state burns service;
- state rehabilitation service;
- emergency department and major trauma centre;
- comprehensive cancer services including radiotherapy treatment facilities, medical oncology and haematology;

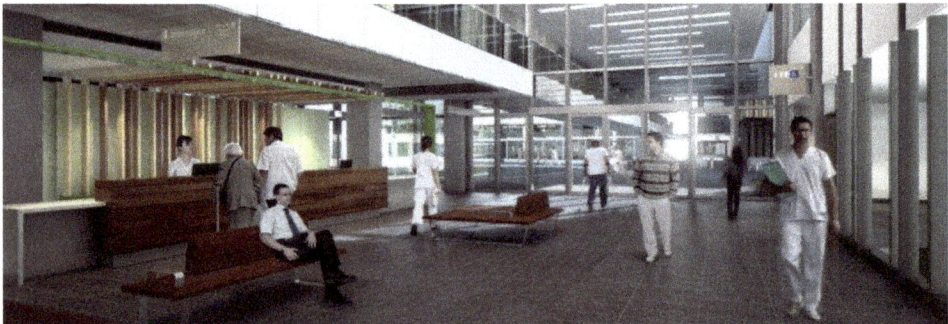

5. FSH - Atrium.

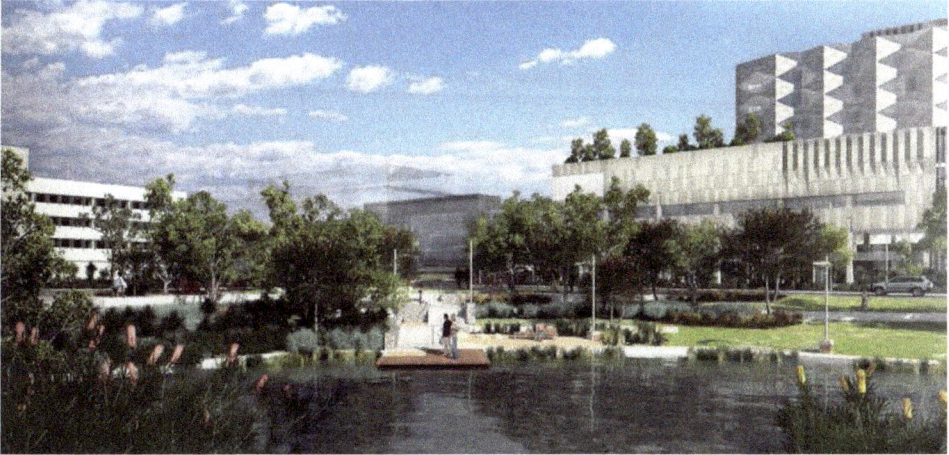

6. FSH - View from the Lake Park.

119

- renal transplantation and dialysis services;
- mental health unit with secure wing and mother and baby unit;
- obstetrics and neonatology services;
- pediatric services;
- pathology, bio-medical engineering and cell tissue manufacturing;
- medical imaging centre;
- medical research through the Western Australian Institute for Medical Research.

Planning & Design Principles

The following planning and design principles were adopted for this project:

- patient-centered care;
- maximized use of single beds for acute patient care;
- clinical services grouped into functional clusters;
- future-proofed to permit future adaptation;
- maximized access to natural daylight, views and access to external areas;
- maximized replacement of landscape;

- separation of front-of-house and back-of-house activities;
- clear wayfinding – East-West Connector;
- information, technology and communications enabled;
- research and education facilities highly visible;
- ease of access to parking.

Planning and Design issues illustrated by FSH

The financing of the Fiona Stanley Hospital has been fully funded by the State Government. It was not a Public Private Partnership although PPPs are used in other States. The Fiona Stanley Hospital project is a good example of an evidence-based design approach.

Professor Roger Ulrich was used as a consultant and his input resulted in the percentage of single-patient rooms being increased from 27% to 83%.

In 2006, a national research centre in Australia established the Australasian Health Facility Guidelines, which were used on Fiona Stanley Hospital.

TESIS Inter-University Research Centre "Systems and Technologies for Social and Healthcare Facilities"
University of Florence, Italy

1. Eye Hospital for Puyang, collaboration between universities and teaching firm.

You are cordially invited to a collaborative presentation of architectural models and drawings for an
我们诚挚地邀请您出席建筑合作设计项目演讲:

"Eye Hospital"

for
Puyang, China

中国濮阳眼科医院

Monday, Oct. 31, 2011   1:30 pm - 4:15pm

Location of Presentation:
HKS Architects
1919 McKinney Ave.
Dallas, Texas

Collaborating Universities:
Southeast University, Nanjing, China
University of Oklahoma, Norman, Oklahoma, USA
Texas A&M University, College Station, Texas, USA

合作学校:
东南大学, 南京, 中国
俄克拉荷马大学, 诺曼, 俄克拉荷马, 美国
德克萨斯A&M大学, 科利奇站, 得克萨斯, 美国

Collaborating Teaching Firms:
IPPR - Institute for Project Planning & Research, Beijing, China
HKS - Shanghai, China & Dallas, Texas, USA
Miles Associates, Oklahoma City, Oklahoma, USA

合作公司:
中国中元国际工程公司, 北京, 中国
HKS建筑师事务所, 上海, 中国＆达拉斯, 德克萨斯, 美国
Miles Associates, 俄克拉荷马市, 俄克拉荷马, 美国

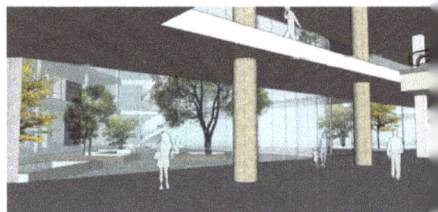
Entrance ha

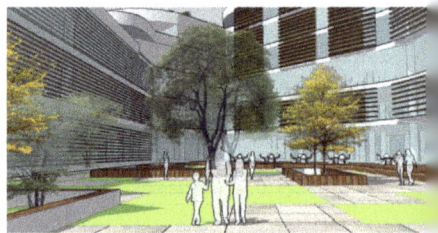
courtya

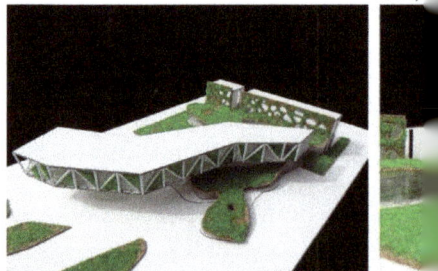

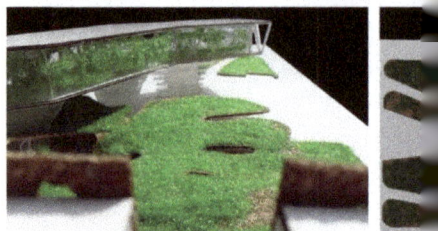

Hospital Planning and Building
"How Do They Do It in China?"

Dr. Xi Qiu Huang
Chief Architect, IPPR (Institute of Project Planning & Research)
Beijing, China
Official Representative of China to UIA - PHG

George J. Mann
AIA, Professor
The Skaggs - Sprague Endowed Chair of Health Facilities Design

121

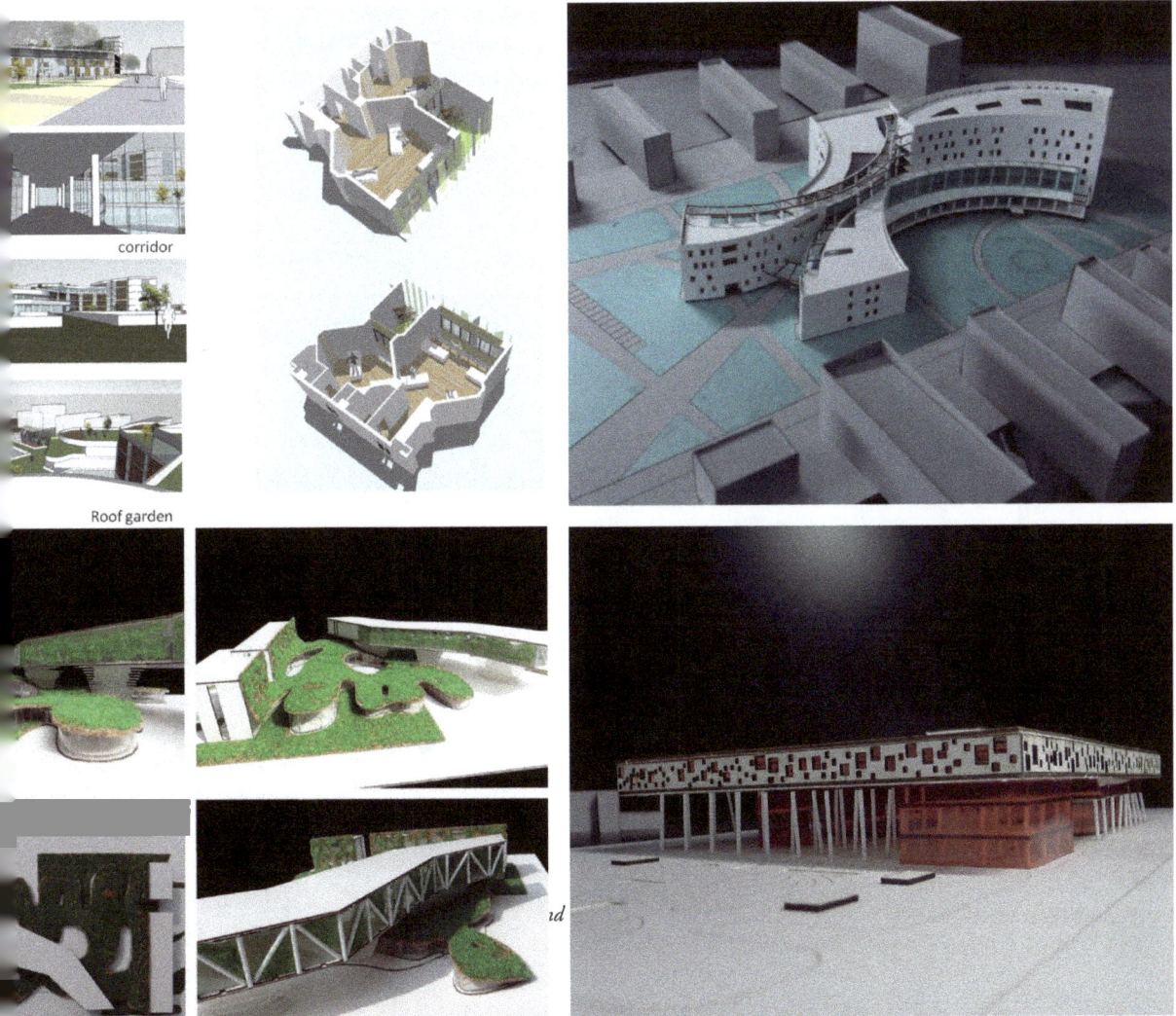

corridor

Roof garden

Designs for an eye hospital in Puyang, China, created by students in a Texas A&M University "Architecture for Health" research and design studio in collaboration with students at Southeast University in Nanjing, China, and the University of Oklahoma, were undertaken in the fall of 2011.

During the semester-long, international collaboration on the project, Texas A&M students used video, teleconferencing, email and web blogs to communicate with their counterparts in China and Oklahoma. Their efforts were guided by three design firms that specialize in healthcare architecture: China - IPPR - International Engineering Corporation, one of China's largest health facilities design and construction firms; HKS Inc. in Shanghai and Dallas; and Miles Associates in Oklahoma City.

Additionally, the project was informed by a weekly lecture series ("China: Toward Improved Health Care and Health Facilities in the Future") that brought healthcare design experts from China and the U.S. to Texas A&M to discuss China's rapidly changing healthcare needs.

The design studio mirrored industry practices in which architects, constructors and clients collaborate electronically over long distances with people they never actually meet in person. Invaluable assistance and advice for the project was provided by Texas A&M faculty members Dr. Zhipeng Lu and Dr. Xuemei Zhu, both of whom are graduates of Southeast University in Nanjing, China. The eye hospital is for the city of Puyang, in the Henan province in China. The hospital included phase one, comprised of an outpatient and inpatient care centre, and phase two, made up of more inpatient rooms and administration and research. Neither phase could exceed 25,000 square metres; the hospital site was 36,000 square metres.

By collaborating with their Chinese counterparts, students gained access to site photos and received useful feedback on topics of regional concern such as

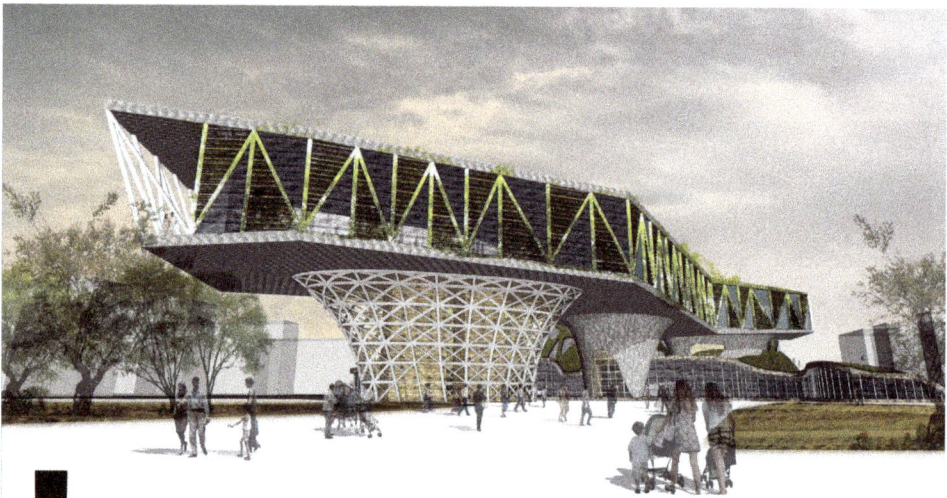

2. Eye Hospital, Puyang: Southeast University Proposals, students Xiang Guo and Baddy Wang.

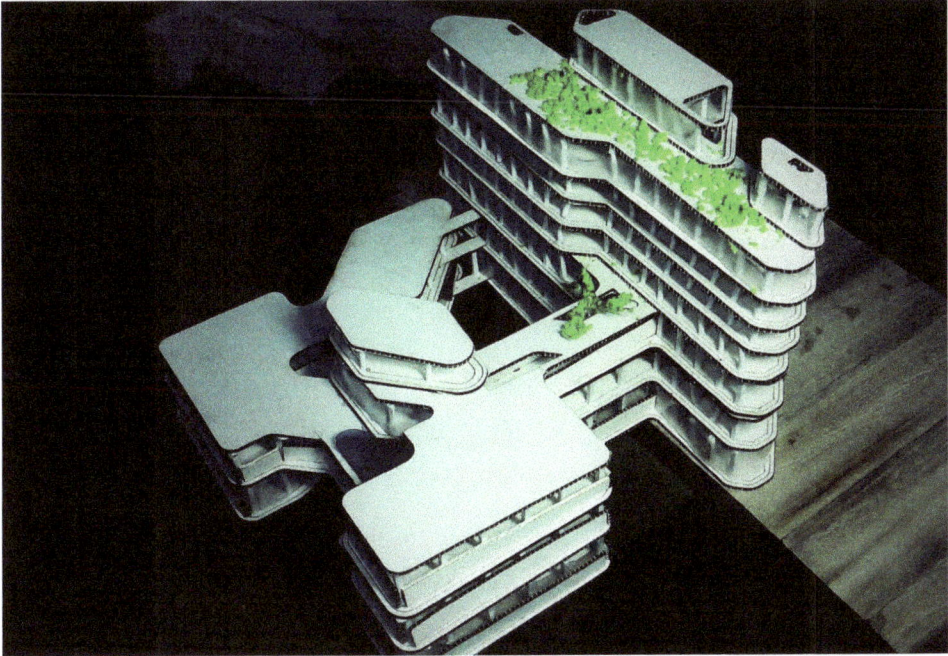

3. Eye Hospital, Puyang: Southeast University Proposals, Touch light students Tina Chai and Ivy Zhang.

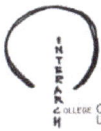

4. Eye Hospital, Puyang: University of Oklahoma Proposals, students Jackie Hood, Jason Clements, Laurie Murphy, Marsi Puente.

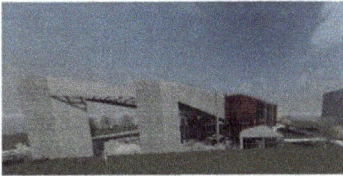

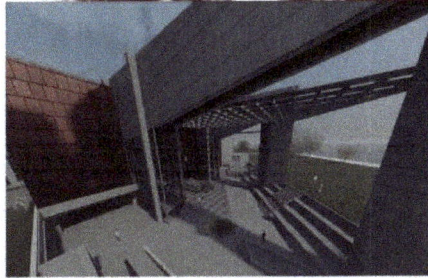

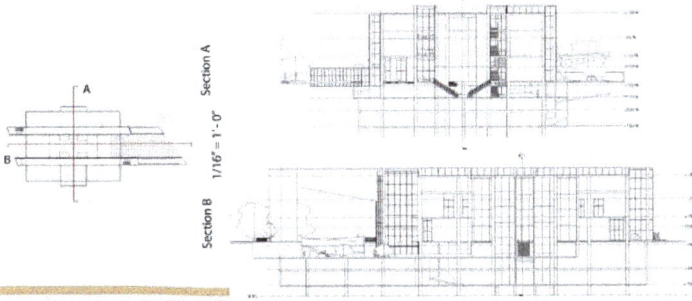

124

5. Eye Hospital, Puyang: University of Oklahoma Proposals, students Jenna Ross, Sarah Corbell, Ping Lu, Kevin Ku.

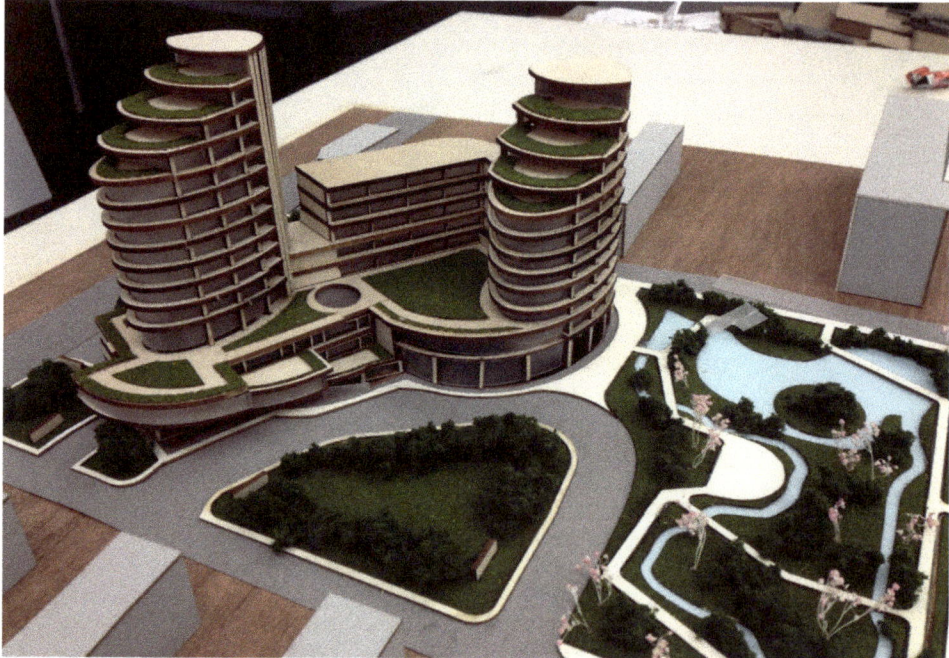

6. Eye Hospital, Puyang: Texas A&M University Proposals.

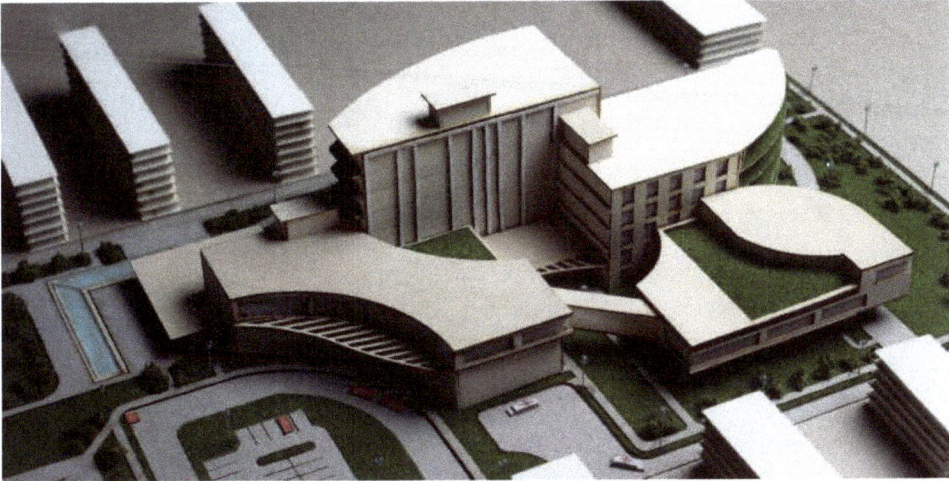

125

7. Eye Hospital, Puyang: Texas A&M University Proposals, students Clara Doyle and Marny Itzkowitz.

Chinese medical practices and the use of 'feng shui' design principles.

In Chinese thought, feng shui is a system of laws considered to govern spatial arrangement and orientation in relation to the flow of energy, or "qi". The resulting favourable or unfavourable effects of feng shui are taken into account when siting and designing buildings.
The collaboration also benefited from the unique perspective brought by interior design students on the OU team. (Interior design is not offered as a degree at Texas A&M.)

Because many foreign design firms are doing more work in China than elsewhere in the world, this Chinese project offered some students a preview of the work they will be doing once they graduate and join a large firm. Craig Beale, FAIA, Executive Vice President, Healthcare Group Director, HKS Dallas and Shanghai, sponsored the visit of Dr. Ying Zhou and three students from Southeast University to visit Texas A&M University and HKS in Dallas in late October. Ronald L. Skaggs, FAIA and Joseph G. Sprague, FAIA closely advised on the design of this project as well as provided funds from their Endowed Chair funds for Dr. Xi Qiu Huang, Chief Architect for IPPR to come to the USA to lecture on IPPR's work, and for the lecture series. Representing Miles Associates was Davene Morgan, a graduate of Texas A&M University.
In October 2010, a delegation of the project faculty from Texas A&M and OU (Professors George J. Mann, James R. Patterson and Prof. Hepi Wachter) travelled to Southeast University in Nanjing and IPPR in Beijing to lecture and present student work on the eye hospital project for faculty and student review. Prof Dave Boeck of the University of Oklahoma also assisted in the project design.

At another project review, hosted on 31 October by the Dallas office of HKS, Texas A&M and OU students and the faculty were joined by three students

TESIS Inter-University Research Centre "Systems and Technologies for Social and Healthcare Facilities"
University of Florence, Italy

TESIS

from Southeast University, their design professor, Dr. Ying Zhou, Dr. Huang Xi Qiu, Chief Architect, IPPR in Beijing and other representatives from IPPR in Beijing.

The entire project involved more than 67 students, six faculty advisors from three universities, and numerous architectural professionals from IPPR, HKS and Miles Associates.

126

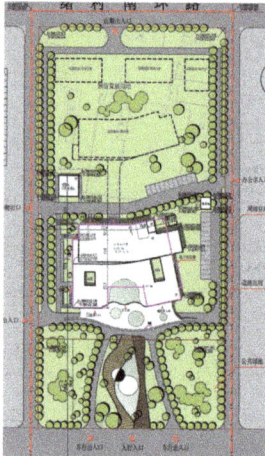

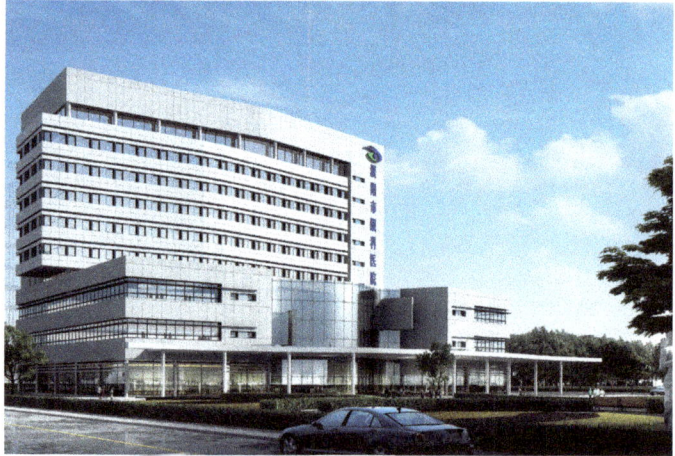

8. Puyang ophthalmology hospital, general layout and perspective.

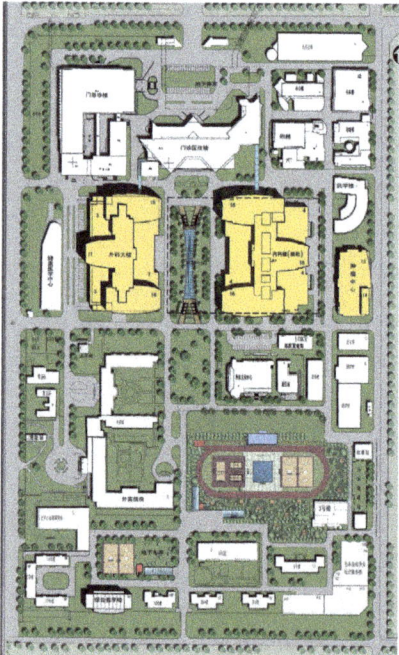

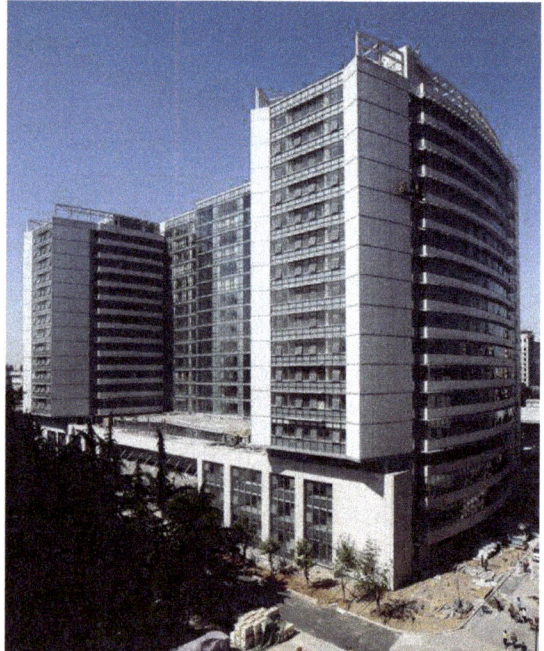

9. Brief introduction of IPPR projects, Surgery Building China PLA General Hospital, Beijing, building area 11,000 m2.

This collaborative experience between universities and between architectural firms in different parts of the world will be a model for how architectural design studios will be taught in the future.

The three universities and the three firms are undertaking another collaborative "Architecture for Health" design project in China to design a Rehabilitation Hospital for Cancer Patients within a major Cancer Medical Centre during the fall of 2012.

127

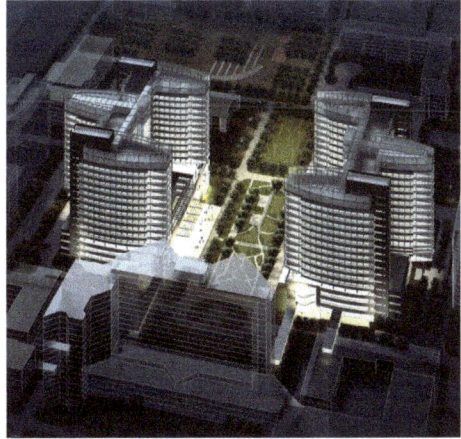

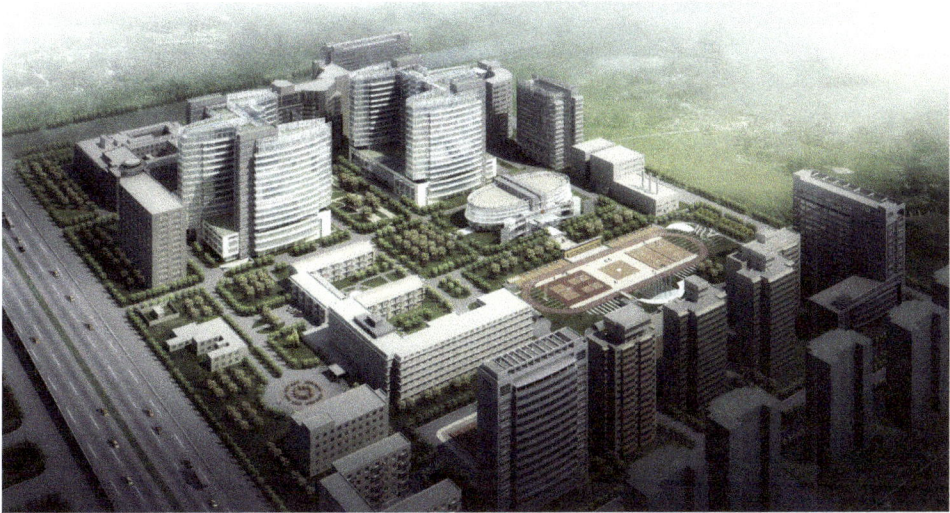

10. *Surgery Building, China PLA General Hospital.*

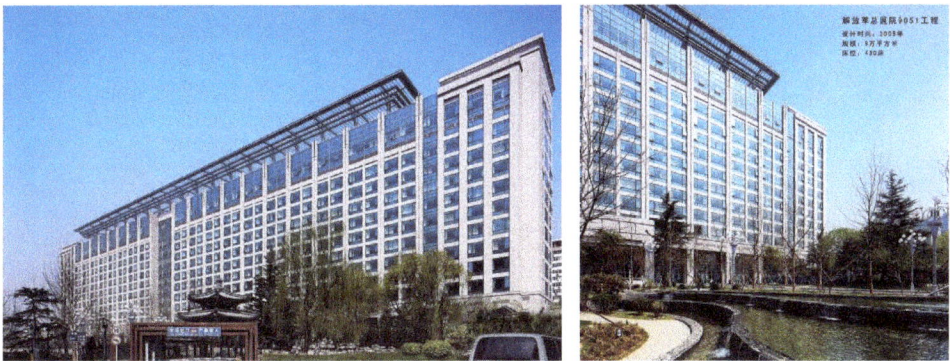

11. *West Campus of China PLA General Hospital, Beijing, building area 90,000 m2.*

TESIS Inter-University Research Centre "Systems and Technologies for Social and Healthcare Facilities"
University of Florence, Italy

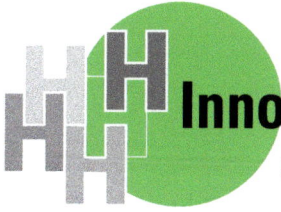

Innovative technologies

Session introduction

The use of the latest technologies available can help to improve the quality of healthcare facilities: new technologies can be instrumental in reducing energy consumption, they can enhance and reduce the time required for the construction process and they can be used to allow user participation in all project phases.

· · · · · · · · · · ·

Robert Martinez's paper outlines strategies for energy efficiency in healthcare buildings based on the actual energy demand of the different environments that comprise the hospital. Once the profiles and needs of the different environments have been defined, it is possible to provide energy for lighting and air conditioning calibrated according to the use, function and times of use for each environment so as to avoid waste that could result from the undifferentiated treatment of the various areas of the hospital.

Robert Martinez p. 131

Philip Patrick Sun describes the strategies for the optimization of cost in the design and construction of healthcare environments. Based on his experience acquired over his thirty-year career as a designer and a client he explains the choices in the organization of buildings, materials and typological aspects that may affect the cost of the facility and improve functional efficiency. The use of prefabricated technologies helps to control the cost of new buildings. In the specific case of the new hospital in Joplin, MO in the Delta Region of the Mississippi, construction costs were reduced through the use of prefabricated elements.

Philip Patrick Sun p. 141

The case study presented by Helina Kotilainen describes the characteristics of a virtual laboratory as a tool for user participation in the design process. The virtual model is set up in a room where there are walls, a ceiling and a floor. The model is a virtual aid that helps to monitor and record user preferences in all design stages. The images generated by computer graphics form a three-dimensional environment in real scale. An essential feature of this technology is the semblance of the simulated environments to real ones, and this allows users to express their points of view in every phase of the design process.

Helina Kotilainen p. 155

TESIS Inter-University Research Centre "Systems and Technologies for Social and Healthcare Facilities" University of Florence, Italy

TESIS

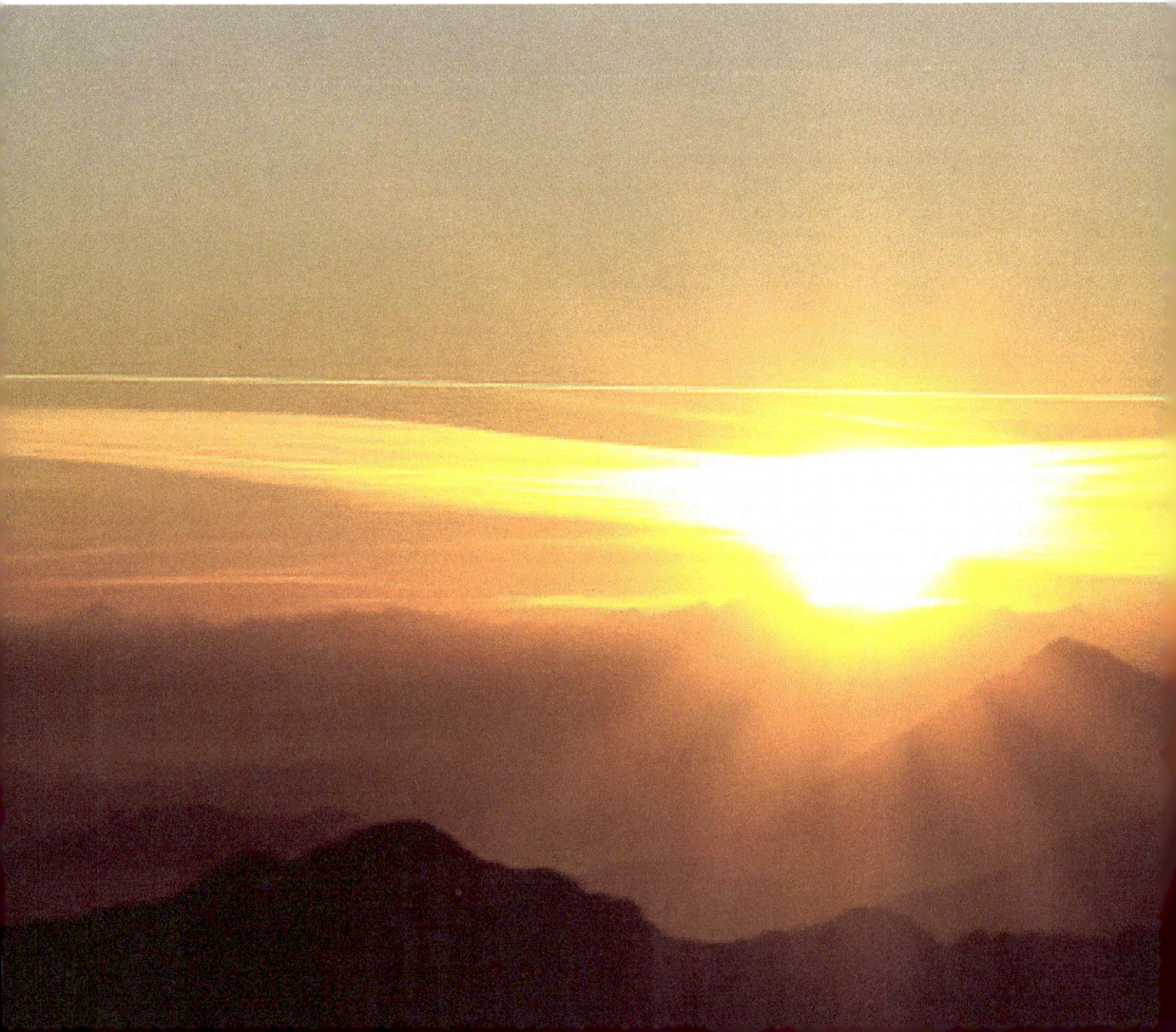

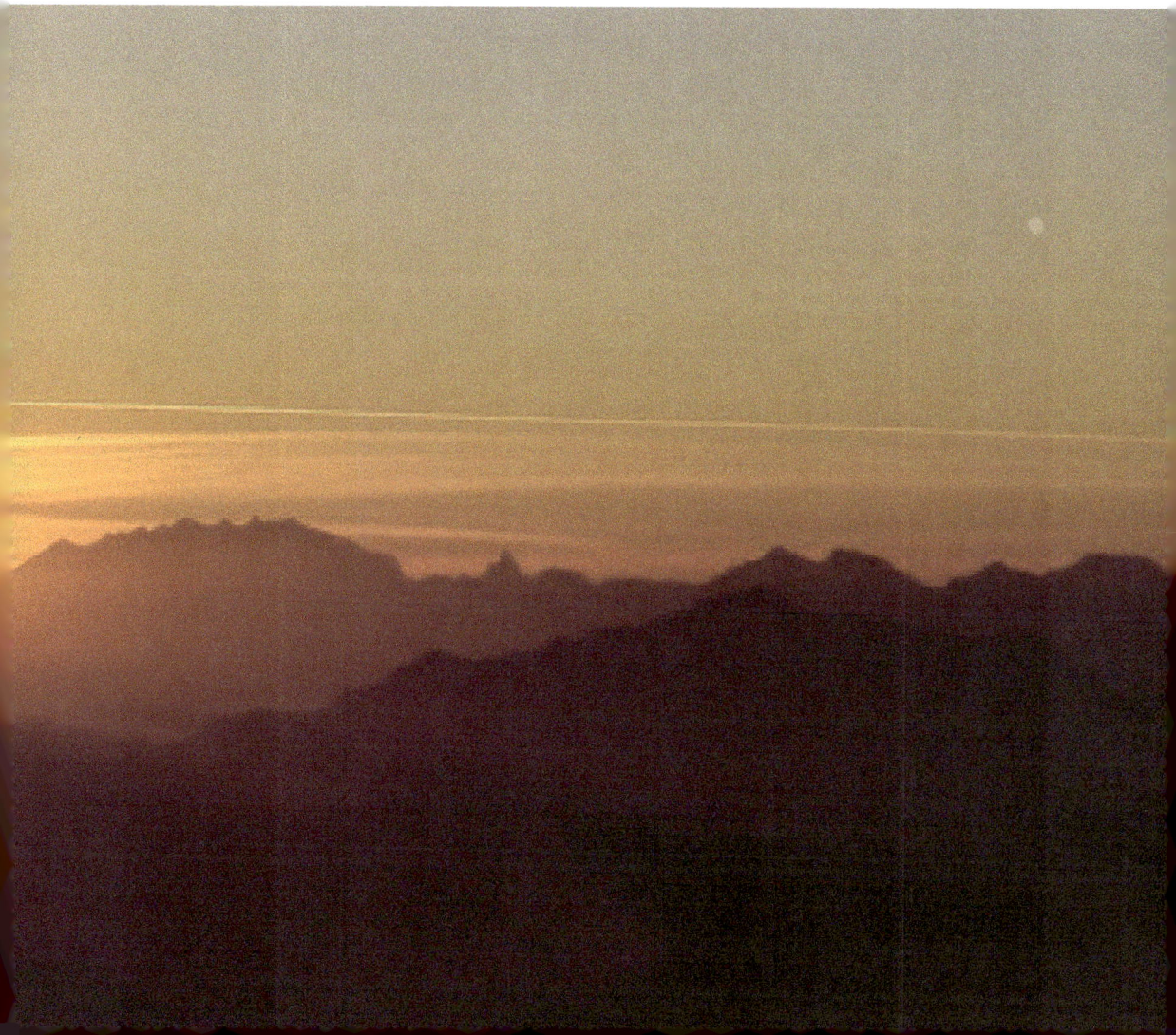

Energy on Demand
Hospital Design for Flexible, Demand-Controlled Energy Usage

Robert Martinez
Norconsult AS & Low Energy Hospitals Project

131

Low Energy Hospitals

Low Energy Hospitals is an innovation project which aims to find and promote feasible design measures that can halve the energy consumption of new hospitals built in Norway.

Led by Norconsult AS, Norway's largest multi-disciplinary consulting engineering firm, it is supported by the Norwegian Research Council and matches funds from private sector partners:

• Helse Sør-Øst – Norway's largest regional health authority; Narud Stokke Wiig – a leading architecture firm in Norway;
• GK-Norway – a large supplier of HVAC equipment and services in Scandinavia;
• SAAS – designs and delivers complete building automation systems; Siemens Healthcare – global supplier of medical equipment;
• Norconsult Information Systems – provides IT solutions for the building sector in Scandinavia.

Organization – Projects

Phase 1 involves a review and consists of the following sub-steps: functional planning, building envelope, hospital equipment, HVAC, integration & control.

Phase 2 involves analysis (until December 2013) and consists of modeling and simulation.

Phase 3 involves the validation (until April 2014) of all the sub-steps developed in phase 1. Phase 4 is organized into a number of actions for the communication (until April 2014) and dissemination of the product design through the publication of articles and papers and through conferences.

Motivation: why hospital energy consumption?

Hospital buildings take the lead in terms of energy intensity; even higher energy consumption is seen in regional and university hospitals and more energy is used in acute-care hospitals: 1.6 TWh. En-

	Acute-care		Regional	
	netto m²	Share of total m²	netto m²	Share of total m²
Daytime activity	26 300	38 %	46 400	48 %
Extended daytime	10 900	16 %	2 200	2 %
Activity 24/7	21 600	31 %	21 000	22 %
Mainly daytime, some evening/night duty	10 200	15 %	26 400	28 %
Sum	69 000	100 %	96 000	100 %

1. Demand related to activity and occupancy levels.

ergy costs for the largest regional health authority (HSØ) approach NOK 1 billion and grow by 100 million each year.

Demand profiles

It can be observed that different areas of acute-care hospitals are used at different times of the day as patient rooms, polyclinics/outpatient care, "hot" floors (imaging, operating rooms, etc.) and technical floors.

The use of these areas is different during the day and night, on weekdays and at the weekend: entire zones are affected and although activity patterns are relatively regular they are different for different zones.

Single rooms and spaces are affected hour by hour; the pattern is irregular and simultaneous occupancy is less than 100%, but different for different zones.

Demand for lighting, ventilation and air cooling/heating is strongly related to activity and occupancy levels and most hospital areas are daytime or extended daytime only.

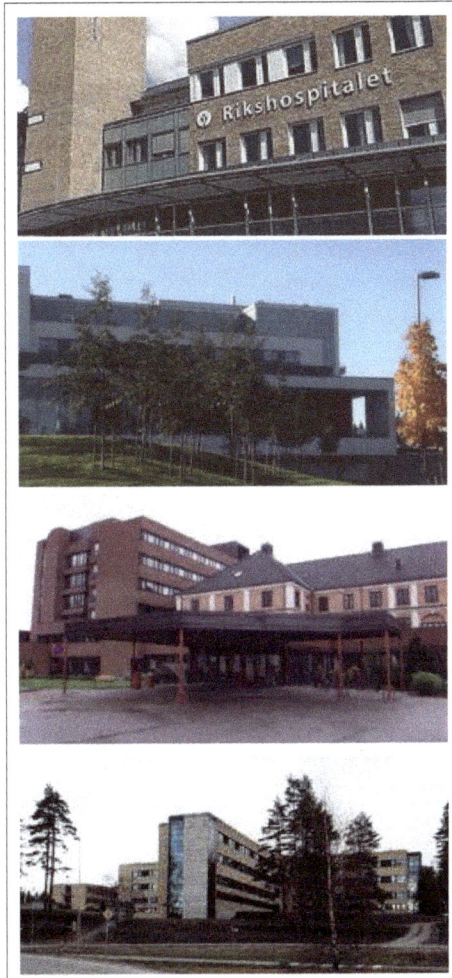

2. *Most hospital areas are daytime or extended daytime only.*

133

Functional area	Activitity level	Area (m2)	% total
Polyclinic , day areas	Daytime activity	6 800	10 %
Intensive care	Activity 24/7	5 400	8 %
Normal bed wards	Activity 24/7	15 700	23 %
Patient hotel	Activity 24/7	3 000	4 %
Operation	Mainly daytime, some evening/night	2 100	3 %
Radiology	Mainly daytime, some evening/night	1.700	2 %
Laboratories	Mainly daytime, some evening/night	6 900	10 %
Sterilisation, kitchens, etc.	Extended daytime	2 000	3 %
Transport, logistic areas	Daytime activity	12 200	18 %
Office areas	Daytime activity	13 200	19 %
Total		69 000	100 %

3. *Day variations by functional area.*

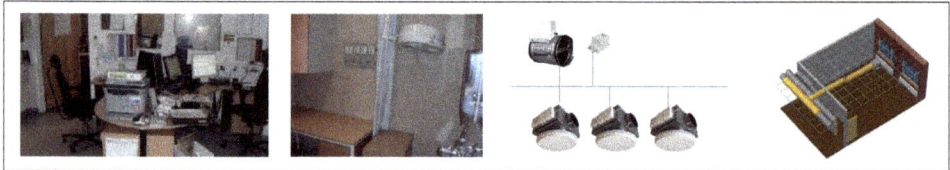

4. Rooms generally devolve from high-tech (treatment rooms) to low-tech (offices or storage spaces). Energy demand-control at room level is needed.

Treatment areas

Data shows that even acute-care hospitals have large variations in activity (area in use) and maximum occupancy levels of less than 100%, with weekly variations of about 40% and daily variations of about 70%, measured by the area in use.

Maximum simultaneous occupancy levels for the daytime are around 55-65% and even lower for non-clinical rooms at around 35%.

If we consider, for example, data from a newer acute-care hospital we may find that the baseload power is 1800 kWh per hour at midnight and the peak load is 2000 kWh per hour at 11 a.m. The variation is only 20% over the day, and there is little variation between weekdays and weekends.

There is great potential for treatment areas to control the energy demand by exploiting usage variations.

Patient areas

Data from a newer acute-care hospital shows that the weekly variation is around 35% (area in use) and the daily variation is around 15% (area in use); the baseload is 800 kWh per hour at midnight and the peak load is 1200 kWh per hour at 10 a.m. In conclusion, patient areas have the potential to control demand (but less potential than treatment areas).

	Dagområde m/poliklinikk	Intensiv	Normal senge-område	Pasient-hotell	Operasjon	Radiologi
1a. Romoppvarming		yellow	brown	yellow		
1b. Ventilasjonsvarme		brown	yellow			
2. Varmtvann	brown					
3a. Vifter		brown	yellow		brown	
3b. Pumper						
4. Belysning			brown	yellow	brown	
5. Teknisk utstyr	brown	yellow			brown	brown
6a. Romkjøling					brown	
6b. Ventilasjonskjøling	yellow			yellow		brown

5. Examples of benchmarking functional areas.

134

Controlling energy demand

Most existing hospitals have limited potential to control demand because they feature constant flow ventilation systems (CAV), have few automated lighting systems and are far behind offices and hotels in demand-control technology.

Nevertheless, today many hospitals practice simple zone-based demand-control. Even newer, large hospitals are divided into only a handful of control zones, and this leaves much potential for more fine-tuned demand-control. Some newer hospitals have variable air volume (VAV) in some areas, but even this system is often controlled by zones.

Over time, zones become a "swiss cheese" of smaller areas and rooms with varying demands, and this implies that rooms are re-purposed without new HVAC commissioning and generally devolve from high-tech (treatment rooms) to low-tech (offices or storage spaces). This creates problems for simple zone-based demand-control because rooms are over-supplied with energy, mostly ventilation and lighting.

It is necessary to control energy demand at room level for several reasons: it follows occupancy and activity; it can be reprogrammed for new supply levels; sensors and controllers can be grouped into a single ceiling unit to control ventilation, lighting, cooling and other equipment. The flow of energy to a zone is commanded by the central building automation system: the philosophy of zone control is "Always ON until turned OFF". The flow of energy to a room or space is determined by the activity level of the occupants: the philosophy of demand-control is "Always OFF until turned ON".

Ventilation and lighting have the most potential for room-based demand-control and together account for around

135

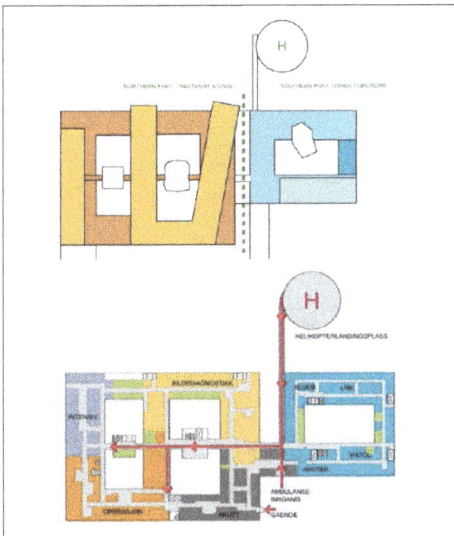

6. *New Molde hospital design, NSW, 2011.*

Specific energy (kWh/m2)	
1a Local room heating	14 %
1b Ventilation heating	28 %
2 Hot water	5 %
3a Ventilation fan motor	13 %
4 Artificial lighting	13 %
5 Techn. equipment	16 %
6 a Room/process cooling	9 %
6b Ventilation cooling	4 %
Total net energy	100 %

7. *Energy demand-control, specific energy.*

TESIS Inter-University Research Centre "Systems and Technologies for Social and Healthcare Facilities"
University of Florence, Italy

TESIS

55% of the total energy consumption in modern acute-care hospitals. Ventilation consumes thermal energy for heating/cooling as well as electrical energy to power fan motors. Ventilation energy accounts for around 44% of the total energy consumption in modern acute-care hospitals and the demand-control of ventilation (DCV) therefore has the largest energy potential.

How can new hospitals be designed for full energy demand-control?

First of all, division into functional areas, good hospital logistics and patient flows will generally also enable good demand-control. Similar functions are usually grouped together and this enables better zonal control, especially for corridors and other connecting areas in hospitals (of which there are a lot). Moreover it is easier to maintain the correct control of ventilation while facing the challenge of maintaining flexibility.

Identify the smallest spaces for room demand-control

A suggestion for the improved control of energy in small spaces (such as patient rooms, bathrooms, treatment rooms, meeting rooms) involves attaching a schedule for occupancy and equipment usage for each room in the room program; this will help HVAC designers. In addition it is important to choose an optimal control strategy for each room/space.

The room type will determine control variables such as the time of day, CO_2, or presence detection; patient rooms and other small rooms controlled by the presence detector, with modulated temperature; CO_2 sensing but not in treatment rooms or operating rooms due to high ventilation rates. New sensing methods are coming, and their installed costs are being reduced; they may have applications in technical areas, labs, etc.

	Today's energy consumption (kWh/m2)	Demand-controlled (kWh/m2)	Reduction
1a Local room heating	55	47	
1b Ventilation heating	110	22	80%
2 Hot water	20	20	
3a Ventilation fan	50	25	50 %
4 Artificial lighting	50	40	20 %
5 Techn. equipment	65	65	
6 a Room cooling	35	26	
6b Ventilation cooling	15	15	25 %
Total net energy	400	260	35 %

8. *Ventilation and lighting have the highest potential for demand-control.*

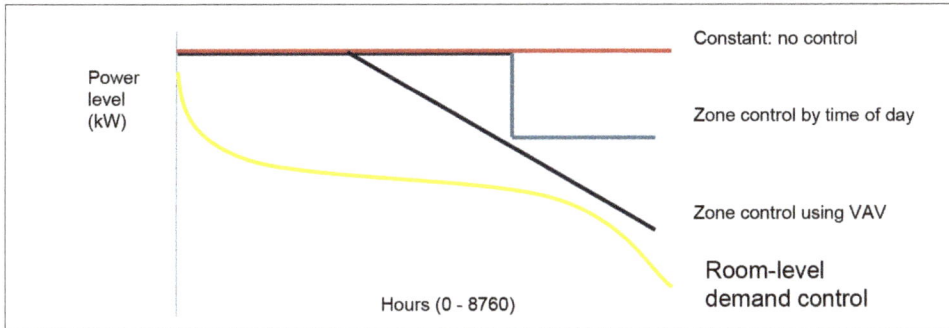

Power level (kW)

Constant: no control

Zone control by time of day

Zone control using VAV

Room-level demand control

Hours (0 - 8760)

9. Energy flow.

Engineers and even some architects will consider thermal energy demands when placing very large imaging equipment.

This design method can be extended to other functional areas and the suggestion is to develop energy signatures for each functional area. This helps in the energy classification (benchmarking) of each area, and goals for energy management. The health authority seeks ISO 14001 certification. An initial step is benchmarking 13 functional areas (out of a total of 81).

Degree of decentralized air handling

Decentralized air handling generally allows better demand-control and it can follow daily variations in different areas,

provide correct temperature and flows. Systems are becoming more price competitive and more robust, but more installed power in air handling units may still be required.
Centralized systems can be dimensioned for higher simultaneous occupancy levels.

Lighting

The potential for energy demand-control could be ensured by presence detectors (on/off) and/or dimming based on daylight levels, and combined with task-oriented lighting design; larger rooms divided into zones to exploit daylight, for example in the early morning; zones near windows dimmed to 0%, middle zones at 30%, and rear zones at 60%.

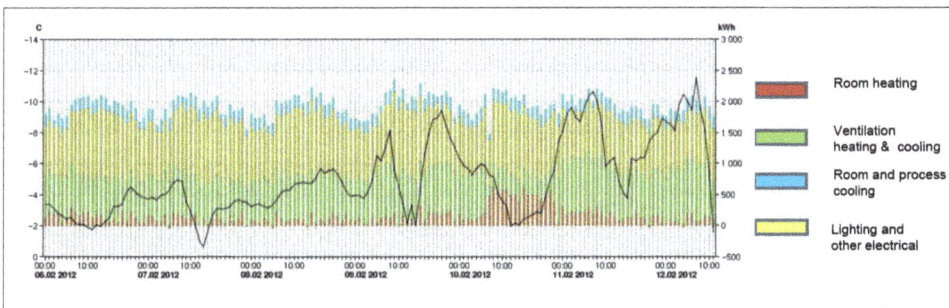

Room heating

Ventilation heating & cooling

Room and process cooling

Lighting and other electrical

10. Treatment areas have great potential for energy demand-control, by exploiting usage variations.

TESIS Inter-University Research Centre "Systems and Technologies for Social and Healthcare Facilities"
University of Florence, Italy

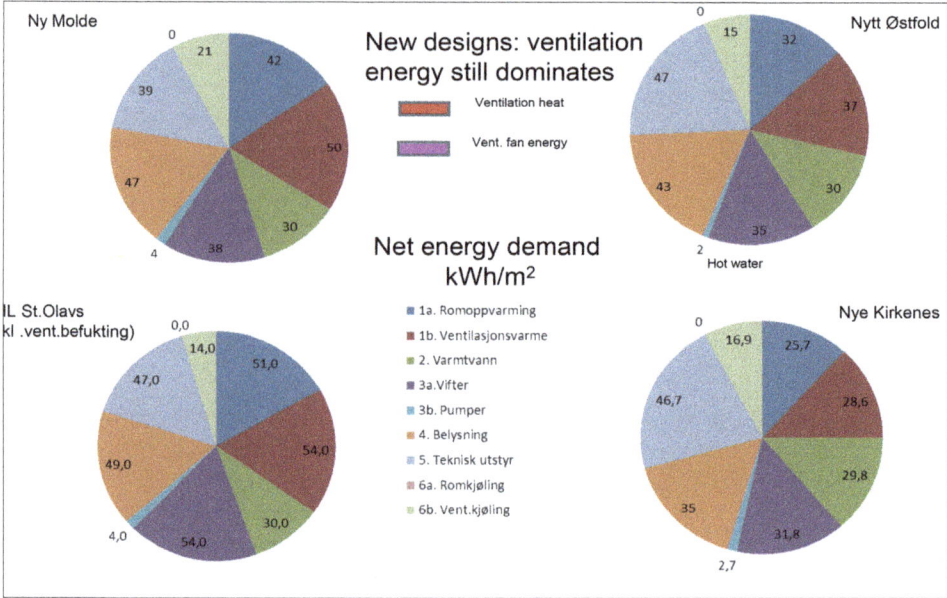

New designs: ventilation energy still dominates

- Ventilation heat
- Vent. fan energy

Net energy demand kWh/m²

- 1a. Romoppvarming
- 1b. Ventilasjonsvarme
- 2. Varmtvann
- 3a.Vifter
- 3b. Pumper
- 4. Belysning
- 5. Teknisk utstyr
- 6a. Romkjøling
- 6b. Vent.kjøling

11. Potential for energy demand-control.

	Ventilation with demand control %	Water-saving faucets %	T8 light fixtures %	Occupancy detector %	Daylight sensor %
Hospital	0,4	0,4	15	1	0
Office building	18	1	40	3	28
Hotels	23	59	17	8	7

12. Based on the percentage of the area heated, Enova Bygningsnettverk, 2008.

What is the potential for room-based energy demand-control?

Ventilation and lighting have the highest potential for demand-control:

- it is more difficult to control the demand for local room heating (1a) due to the time lag;
- domestic hot water (2) is already on-demand, and water-saving taps can be installed;
- most hospital technical equipment (5) is already on-demand; room cooling (6a) is fixed by continuous process and IT equipment demands.

Ventilation

There is a 50% energy saving potential for demand-control at room level. Heating is decoupled from air handling because, much like driving with foot gas and brake pedals at the same time, while large ventilation air flows have a cooling effect they are counteracted by room heaters.

Lower airflows have important side-effects which implies lower fan power (power varies according to speed) and more effective heat recovery. This is very important in hospitals which have only a 55% recovery rate. Good results have

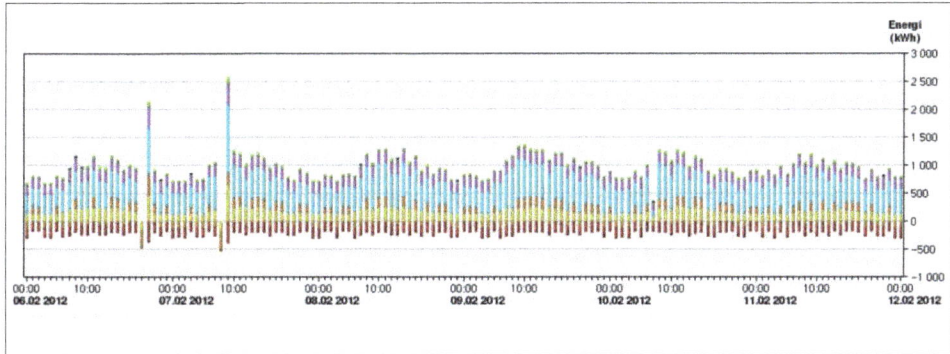

13. *Patient areas have the potential for demand-control, but less potential than treatment areas.*

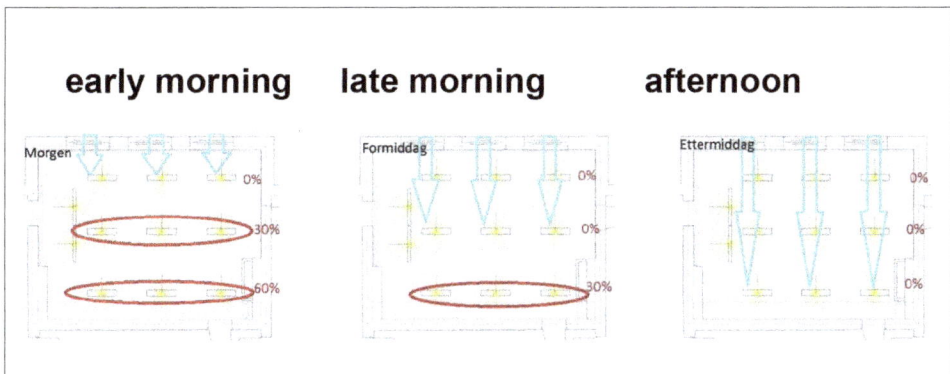

14. *Swegon's WISE system 2011, and lighting at different times of the day.*

been obtained with DCV in Borås hospital, which contributes to its very low energy consumption (105 kWh/m² in building energy). DCV will become more important in the shift from "passive house" hospitals towards large demand for cooling.

Lighting

Fixtures and light sources for 1 year's typical energy consumption represent 20-35% of all electrical energy consumption in hospitals. Demand-control saves electricity and maintenance time. Cooling energy is saved, but even cold climate hospitals have space cooling baseloads in summer. 20% of lighting energy becomes cooling energy. In winter not all heat energy from lighting displaces room heating.

BONUS theme: Medical technical equipment

MTE consumes 15-20% of electrical energy in newer hospitals and this figure is growing. Is it possible to control demand? More research is needed with the aim of reducing standby power and the large baseload power required to cool this equipment.

1. Sunset Mississippi.

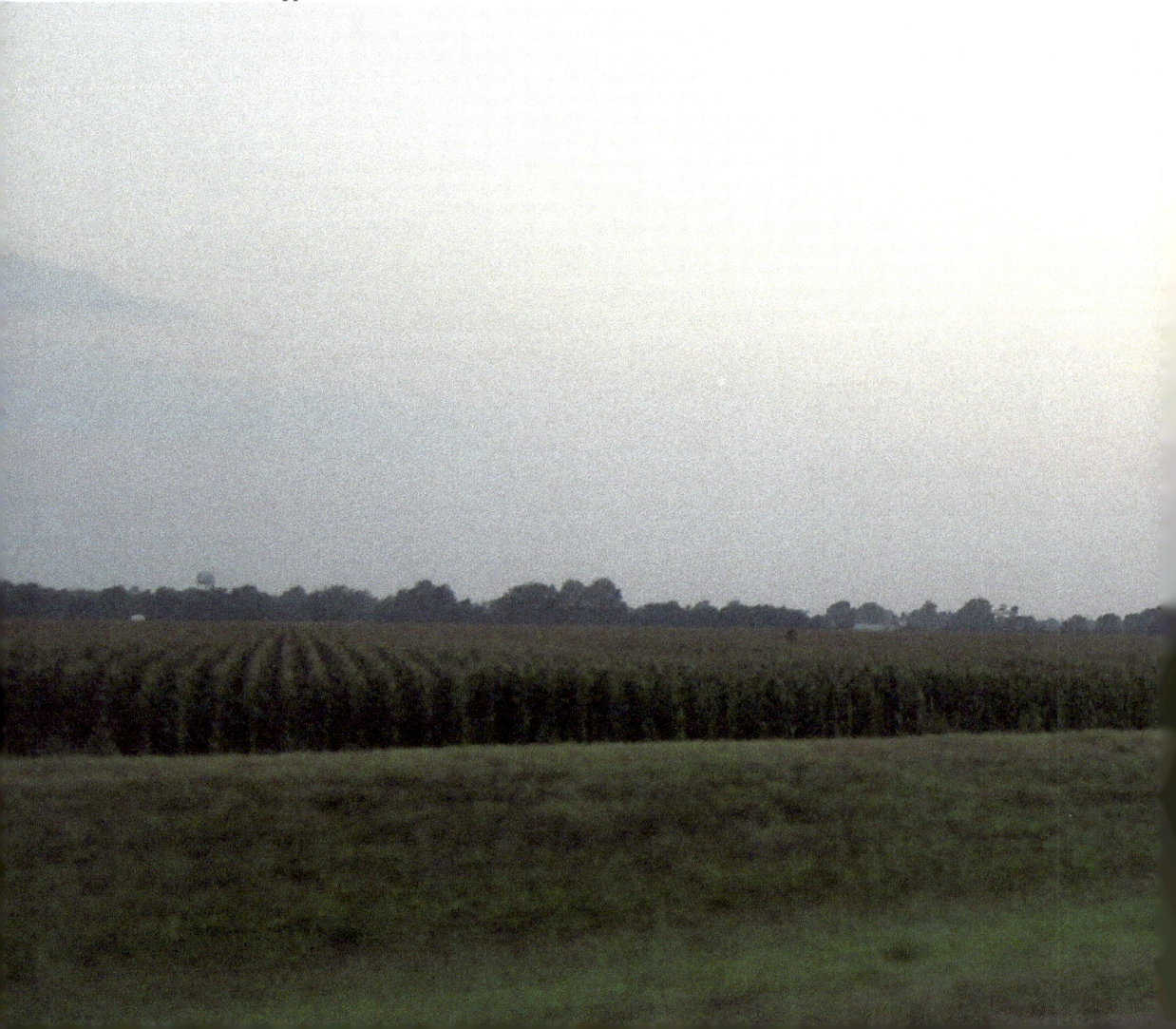

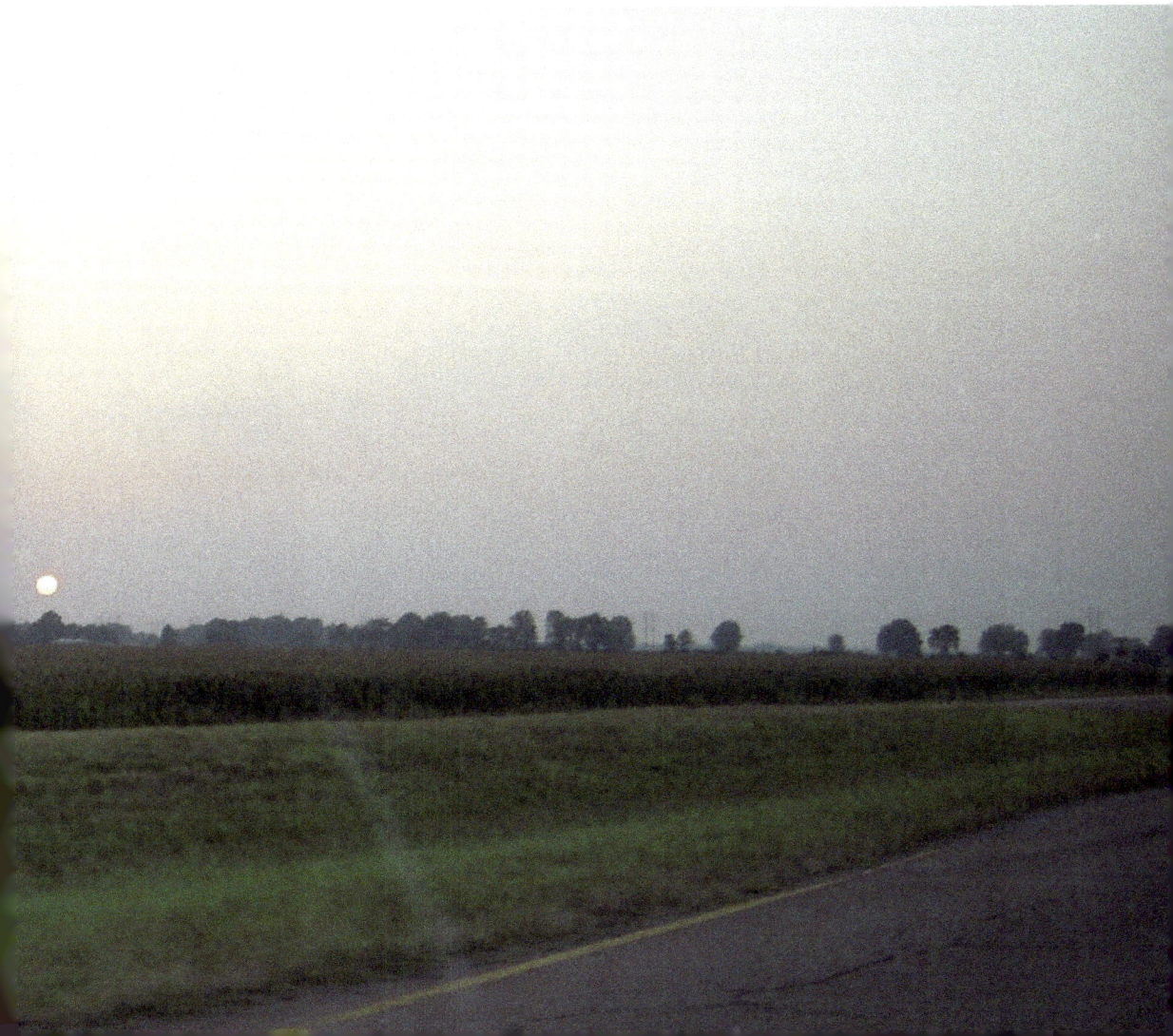

Better, Faster, Smarter
Planning for Underserved Clinical Settings

Philip Patrick Sun
AIA, ACHA, NCARB

The delivery of healthcare globally has not been without planning, political and demographic challenges. This is world-wide. While some counties have had the benefit of technological advances these benefits have not necessarily resulted in a system of care that addresses an entire population or that has created a healthy environment. Part of the challenge has been the ability or inability for design to help develop solutions that enhance both the creation of healthy environments and curing the sick. Doing this well, quickly and with as few wasted resources as possible is a triple challenge.

This paper is about Better, Faster, and Smarter. Better Value, Faster Delivery and Smarter Operations. It will include a few quotes that may add depth and a bit of levity, starting with the following quote: "It is a lot harder to keep people well than it is to just get them over a sickness." DeForest Clinton Jarvis

The author's career and involvement with healthcare over the past thirty years has been intricate. As an architect and as a client the path was a long journey through public projects, private programs, processes such as design-bid-build, construction management, design build and now integrated project delivery. The net result has been the capture of lessons learned from a few examples of projects and programs which include a major public healthcare system

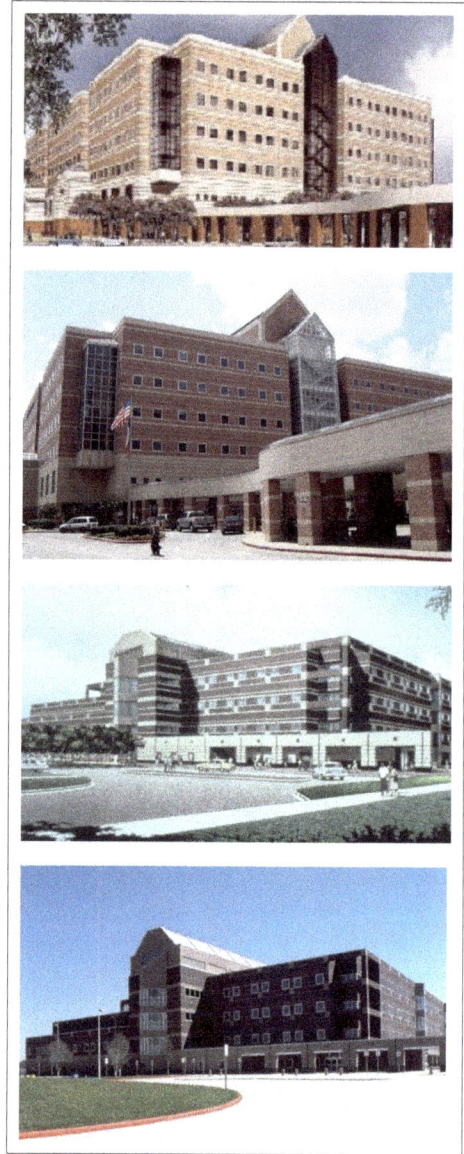

2. *Major Public Healthcare System.*

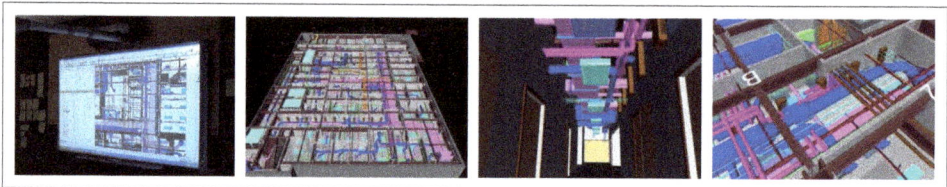

3. *A critical San Francisco Hospital, BIM and IPD.*

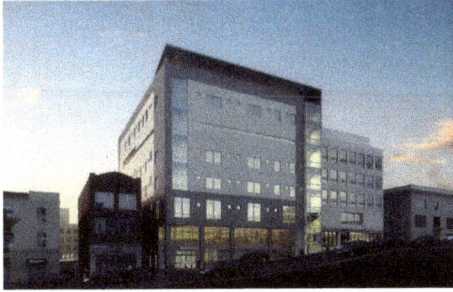

4. A critical San Francisco Hospital, on target for LEED Gold.

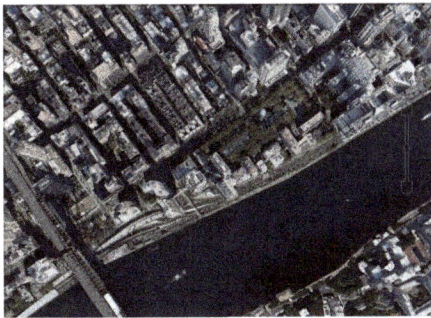

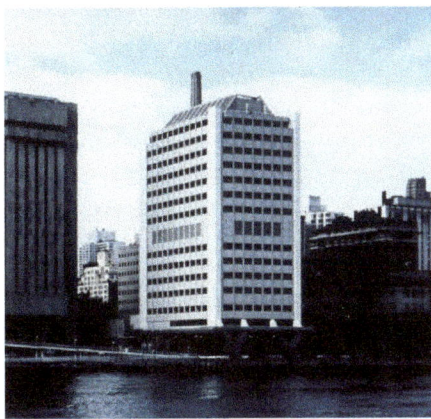

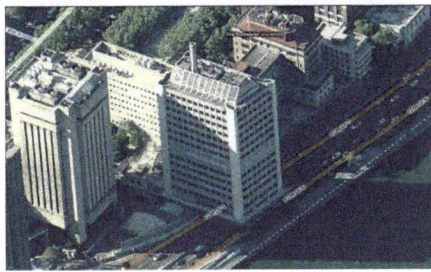

5. Major NY Medical Research Institute.

and the development of two teaching hospitals with no change orders, under budget, on schedule and awarded multiple gold medals, such as the completion of major research centres including one in New York City built over FDR Drive which used Lean techniques. In addition to public projects and research centres lessons have also been learned from a prominent small hospital in San Francisco on a most difficult site where the use of BIM and Integrated Project Delivery is leading to a 35% cost benefit and a fully coordinated project.

143

This paper is about the lessons learned, the process used and the new technology that enables these outcomes, and will talk about the context, process and the solution. First of all it will address the context, healthcare in the United States, starting with a quote:

"Light travels faster than sound.
This is why some people appear bright
until you hear them speak."
author unknown

HEALTHCARE IN THE USA

"A Hospital is No Place to Be Sick"
Samuel Goldwyn

Although there are many statistics that could be given here, the most recent findings are that American healthcare is actually a system of "sick care". This is often underscored by the critically high cost of care (at over 16% of GDP and the highest per capita cost in the world) and the number of people who are not insured and find access to care difficult. It is estimated that 49.9 million people are not insured and many are underinsured. The cost of care is a major source

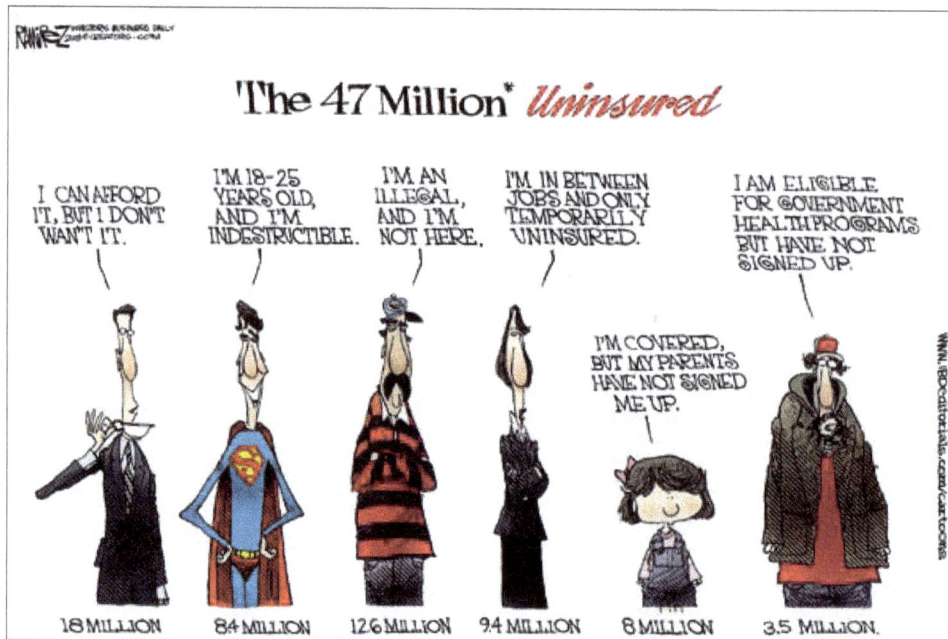

6. Growing numbers of the uninsured. Source: Michael Ramirez, IDB Political Cartoons, 2011.

of economic stress to individuals, families, companies and the economy. The USA is different from the rest of the world in that the system is by and large a private system with heavy reliance on a private profit-oriented healthcare insurance industry.

The quality of care is a related issue. Even with high costs the markers of health outcomes are not favorable as measured by groups such as the World Health Organization (WHO). WHO has ranked the USA 37th in the quality of care. Longevity, disease indicators and other measures show the cost of care and health outcomes have little to do with success in this system.

Surveys have shown individual, public and official governmental displeasure with the current healthcare system and recently new legislation has come into effect: Public Law 111-141; the Patient Protection and Affordable Care Act. One of the directives of the "Act" is to create better access to care. One mechanism is to create better access facilities. As such USD 11 billion is being directed to Community Health Centers across the USA. This is primarily for Federally Qualified Health Centers who apply for and receive grants to help provide care to those who cannot afford it and to subsidize the cost of construction for new and renovated facilities.

The construction costs for healthcare facilities in the USA have increased dramatically. The cost of all construction has increased but that of healthcare more dramatically. This directly affects the cost of care. In addition the planning process can either help or be part of the problem in delivering cost-effective care.

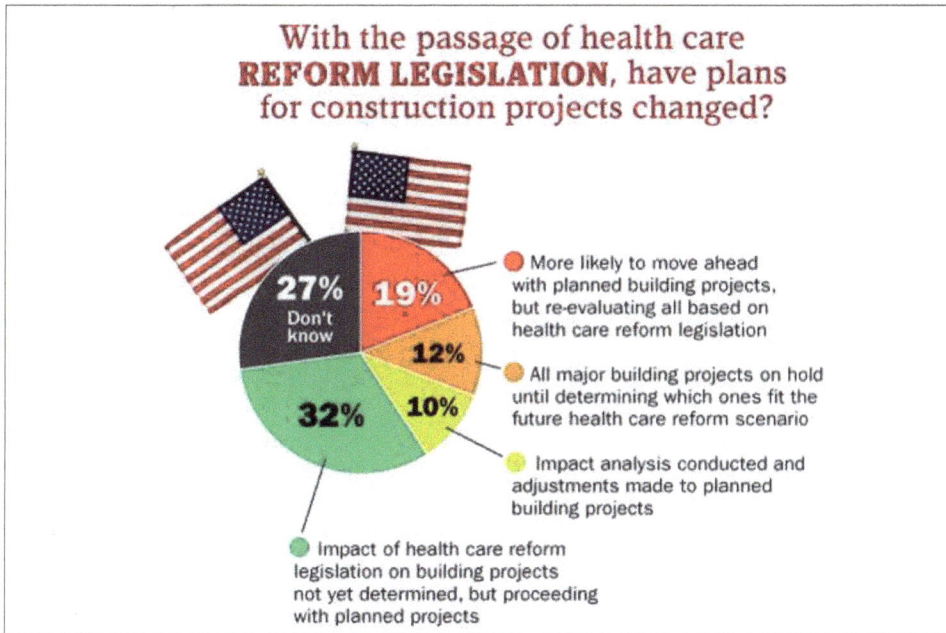

With the passage of health care
REFORM LEGISLATION, have plans
for construction projects changed?

27% Don't know

19%

12%

10%

32%

- More likely to move ahead with planned building projects, but re-evaluating all based on health care reform legislation

- All major building projects on hold until determining which ones fit the future health care reform scenario

- Impact analysis conducted and adjustments made to planned building projects

- Impact of health care reform legislation on building projects not yet determined, but proceeding with planned projects

7. Construction survey. Source: Health Facilities Management/ASHE 2011.

The study area for this paper is the Mississippi Delta, a region of very fertile agricultural lands. This area has fed the USA since the development of the country and has allowed the USA to be independently able to feed itself for the past 200 years. The six major river systems that join the Mississippi have provided the least costly form of transportation over the years allowing the country and region to have benefited from a constant and stable agricultural centre.

However, the region has not only been in decline and has lost and is losing its population but it has also become one of the poorest regions in the country. This area has the lowest income, the shortest longevity, and the highest degree of problems related to heart disease, strokes, diabetes and rampant obesity. It is also culturally the heart of American

Blues Music. In addition the area is historically known as the "south" and has a deep relationship with the continuing memory of a troubled past.

This region is challenged with few construction skilled labor resources. Being primarily agricultural, with few major projects to support a construction industry and few training facilities, the amount of skilled trades and labor is limited. In addition the cost of construction is not low, which is initially counterintuitive.

This study concentrates on this region and the Delta Health Center, the first FQHC (Federally Qualified Health Center) in the USA, started over fifty years ago. This is currently a system of four facilities serving three counties, Bolivar, Sunflower and Washington. Each

145

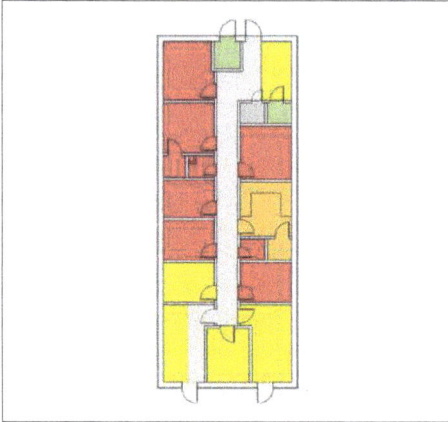

8. *The Moorehead facility.*

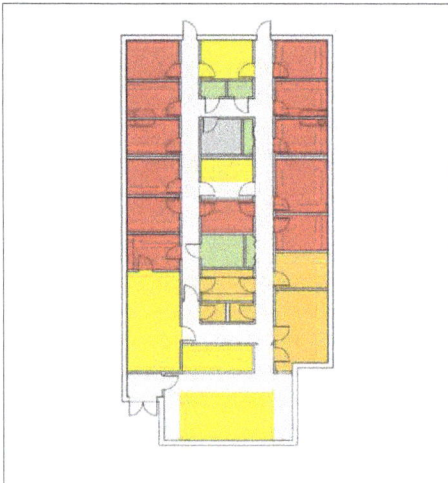

9. *The Greenville facility.*

of these counties has a high degree of poverty with some towns in excess of 50% poverty.

There was an opportunity to organize the challenges into healthcare delivery, regional and local health needs, the limited construction resources, and to recognize that for healthcare facilities:

*Uniquely Complex Requirements
require
Unique Solutions
which require
Unique Design Processes
which in turn require
Unique Management Approaches.*

What's more, importantly, the right problem(s) need to be addressed.

As the contribution provided by construction is the built environment architects and planners must ensure it provides and enhances the solution to the problem rather than creates a greater problem. It is clear that the cost of care and opportunities to provide better patient outcomes are critically important to any measure of success.

Studies by the National Health Service

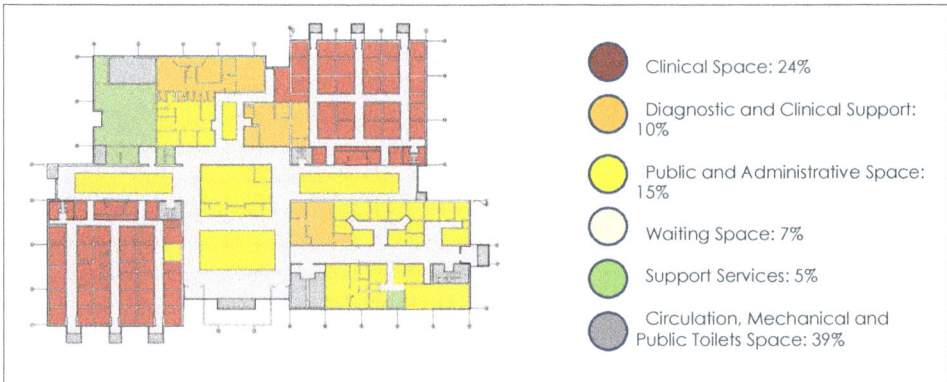

Clinical Space: 24%

Diagnostic and Clinical Support: 10%

Public and Administrative Space: 15%

Waiting Space: 7%

Support Services: 5%

Circulation, Mechanical and Public Toilets Space: 39%

10. *The Mound Bayou facility.*

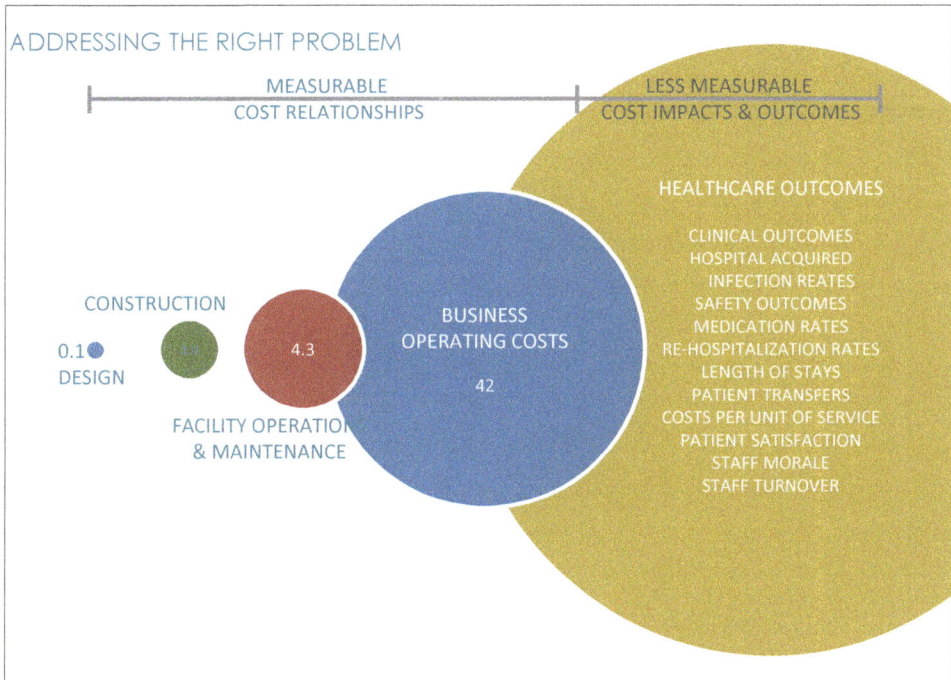

ADDRESSING THE RIGHT PROBLEM

MEASURABLE
COST RELATIONSHIPS

LESS MEASURABLE
COST IMPACTS & OUTCOMES

HEALTHCARE OUTCOMES

CLINICAL OUTCOMES
HOSPITAL ACQUIRED
INFECTION REATES
SAFETY OUTCOMES
MEDICATION RATES
RE-HOSPITALIZATION RATES
LENGTH OF STAYS
PATIENT TRANSFERS
COSTS PER UNIT OF SERVICE
PATIENT SATISFACTION
STAFF MORALE
STAFF TURNOVER

CONSTRUCTION

0.1
DESIGN

4.3

BUSINESS
OPERATING COSTS

42

FACILITY OPERATION
& MAINTENANCE

147

11. Addressing the right problem: measurable cost relationships and less measurable cost impacts and healthcare outcomes.

have shown that if the cost of design is 0.1, then generally the cost of construction is 1.0 as a ratio (that is design and all its related costs come to roughly 10% of the construction cost).

The cost of maintaining and powering these facilities is generally a factor of 4.3. But the real cost or operational or business cost is 42 times the construction cost and 420 times the design cost.

Therefore design has the ability to dramatically affect the operations cost based on how the planning and design are conducted and the resultant facility. Planning and design must therefore look ahead to business operations and beyond peer group awards, "value" engineering exercises, and subjective

aesthetics. It must be understood that efficiency does not necessarily mean a smaller building but a better format for more efficient staffing, lower costs for business operations and better patient treatment, staff satisfaction and curative results. Even beyond this, facilities are seen as a way of improving the difficult to measure but most important world of patient outcomes.

To meet this challenge Lean and Integrated Project Delivery (IPD) techniques have been used.

As for process and research it has been said that: *"To steal ideas from one person is plagiarism. To steal from many is research."* Wilson Mizner
In terms of process and management, re-

fer to the following the three resources:
- Bioteaming Manifesto by Ken Thompson and Robin Good;
- Problem Seeking by William Pena, FAIA;
- The Toyota Way by Jeffrey K. Liker.

Each resource contributes to the manner of thinking and data organization, which leads to decision management and durable decision-making by the owner and the integrated design team.

Lessons learned from these resources and experiences underscore the fact that an integrated team works far more effectively than the traditional "command and control" model. Bioteaming shows that the team should be treated as a whole and living mechanism and that team members should not be treated as technicians with tasks.

Problem Seeking provides a format for data gathering and organization that leads to decision management, the essence of which is to programmatically Establish Goals, Collect and Analyze Facts, Uncover and Test Concepts, Determine Needs (needs are different to "wants" because "needs" are balanced against a budget), and State the Problem (what makes this project unique and different to all other projects).

The Toyota way teaches business and management regarding how to reduce "waste" in the production of the project. Indeed, spending more time on organizing might seem less effective but if the decisions are durable then it avoids changes that would require substantially more time in the long run. The subtlety of "pull" versus "push" and other lessons

148

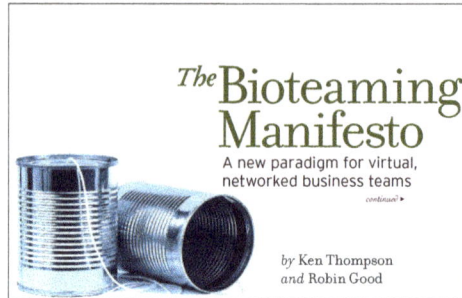

12. *Bioteaming Manifesto by Ken Thompson and Robin Good.*

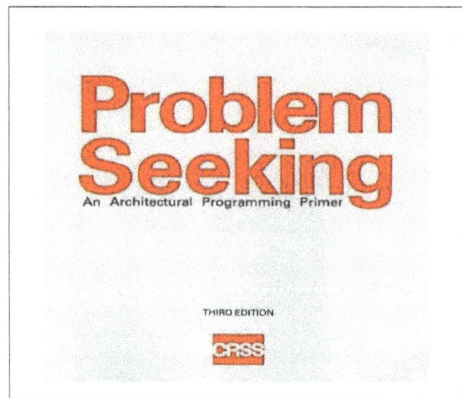

13. *Problem Seeking by William Pena, FAIA.*

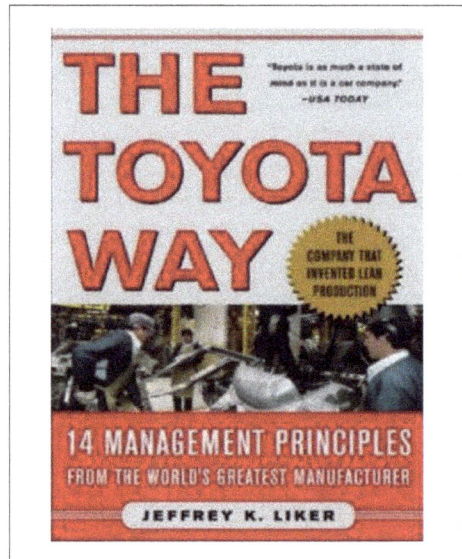

14. *The Toyota Way by Jeffrey K. Liker.*

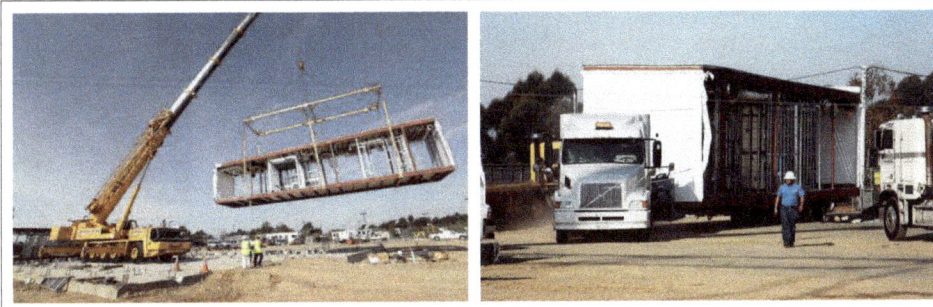

15. Walden Structures: Delivery and assembly.

reveal how Toyota succeeded and how others can succeed as well.

With time and experience the five major areas that have helped to organize and execute successful projects are as follows:

- Process Mapping
- Target Costing
- Set Based Design
- Systems Integration and Optimization
- Decision Management

A major factor is in understanding "decisions" and how decisions manifest themselves and are developed. There are three principal components of decisions related to projects and the groups involved in working on them. First, "memory" and how the same "memory" must be shared and there must be a collective "common memory".

The second is to have "common or collective reasoning". There must be a common understanding of reasoning in the same way, otherwise "two plus two equals five". Without common and collective reasoning the basis for a durable decision will not form.

Finally decisions and durable decisions come from establishing a deep process of engagement which strikes at and

stimulates a variety of cognitive senses. To achieve this there must be common and collective "concept formation". As the group achieves concept formation, the concepts are embedded as are the "decisions". Thus durable decisions develop which effectively reduce waste from change, and thus reduce costs because the major cause of cost increase is change.

There are several graphics that evoke some of the principal programmatic concepts such as access, flow, separation, orientation, integration, security/privacy, relationships and finally prioritization. The ability and need to prioritize is critical to decision management. Prioritization means being able to order priorities as 1, 2, 3, and so forth. It is critically important not have three number 1 priorities.

Setting priorities can be difficult but ignoring or bypassing them is an invitation and investment in disaster.

In the case study the team was integrated as much as possible before there was a project. In this case elements of the team came together because of friendships and working relationships that sought

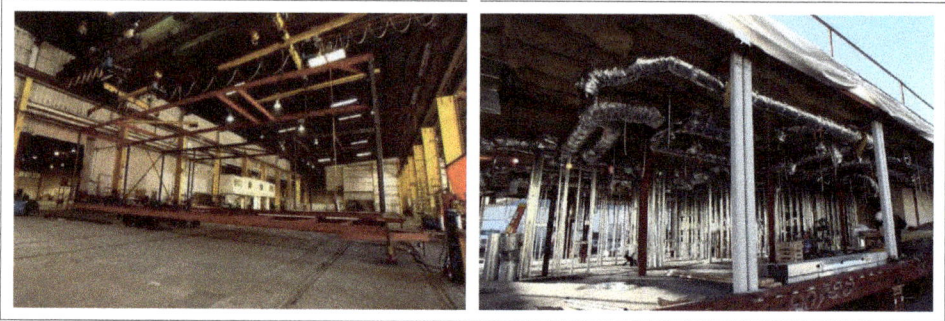

150

16. *Walden Structures: Factory assembly of modular units with systems included.*

to bring together solutions which would benefit healthcare and project delivery. A grant was written for these elements and the grant was awarded from the Patient Protection and Affordable Care Act (PL 111-148) described earlier. The grant pays in part for the design and construction of the project.

The integration of communications and working as a group, in the same space and time, is highly important to successful Integrated Project Delivery or "IPD."

Using the five major elements, the first was process mapping with physicians and staff which helped to create the essence of the types of working environments for the more "efficient and improved patient outcome model" environments. The exam rooms, for example, are modeled not only around the functional equipment required for each activity, but also around the philosophy of services to be provided.

In this case healthcare goes beyond "sick care" and the exam room has two environments: a "clinical" side and an "education" side. The education side provides an area where the physician or nurse provider can discuss health issues with

the patient at a shared table (in this case a Herman Miller "teardrop" table located in the corner). This helps develop and integrate patient trust and communications and a related interactive computer touch screen monitor is used to provide personal patient information as well as to provide education from tapes, videos and interactive exercises while the care provider might be out of the room.

The room is larger than a typical exam room, but its use eliminates the need for the patient to go to the physician's office for consultation and provides a less stressful interaction for the patient. Education is an important step in the "health" care process and this type of space helps in going beyond "sick" care.

The spatial organization was also developed through process mapping with physicians and staff. Certain programmatic models were discussed and joint concept formation led to the ratio of one office for three exam rooms and two care providers per organized medical pod.

The concept of a prime design and healing environment resulted in the decision to use controlled natural lighting as a major element in plan development.

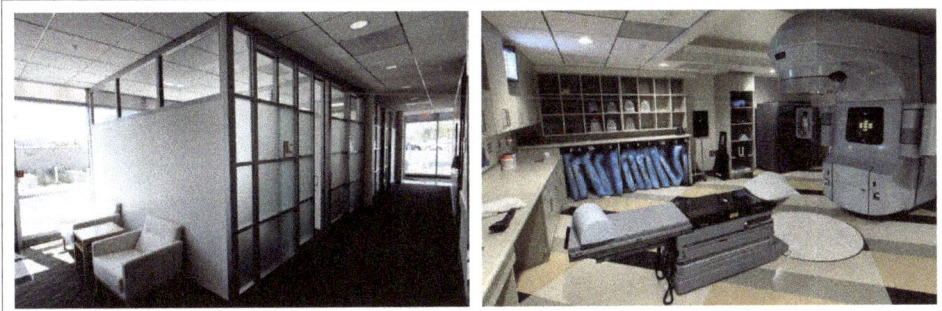

17. Walden Structures: Interior examples.

While the Mississippi Delta has an abundance of natural light, as do many areas of the world, most clinic plans are developed for corridor efficiency such that there are a multitude of anonymous corridors. This has no benefit whatsoever to patients or staff stress reduction. The artificially lit corridors create greater stress and reduce the ability of the human immune system to assist in the healing process.

Think courtyards instead. Even the use of skylights is not as helpful as the use of courtyards. Thus the development of these medical pods comes from the ancient use of courtyards as calming and healing environments. The democratic distribution of natural light along corridors and in waiting rooms is a basic concept for this approach towards building a healthy and a health promoting facility.

The production of the facility and its methodology was based on the availability of construction resources as discussed previously. The critical need is for examination and treatment spaces to be of high quality, reliable and repeatable construction or production. This suggested a manufacturing process such as modular construction off-site. These modules could be built in a repeatable and reliable manner under a weather protected environment at a reasonable cost.

Simple spaces such as corridors and waiting rooms could be built on-site by local labor. This led to the development of the concept of a hybrid combination which maximized the best attributes of local labor and manufacturing to build technically demanding spaces.

An example of the use of modular construction is the recently opened hospital in Joplin, MO. While the Joplin hospital design did not maximize the effectiveness of modular construction, prefabricated modules developed precisely along the lines of dimensions that can be easily shipped and installed. The corridors and waiting room on the other hand can include local influences that respond to regional and climatic needs.

The simple concept is to locally build the foundation, while the modules are being produced off-site (with all their finishes and all mechanical, electrical and plumbing systems), install them on-site and complete the corridors and waiting rooms on-site.

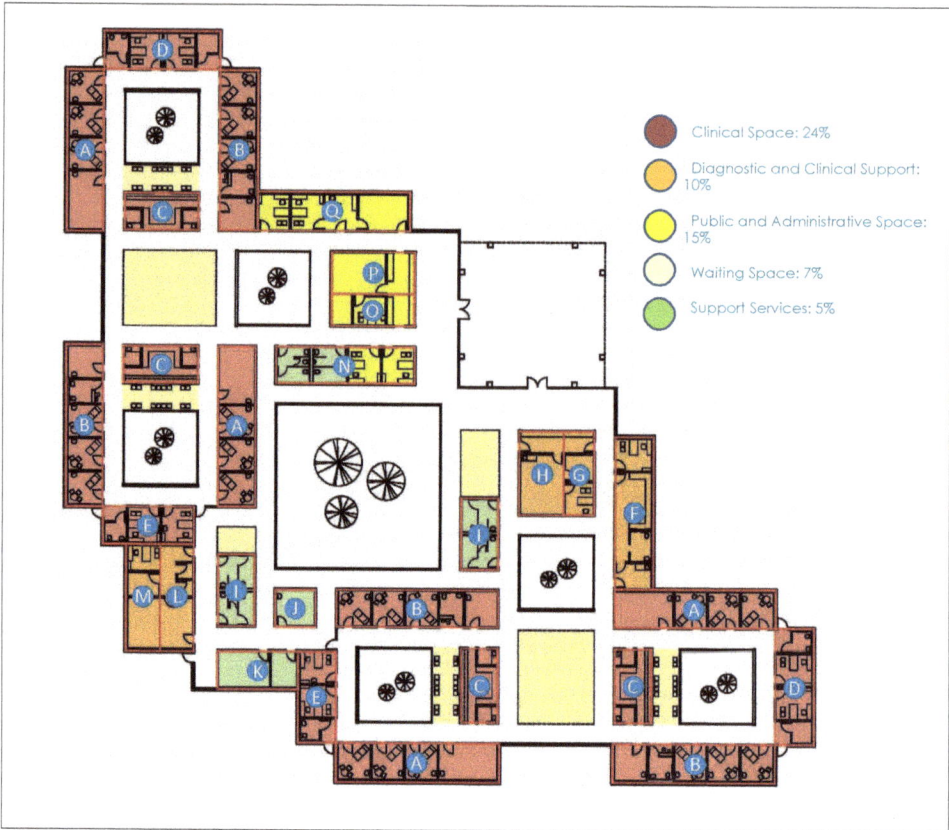

Clinical Space: 24%

Diagnostic and Clinical Support: 10%

Public and Administrative Space: 15%

Waiting Space: 7%

Support Services: 5%

18. New Hospital in Joplin, MO, functional zoning.

All the mechanical and almost all the electrical systems would come with the modules. The HVAC from the modules feed the corridors and waiting rooms from side diffusers.

The time savings alone are expected to create a facility in almost half the conventional construction time.

In addition the use of manufacturing is emphasized by using systems casework and furnishings, thus again maximizing repeatable reliability. The impact on the environment is also reduced by limiting on-site waste and limiting damage to the site by reducing materials and workers on the site.

This total facility is approximately 25,000 square feet, approximately half of which is modular and half of which is comprised of corridors and waiting rooms built on-site. There are 29 units in this plan which anticipates 40,000 to 60,000 visits annually. A larger and a smaller model were developed, and they all use the same modules.

There are other opportunities to perfect concepts such as this, but it is hoped it will be possible to produce a facility in almost half the time, with a high degree

153

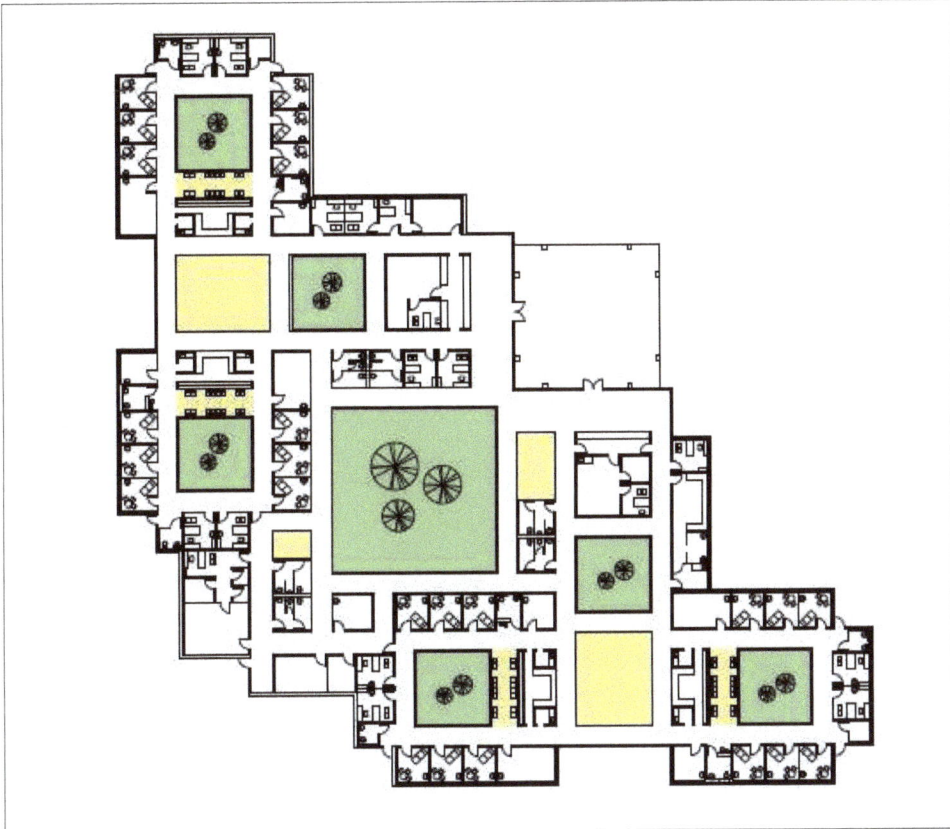

19. New Hospital in Joplin, MO, courtyards bring natural light to corridors and waiting areas.

of quality and an expected cost of 30% below comparable construction, and to benefit the delivery of healthcare. Moreover, to develop a physical plan from process mapping and a systematic view of patient care delivery that emphasizes patient outcomes and "health" care and not just "sick" care, supporting attempts such as this for integrated teams to provide solutions for the care delivery crisis.

As a final quote to remember when seeking solutions:
"Never be afraid to try something new. Remember amateurs built the ark. Professionals built the Titanic."

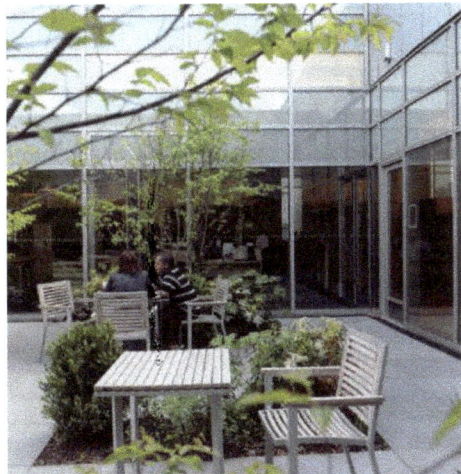

20. Courtyards.

TESIS Inter-University Research Centre "Systems and Technologies for Social and Healthcare Facilities"
University of Florence, Italy

1. *South Ostrobothnia Central Hospital.*

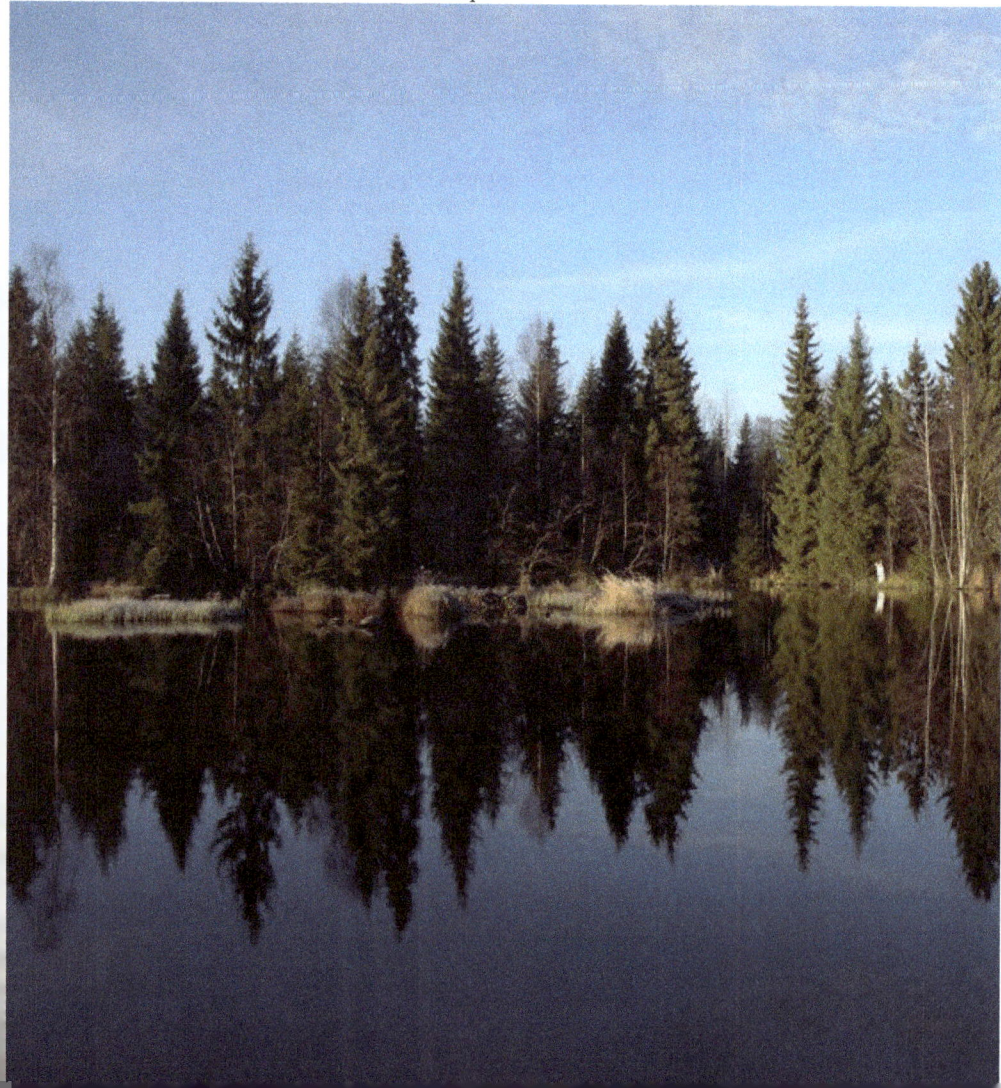

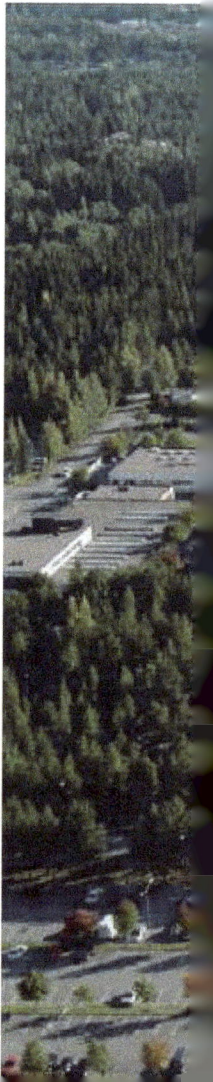

Virtual Design in Hospitals (CAVE)
A Case Study

Helina Kotilainen
Chief Architect, M.Sc.(Archit.), SAFA
The National Institute of Health and Welfare (THL)

155

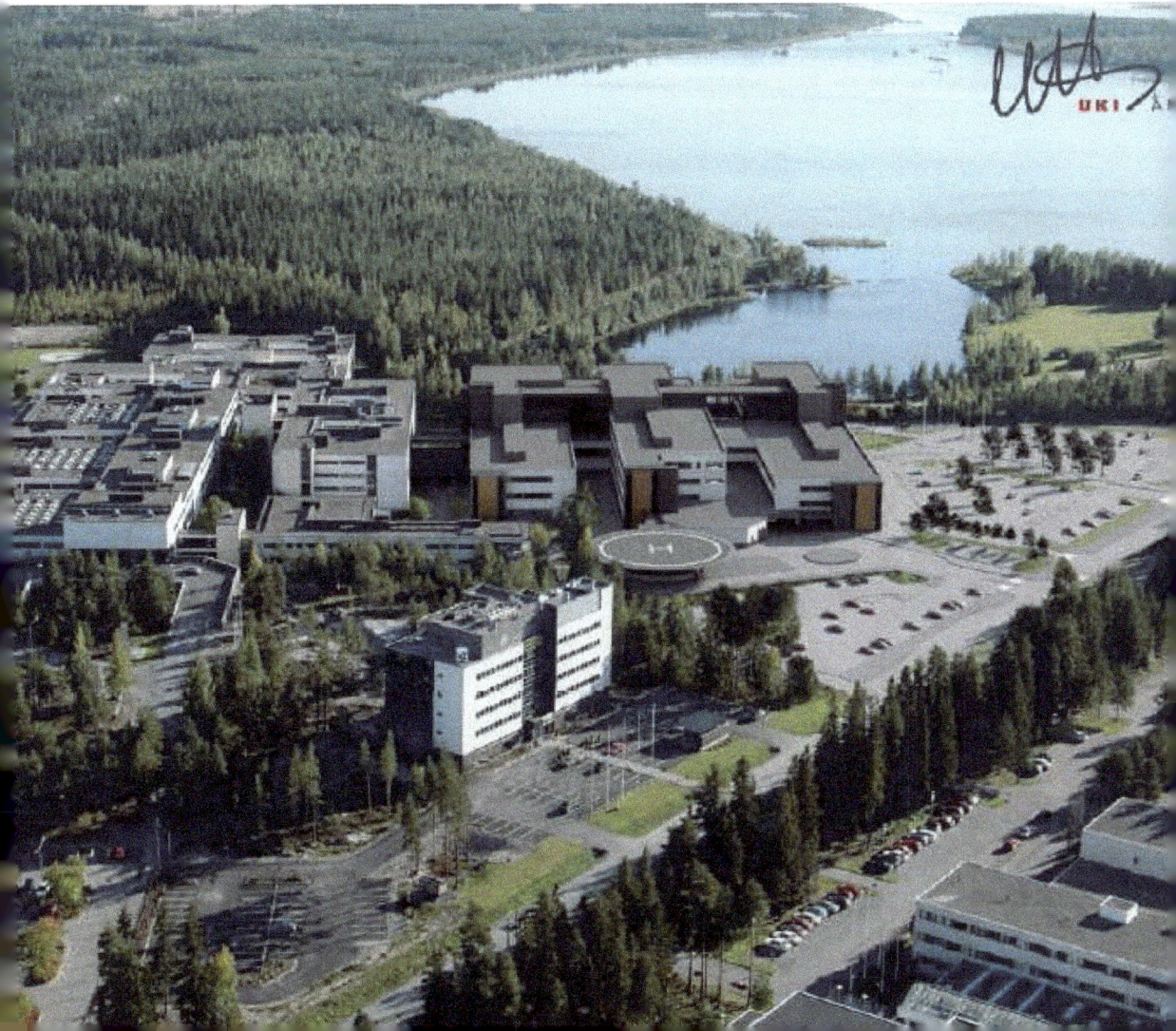

Virtual environment (CAVE) as a tool for end-user participation in emergency unit design, a case study

Abstract

South Ostrobothnia Central Hospital is a secondary health care unit serving a population of 200,000 inhabitants. The hospital was built in several stages. This extension involves approximately 130 beds and facilities for approximately 20 different units. The new building will employ 450 people. Some of the new facilities will be occupied by the primary health care services of the City of Seinajoki. The city is also home to Seinajoki University of Applied Sciences and its virtual laboratory. For the purposes of this project, the South Ostrobothnia Hospital District joined forces with a number of partners to use the virtual laboratory as a design tool to allow end users to participate in project planning. The computer-assisted virtual environment (CAVE) used in the project is a room comprising walls, a ceiling, and a floor. Images generated using computer graphics cards are projected onto these surfaces, which, when viewed through stereoscopic glasses, are transformed into a three-dimensional full-scale environment.

The most important property of a CAVE-type virtual environment is its scale, i.e. the ability of visitors to perceive the environment as almost real. Visitors are able to move to some extent within the space itself and to travel longer distances with the help of a 3D mouse. An examination room, a patient room and the emergency centre were selected because hospitals regularly have multiple identical examination rooms and patient rooms. The emergency centre is a new kind of unit, and its design involved several functional issues.

The end users visited the environment in small focus groups. All conversations that took place in the virtual environment were recorded and videotaped and later analyzed. The total number of visitors in the virtual environment was just over 280. A total of 34 recordings were made of group interviews. The content analysis revealed a total of 14 primary themes and 26 secondary themes. Layout was the most important theme identified with regard to the emergency centre.

The number one secondary theme was functionality, followed by the positioning and expediency of different elements. As regards the use of the virtual environment, the emergency centre attracted the most comments on functionality as well as the usefulness of the virtual environment. Valuable information was gained on situations assessing interaction between staff and patients. This is interesting as visitors were required to visualise and move around a relatively complex space. A total of approximately 90% of the visitors considered commenting on the environment easy or relatively easy.

The potential use of virtual environments at different stages of the design process offers exciting vistas. Technological development can also enable more extensive use of virtual environments in the future.

South Ostrobothnia Hospital District

The catchment area of the South Os-trobothnia Hospital District is approximately 200,000 people. The specialized healthcare hospital has a capacity of 482 beds, 265,000 outpatient visits per year and 20,000 surgical operations per year.

The main hospital was built in 1977 and over the years several extensions have been added. The latest one, Y-building, was commissioned in autumn 2012.

Computer-Assisted Virtual Environment CAVE

The Computer-Assisted Virtual Environment CAVE is a "glass box" measuring 3 x 3 x 2.5 m with a ceiling, floor and three walls. The images, generated using computer graphics cards, are projected onto the walls in a darkened room with several projectors.

Modeling is based on Autodesk 3DS Max software and viewers wearing stereoscopic glasses (with a tracking system) either move short distances by themselves or longer distances using a 3D mouse.

Visits to CAVE

A patient room, an examination room and part of an emergency centre (1000 m²) were modeled into the CAVE.
Altogether over 280 visitors had the chance to visit the virtual model: they were the board of the Y-house, designers, planners, engineers, contractors, the accessible building committee and end-users from the health centre and specialized healthcare.

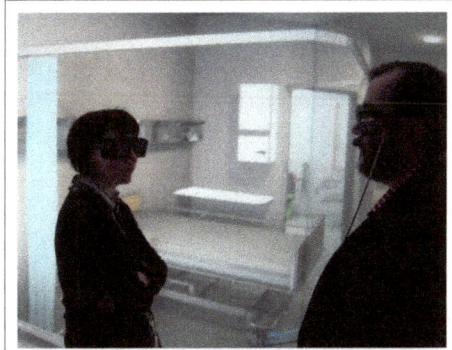

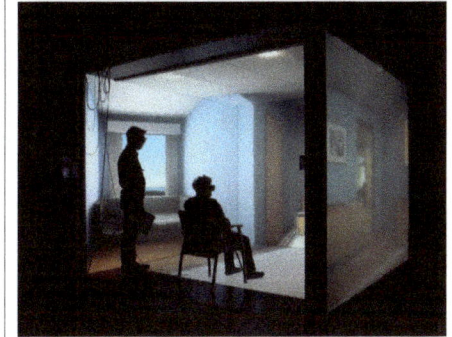

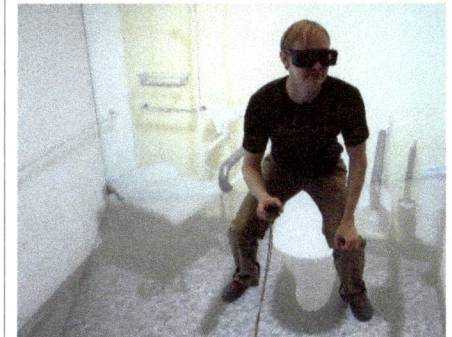

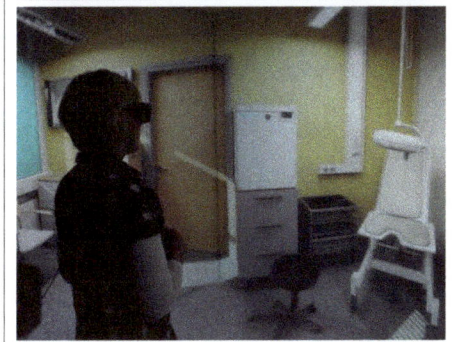

157

2. Computer-Assisted Virtual Environment CAVE.

TESIS Inter-University Research Centre "Systems and Technologies for Social and Healthcare Facilities"
University of Florence, Italy

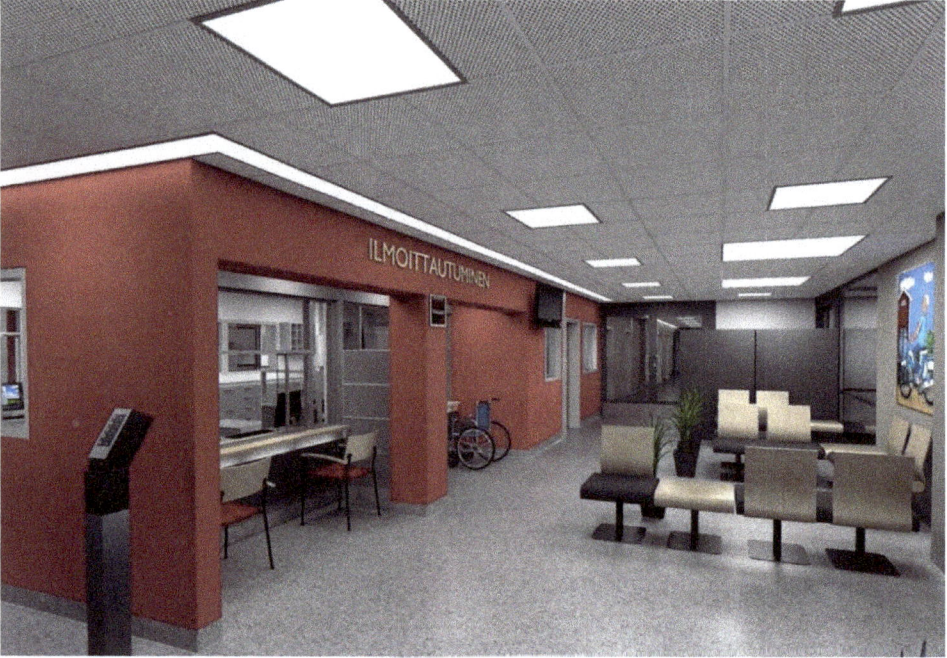

3. Virtual model of an emergency centre, approx. 1000 m².

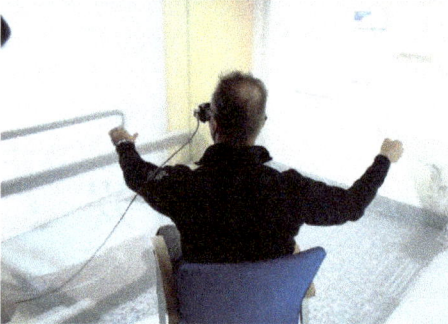

4. Virtual model of a patient room.

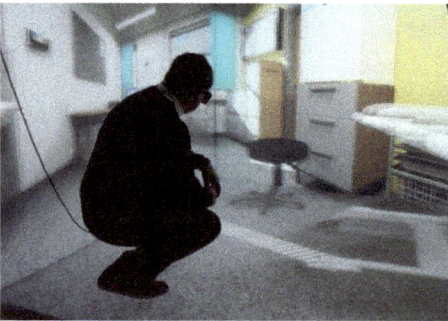

5. Virtual model of an examination room.

After the visits questionnaires were distributed to the end-users and 187 of them were returned. Four of the visitor groups tested the signs and guidance.

Content of the CAVE studies

Research material consisted of recorded and decoded discussions, video recordings, photographs and questionnaires.
The following research methods were applied: thematic contents analysis (decoded discussions) and SPSS software (questionnaires).
A thematic contents analysis on interviews in CAVE produced altogether approx. 4600 findings.

They were grouped into 14 primary themes (layout, accessibility, furniture, accessories, materials, durability, ergo-

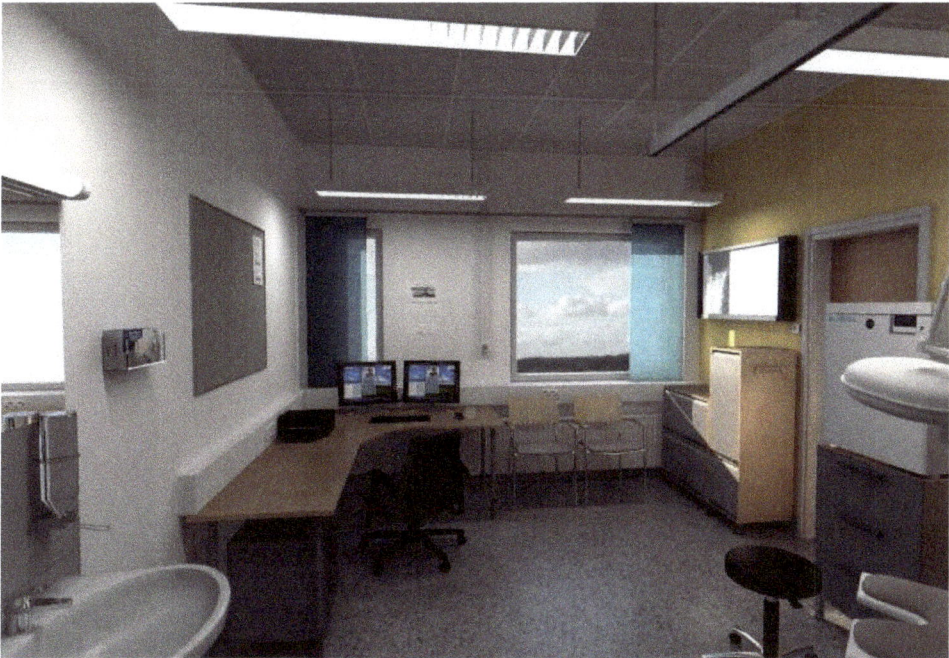

6. Virtual model of an examination room.

nomics, hygiene, safety, lighting, colours, blinds/curtains, aesthetics, virtual environments) and 23 to 25 secondary themes (accessibility, ergonomics, aesthetics (art), hygiene, practicality, easy-to-open windows, furniture, touchability, positioning, needs, dimensions, layout, functionality, safety, type, accessories, lighting, daylight, blinds/curtains, attractiveness, colours, privacy, acoustics, view, durability, ease of maintenance, materials, appeal).

A part of the emergency centre (approx. 1000 m²) was modeled into the CAVE. As an example of the research material the interviews of 17 groups that visited the virtual emergency centre produced 1992 findings and 65 questionnaires.

The spaces modeled into the CAVE were registration, triage, waiting areas, corridors and observation rooms.

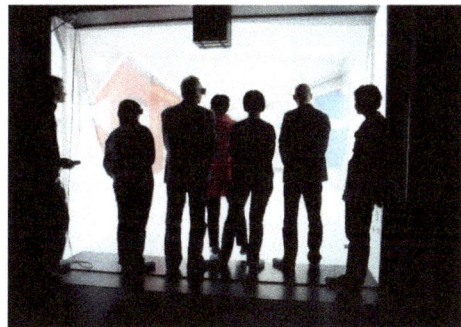

7. Research material: interviews with 17 groups.

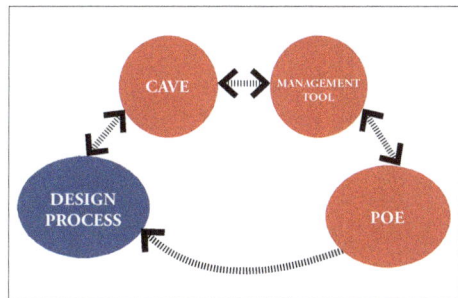

8. Design process / learning organization.

TESIS Inter-University Research Centre "Systems and Technologies for Social and Healthcare Facilities"
University of Florence, Italy

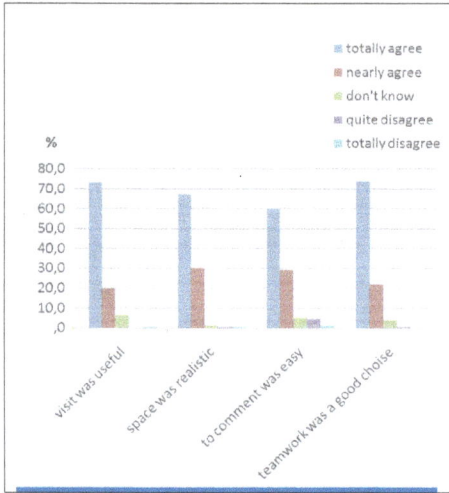

9. *Emergency centre, primary themes.*

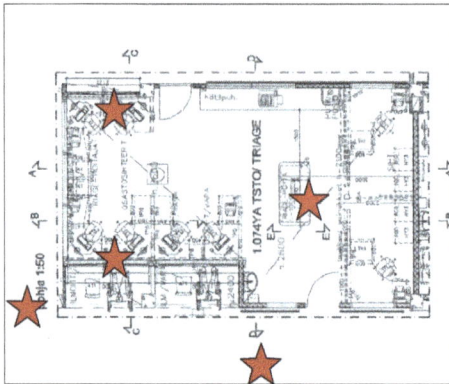

10. *Triage comments in CAVE.*

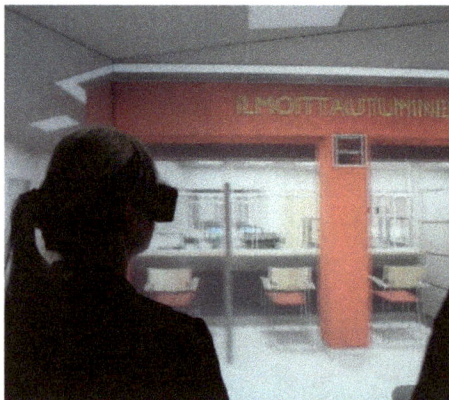

11. *CAVE allows a virtual walk-through of the rendering and interaction with 3D objects.*

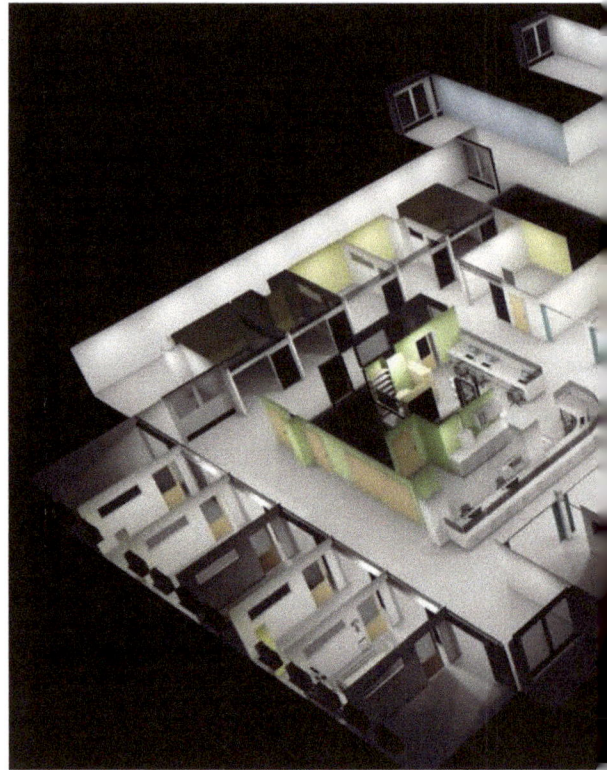

12. *Virtual model of the emergency centre (a part).*

The visitors especially commented on the entrance to the emergency centre, patient/staff contact, working in triage/ privacy, safety, accessibility and guidance.

SUMMARY, issues mentioned most often

In the examination rooms most attention was paid to the furniture, accessories and layout. In patient rooms accessories were the priority, then furniture and layout.

In bathrooms the most important issues were accessories and then layout and accessibility. In the emergency centre most discussions focused on layout and after that accessories and furniture.

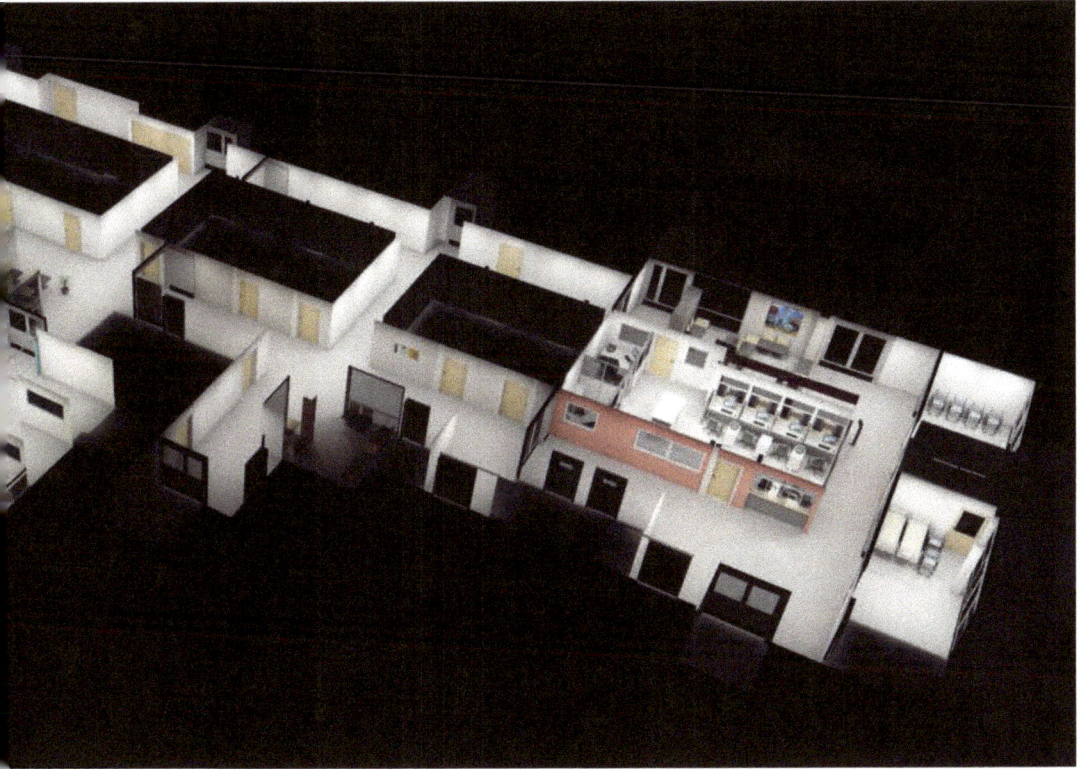

Interaction between staff and patients was analyzed in relation to functions in the examination room, interaction around the examination table, functions in the patient room, assisting the patient at the bedside and in the bathroom, monitoring the patient in the emergency centre and controlling visitors in the unit, triage functions, patient registration, and control of the arrivals area.

CAVE can be used in different planning phases: project planning/alternative space requirements, complex departmental entities, drafting phase, space models, size, fit to functions (repeated spaces), later phases, and focusing on details to produce vivid alternatives easily and to produce alternatives before the architectural drawings.

How it works

CAVE allows you to walk through your rendering, experience your designs in full scale and explore arbitrarily large spaces in stereoscopic 3D vision.

Design process / learning organization

CAVE is a virtual environment tool that can be used together with a requirements-based management tool and a web-based post occupancy evaluation, which were developed simultaneously in this project for the Y-building of South Ostrobothnia Hospital District.

TESIS Inter-University Research Centre "Systems and Technologies for Social and Healthcare Facilities"
University of Florence, Italy

TESIS

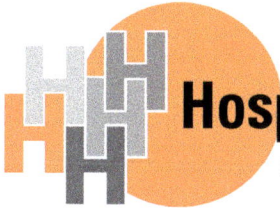

Hospital Planning Evaluations

Session introduction

The session addresses research issues concerning the assessment of costs in the design of healthcare buildings: time, design quality and cost control. The three issues are closely related as they affect each other in a relationship of continuous interconnection.

. . . .

Hans Eggen's paper describes the INO hospital in Berne. The case study shows how the design of a healthcare facility is a process that can take a long time. The INO building in Berne represents an occurrence of advanced design from the point of view of functional and technological choices, which uses the pre-existing buildings as an irreplaceable support for the care activity.

The case study highlights how it is possible to improve the quality of built environments optimizing the cost and construction time through interventions limited to a single building and not the entire healthcare complex.

Hans Eggen
p. 165

The paper by Hilde Vermolen and Margo Annemans highlights how design costs have a lower incidence rate than the maintenance, management and running costs of healthcare facilities. On the other hand, however, good quality design can have a significant impact on the perception of the environment by the staff, patients and visitors. In light of the above, it is twice as convenient to invest in the design phase due to the low incidence of the design costs on the overall cost of the project and the benefits that can affect the users regarding the use of the spaces.

Hilde Vermolen e Margo Annemans
p. 183

Finally, another important factor in the design and construction of healthcare facilities is cost control in the planning and design of works. Karin Imoberdorf's paper describes the operation of a tool for cost control, the Benchmarksystem created by Lead Consultants Inc. This tool allows the cost items to be defined in all phases of the design, helps to predict whether the investments will be covered and if necessary allows the changes to be evaluated through simulations.

Karin Imoberdorf
p. 195

TESIS Inter-University Research Centre "Systems and Technologies for Social and Healthcare Facilities"
University of Florence, Italy

TESIS

1. *Swiss university hospital "Insel" in Berne.*

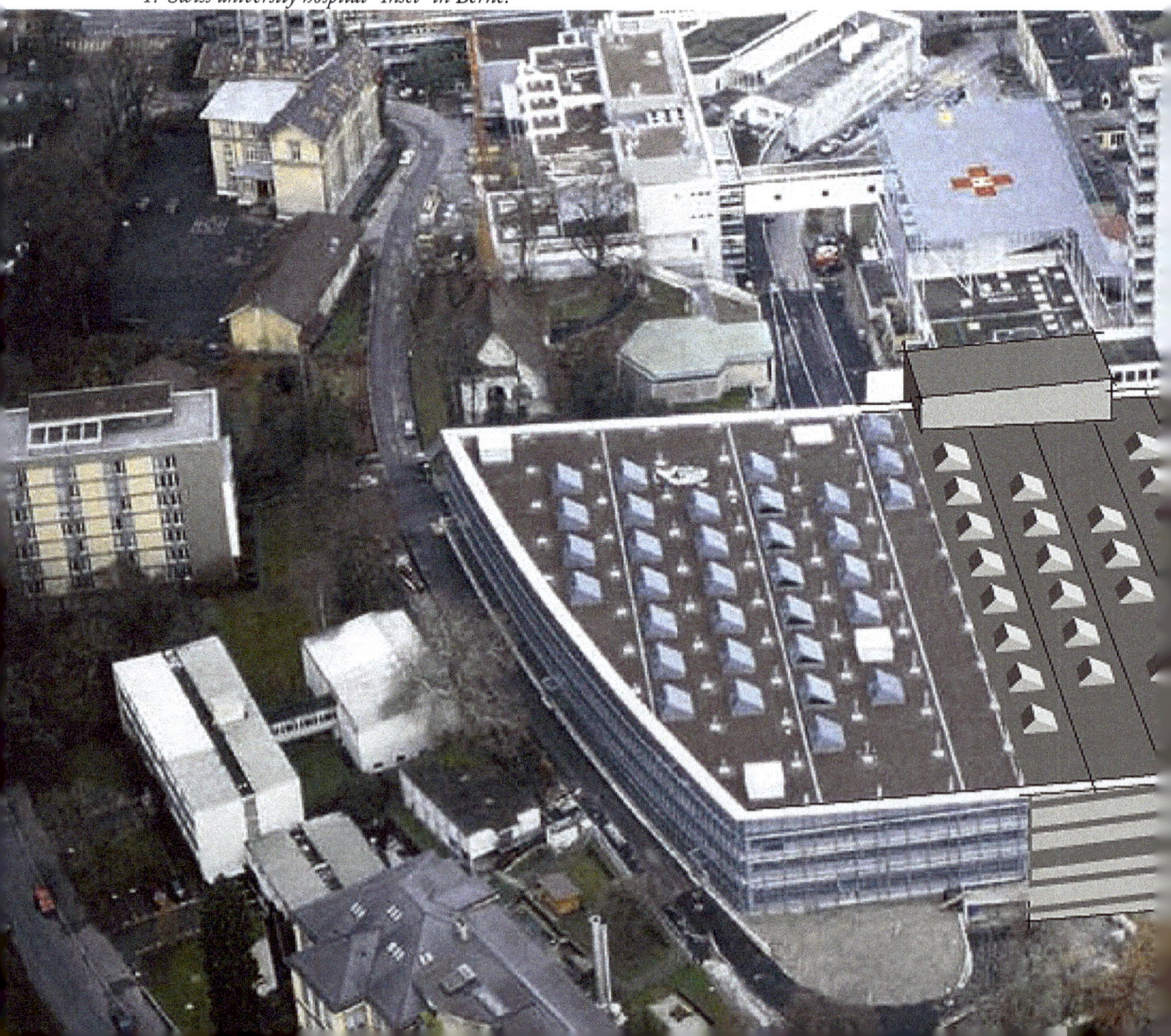

Financial Reasons
Why University Hospitals Cannot Change Sites
Quality Improvement Everywhere but Less and Less Funding
Available

Hans Eggen
Director of the UIA Work Programme Public Health

165

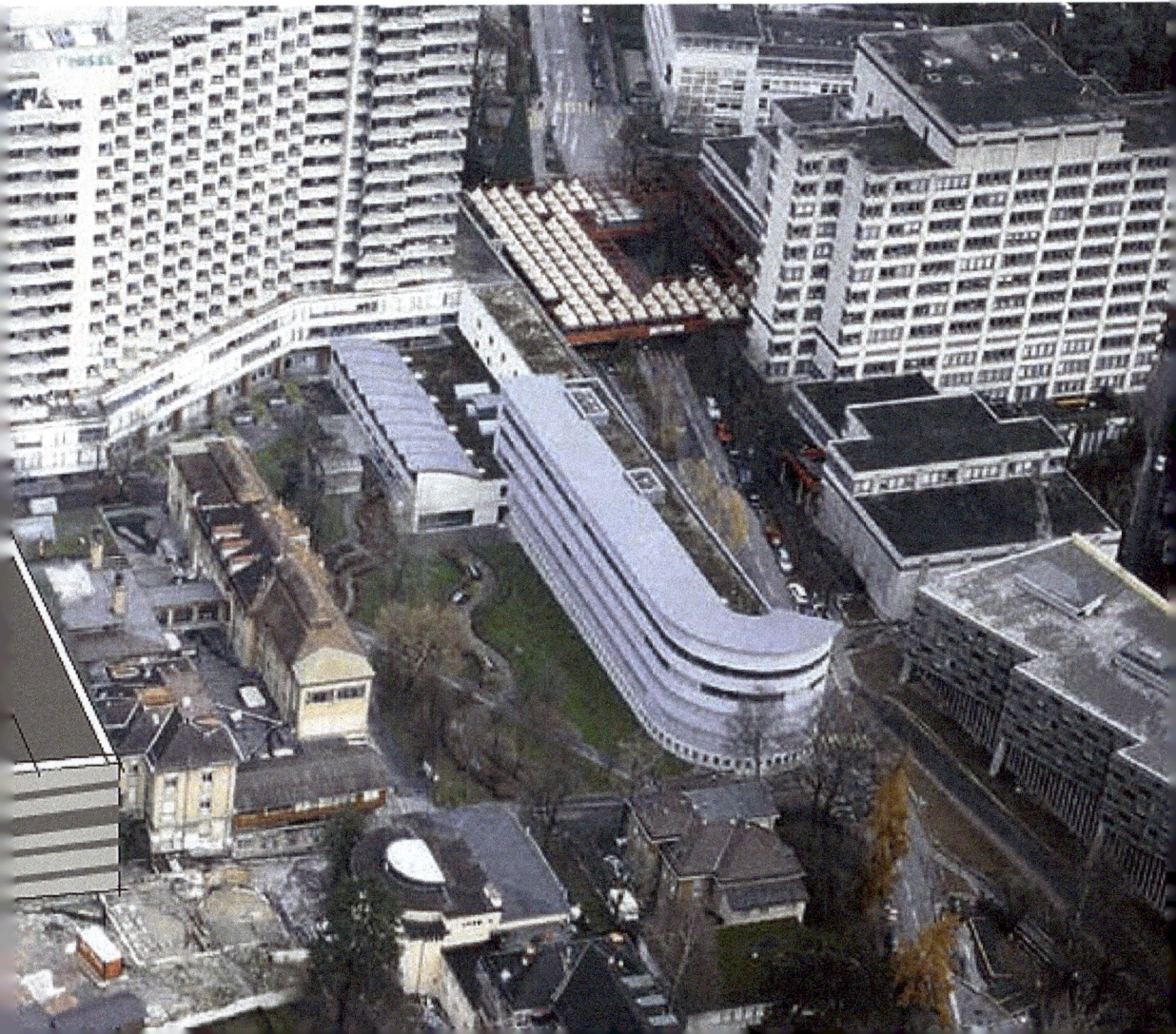

This paper deals with the case study of the Swiss university hospital "Insel" in Berne.

It covers aspects of master planning related to financial implications. On this large site the buildings marked with a red dot (image 2) were all designed by Hans Eggen's former company, Itten+Brechbühl AG, since 1973.

166

It is important to remember that for almost every building the company had to participate in an architectural competition and win. The buildings marked with a blue dot are those for which they only received second prize. The article focuses on the INO treatment building after providing a historical background.

History

One of the first site plans dates back to 1884, which means that a large hospital can remain on the same site for centuries. Will this be possible in the future too?

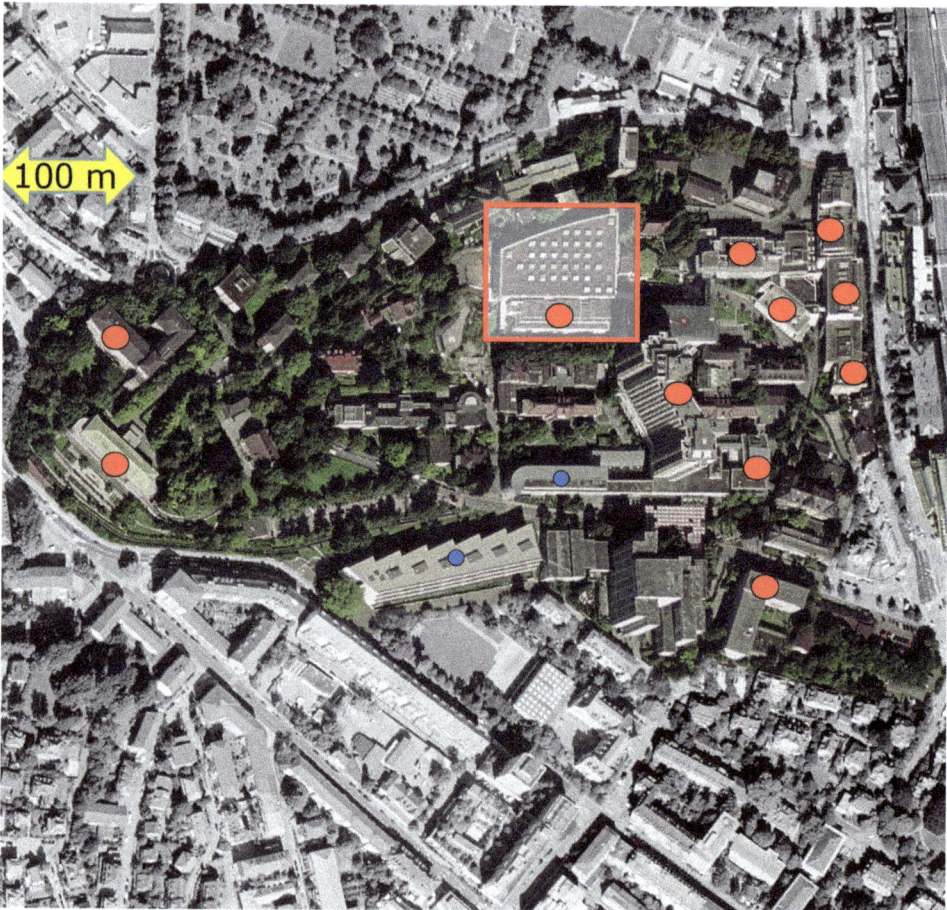

2. The buildings with a red dot were all designed by Hans Eggen's former company, winning first prize in design competitions. The blue dots indicate second prize.

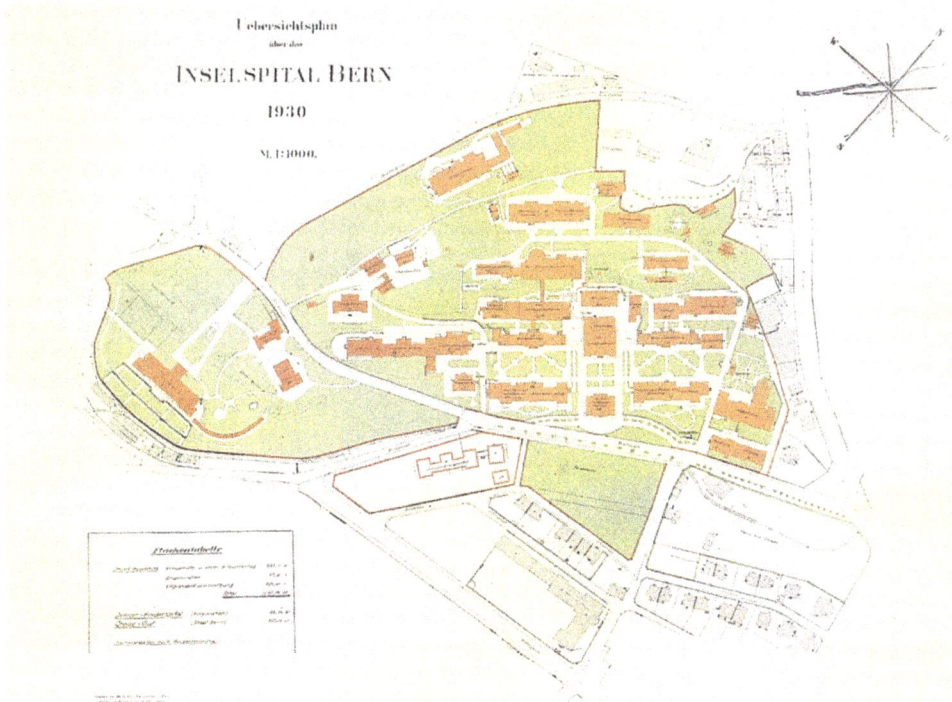

3. In 1924 two architects won a competition for a new hospital building which was constructed in this corner of the site.

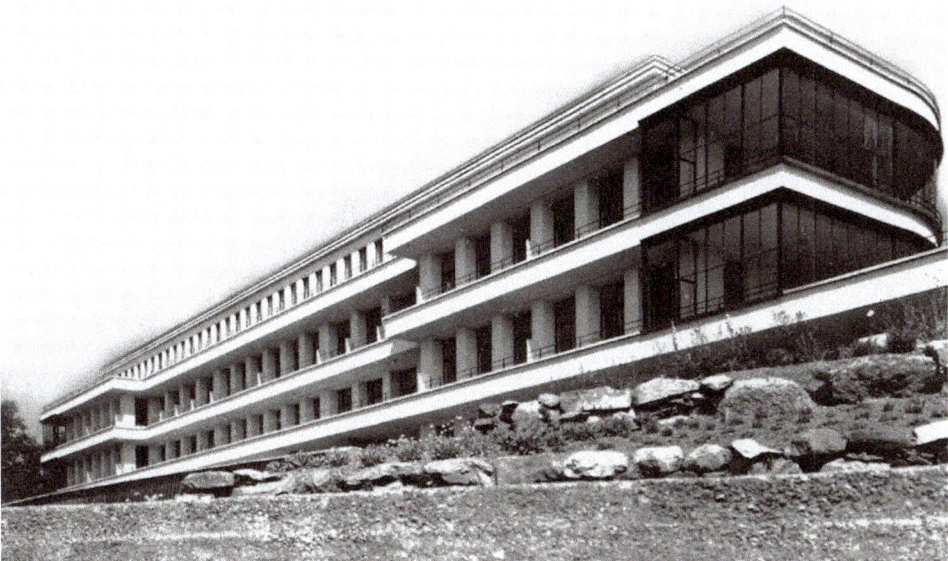

4. Lory Hospital, completed in 1929.

TESIS Inter-University Research Centre "Systems and Technologies for Social and Healthcare Facilities"
University of Florence, Italy

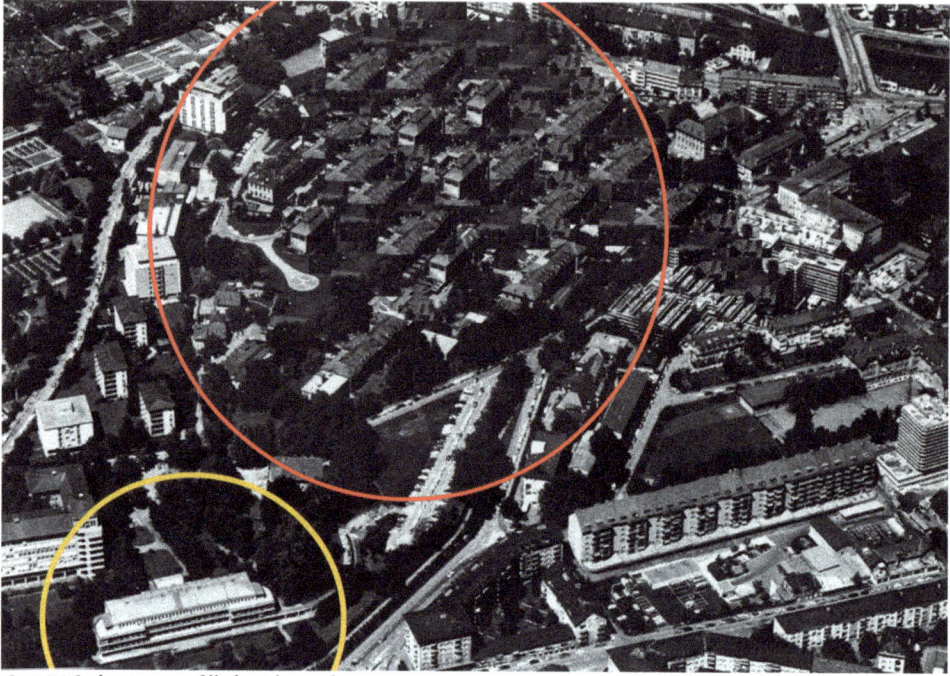

5. 1956, the site was filled with pavilions.

At the beginning each building had a distinct function and over the years more and more specialized pavilions were added.

In 1924 two architects won a competition to create a new hospital building which was constructed in this corner of the site and completed in 1929. This building was the start of Salvisberg and Brechbühl in Switzerland. Publications on the concept and the architectural impact opened the field for many more hospital projects all over the country.

In 1956 the site was filled up with pavilions. It is possible to recognize the Lory Hospital in the front left-hand corner. In this year Itten+Brechbühl was awarded the design contract to develop a new university hospital. Since all the land was fully occupied a new concept was required.

A collage created in Photoshop shows the change to a vertical concept (images 5-6). What can be observed in these two images actually took 17 years to achieve.

In 1973 the new university hospital was completed. It was situated right in the middle of the old pavilion campus and the intention was to replace all the remaining units. Some of them are partly still in use to this day. This university hospital is one of five in Switzerland serving a population of more than 1 million people.

While the politicians where convinced in 1973 that nothing else would ever be needed, there was however the opportunity to consider future development.

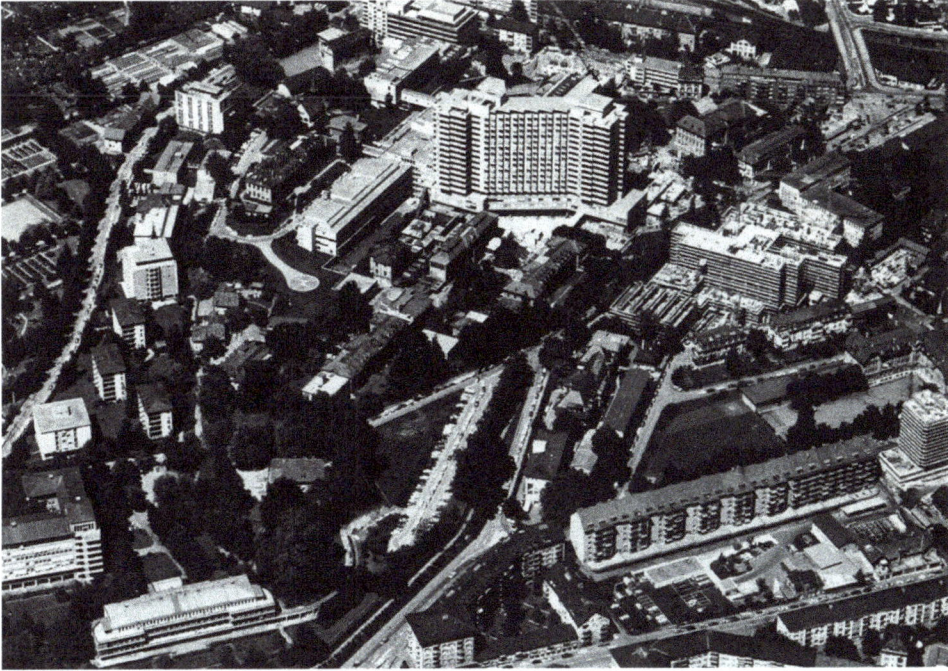

6. *The university hospital was completed in 1973. It was situated in the middle of the old pavilion campus.*

The first master plan

Here are a few conclusions the author deems valid for any hospital site:

- new treatment services must be adapted and extended continuously, and if possible they must be directly adjacent to the existing facilities;
- it is therefore absolutely vital to have free land available directly adjacent to the corresponding building;
- there must be appropriately sized free plots on which a new project could be realized within 3 years (see the yellow dots).

The first master plan explained the idea that it is important to know where extensions can be concentrated but at the same time to show where "obsolete old buildings" should be torn down and removed in order to obtain an open field for the future.

The cleared land could be used as a hospital garden. However this did not happen at all over the last 40 years as it is so much easier just to fill up every empty corner – but this is the wrong approach. This first master plan from 1973 already shows the idea of a large treatment building. This is the current location of the INO building, which will be completed in 2012.

INO (Intensive care emergency and operation centre)

1998 saw the result of a first conceptual competition based on the idea of producing an empty structure as a primary

TESIS Inter-University Research Centre "Systems and Technologies for Social and Healthcare Facilities"
University of Florence, Italy

TESIS

170

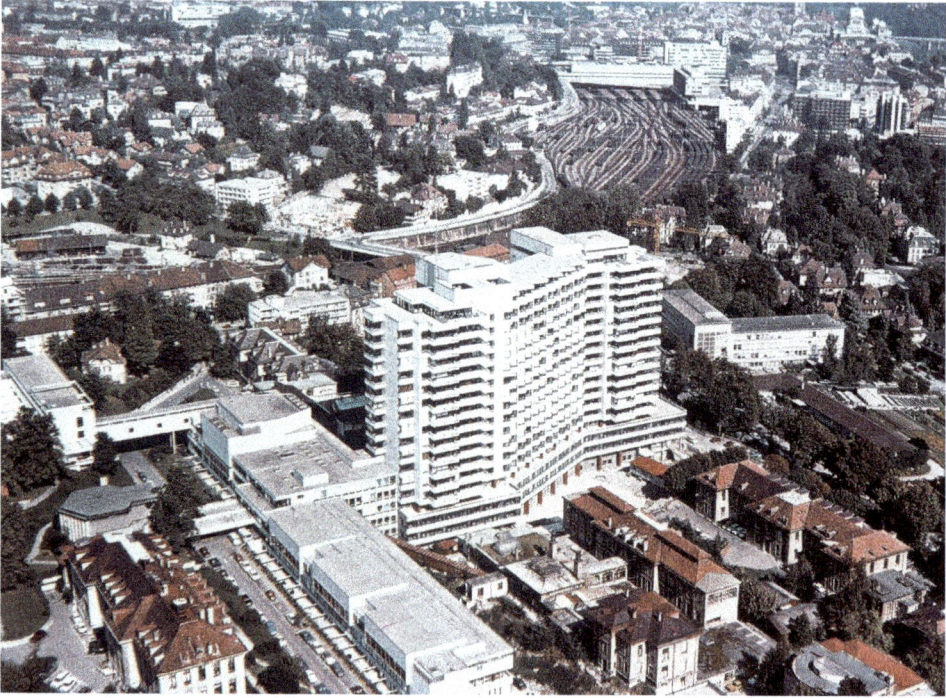

7. *1973, a large treatment building.*

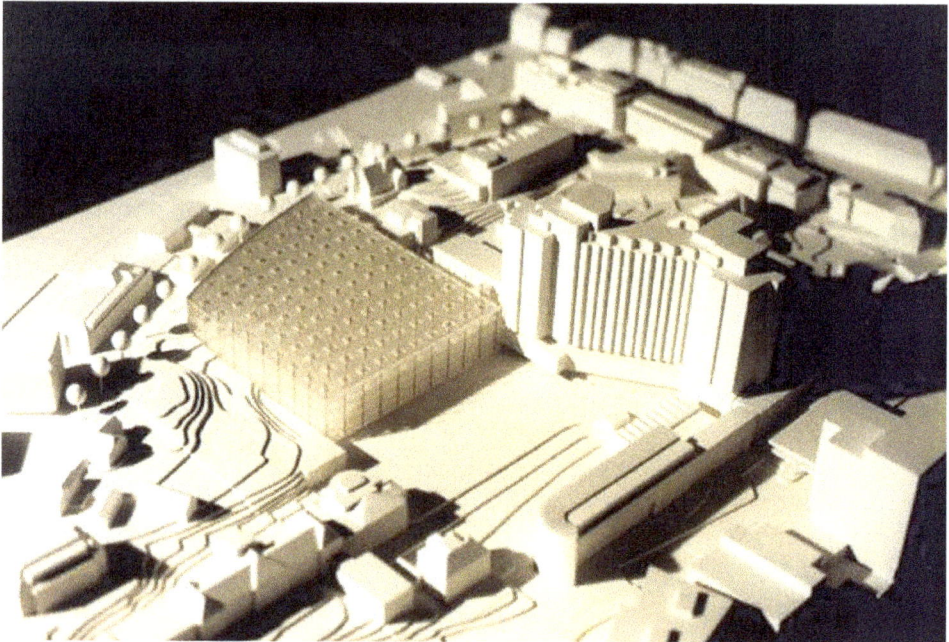

8. *1998, the result of a first conceptual competition.*

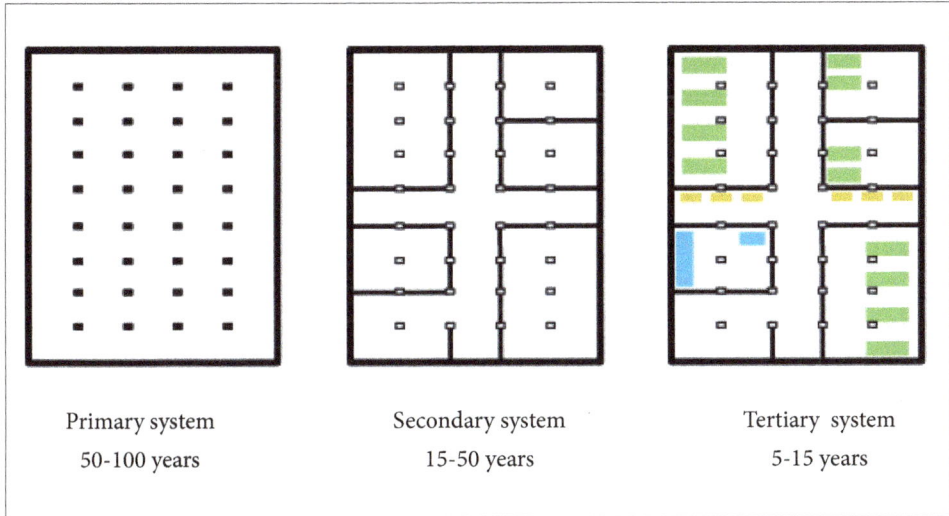

Primary system	Secondary system	Tertiary system
50-100 years	15-50 years	5-15 years

9. *The separation of systems as a design concept.*

171

system to be built while the competition for the next structure for the secondary system could be launched. In short, Itten+Brechbühl AG won the second competition for the secondary system in 1998.

The basic idea given by the client stipulated that such a primary system would perhaps have a life expectancy of 50 to 100 years.

A primary system is basically an empty structure. This basic idea was imposed on all participants of the second competition in order to produce a flexible layout. When architects took over the primary system it was in this stage of completion. The idea is that the internal separation walls, the technical installations and all the finishes have a shorter life expectancy of 15 to 50 years. Finally the equipment, as a tertiary system, has a life expectancy of only 5 to 15 years. The client reasoned that equipment could simply be added at the end like the furniture.

It is without doubt an intelligent con-cept, however architects questioned the procedure of giving separate contracts to 3 independent teams, thinking that this would separate the systems more effectively. This it does, but it was much more complicated to unite the 3 systems and have them function properly together compared to just keeping them separate. Furthermore the primary system already contained some basic defects due to the fact that the client and the architects who invented this idea of separation had no idea what a treatment building would really require, such as floor-to-floor spacing, anticipated floor loads, etc.

Itten+Brechbühl architects preferred to concentrate on the positive aspects, i.e. the flexibility of the design.

Image 12 shows the surgery floor level. The winning concept proposed the new idea of grouping operating theatres into clusters of 4. This idea of grouping operating theatres together in the form of a cluster had never been done before. The architects proposed 6 such clusters with

172

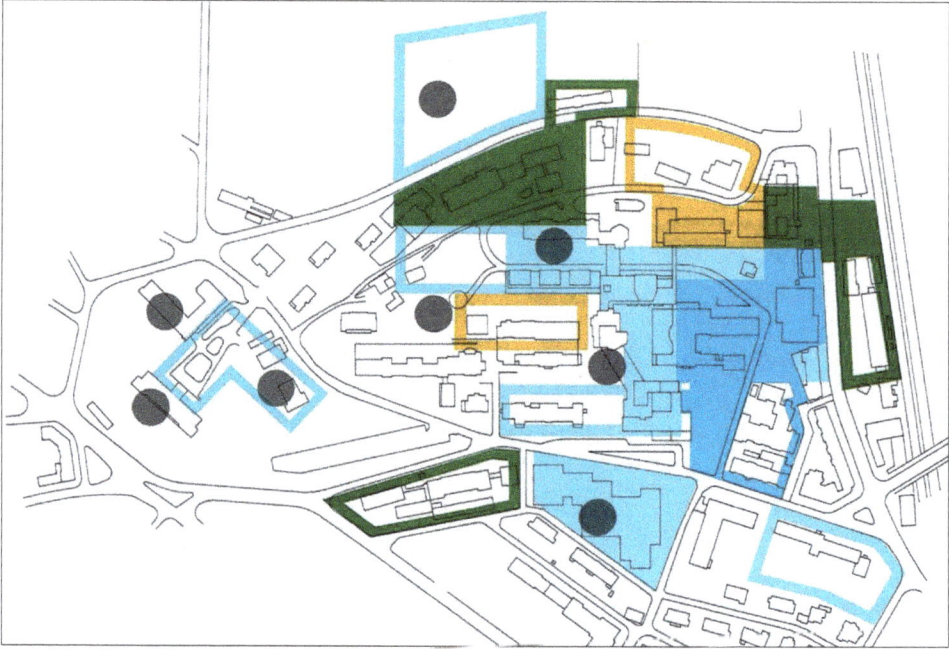

10. *Ideas for the first master plan.*

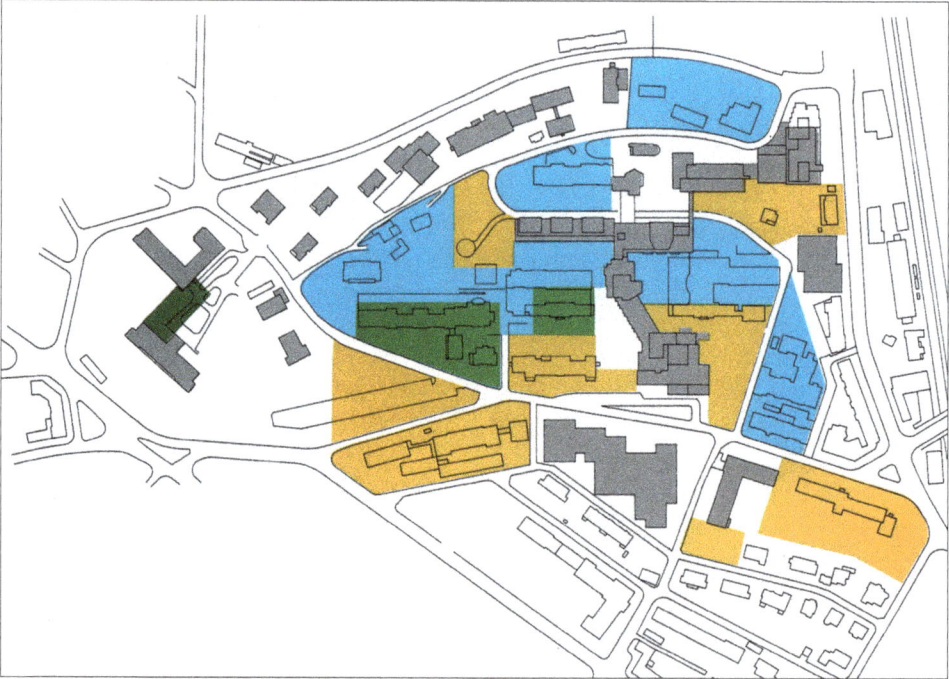

11. *In 1973 there were still many free plots, shown in yellow.*

4 operating rooms in each group, all of which could be served from a central holding area. For many years during the design phase the surgeons did not accept this cluster idea and finally the architects were forced to return to a conventional system. Without going into the details of the discussion, the 2 completely different layouts prove the flexibility of the basic concept.

A further positive idea is that of grey zones. The basic concept contained the idea that since it takes so many years from the planning stage until completion, extra empty floor areas were included in the primary system by making it slightly larger; this extra space could be used at a later stage.

The cross section highlights that the building was constructed in 3 separate phases, also producing an extension to the surgery department.

The deep plan of such a treatment building has some advantages however there are also some critical defects.

A building of 86 m by 100 m is too deep. The light shafts can only bring natural light into the upper floors; it is doubtful the light will reach further down. However, the deep plan can help to obtain efficient treatment units: intensive care, for example, in order to penetrate even more deeply into the design of this building.

Intensive care

How does the multidisciplinary intensive medicine clinic function in a university hospital?

There are 16 patients on one side. These spaces are reserved for patients coming directly from an intense operation. However they only remain here for a

173

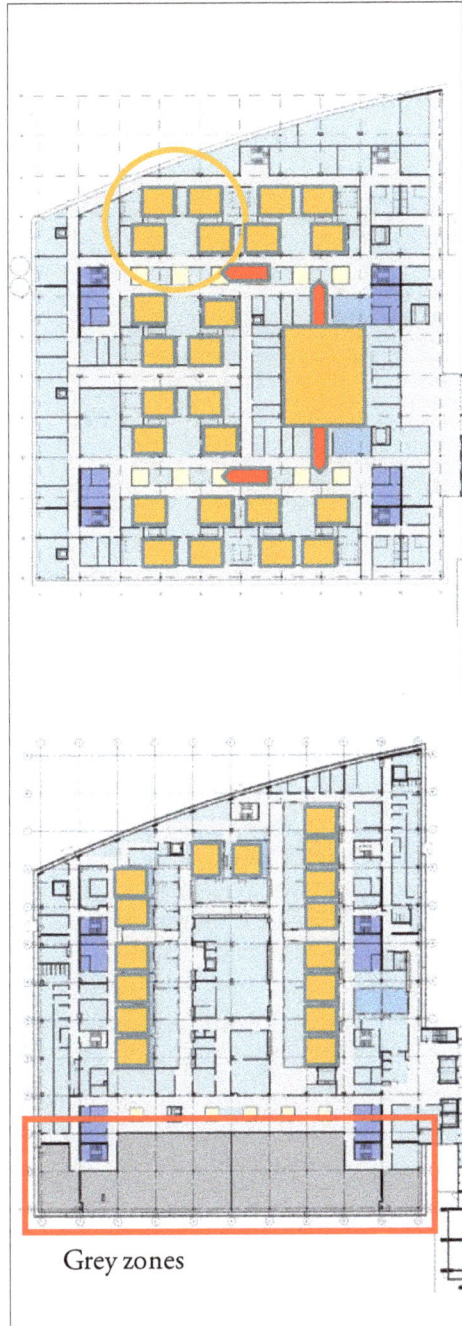

Grey zones

12. INO, 1998 competition, cluster of 4 operating rooms and conventional system.

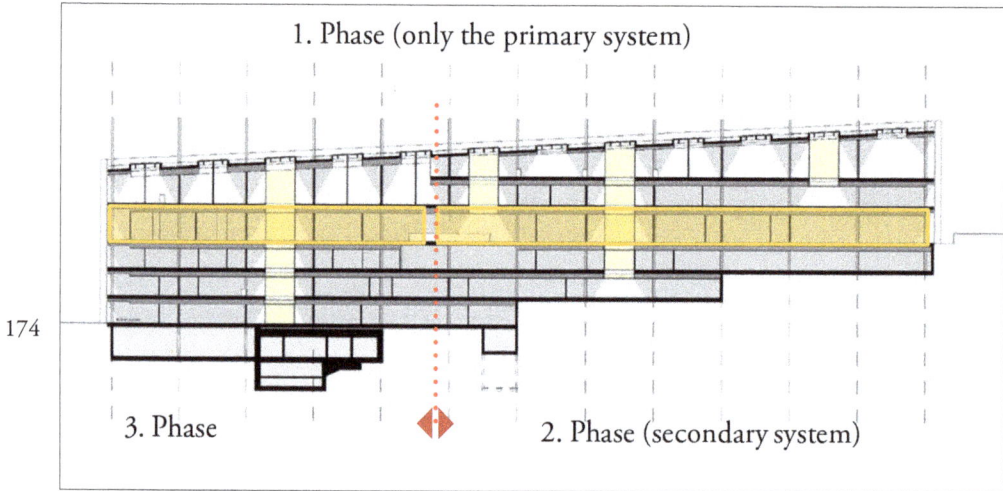

1. Phase (only the primary system)

3. Phase   2. Phase (secondary system)

174

13. INO University Hospital, "Insel" in Berne: the deep plan.

maximum of 24 hours. A further 16 patients are placed on the other side. The client chose a combination of 4-bed, 2-bed and 1-bed units. The staff is divided into 4 teams, each serving 8 patients. They change from one side to the other every 2 months.

This is how it looked in November 2011. This picture (image 19) and the following detail (image 20) show that all the equipment is suspended from the ceiling leaving the floor free and making the layout more flexible.

Image 15 shows how it will look in 1 month. The advantage is that the patient can be placed individually in any position and staff have free access to the patient from all sides.

How can the quality of the ICU be checked?

For many years there has been a continuous cross-check of the benchmark results obtained by the top European university hospitals (perhaps once a month). The hospital in Berne aims to be in the top 3 for each item of comparison.

They have not yet moved into this new

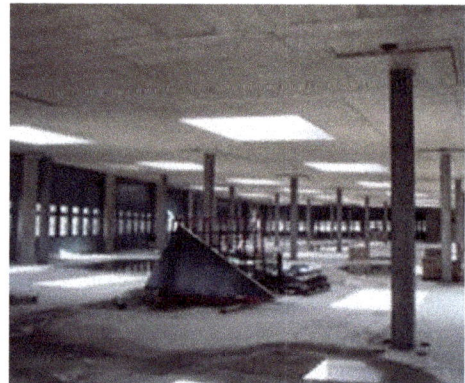

14. Primary system.

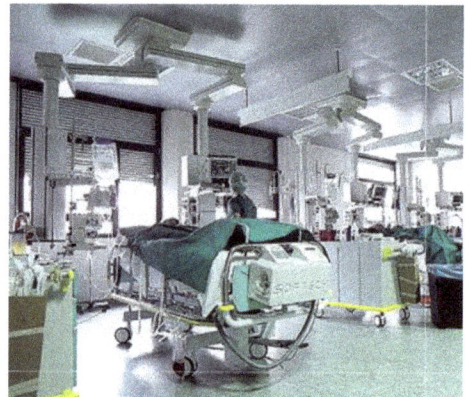

15. Intensive medicine clinic.

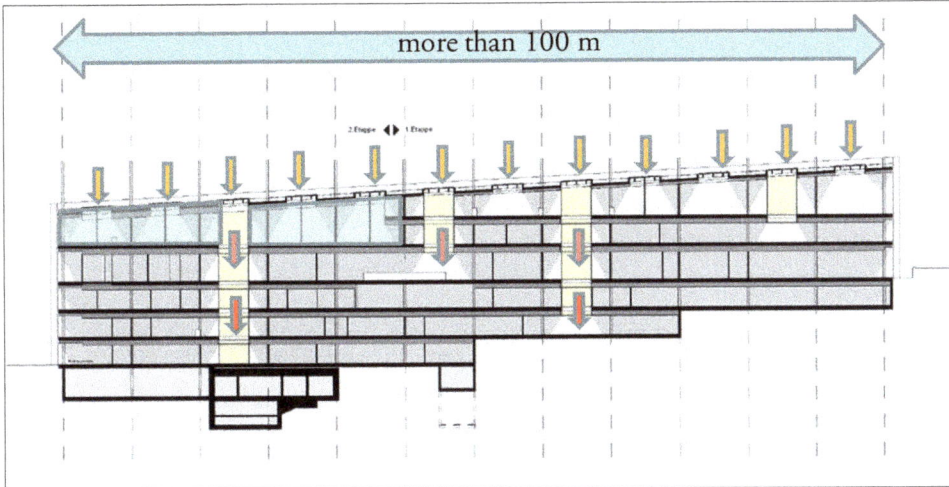

16. *Intensive care unit.*

175

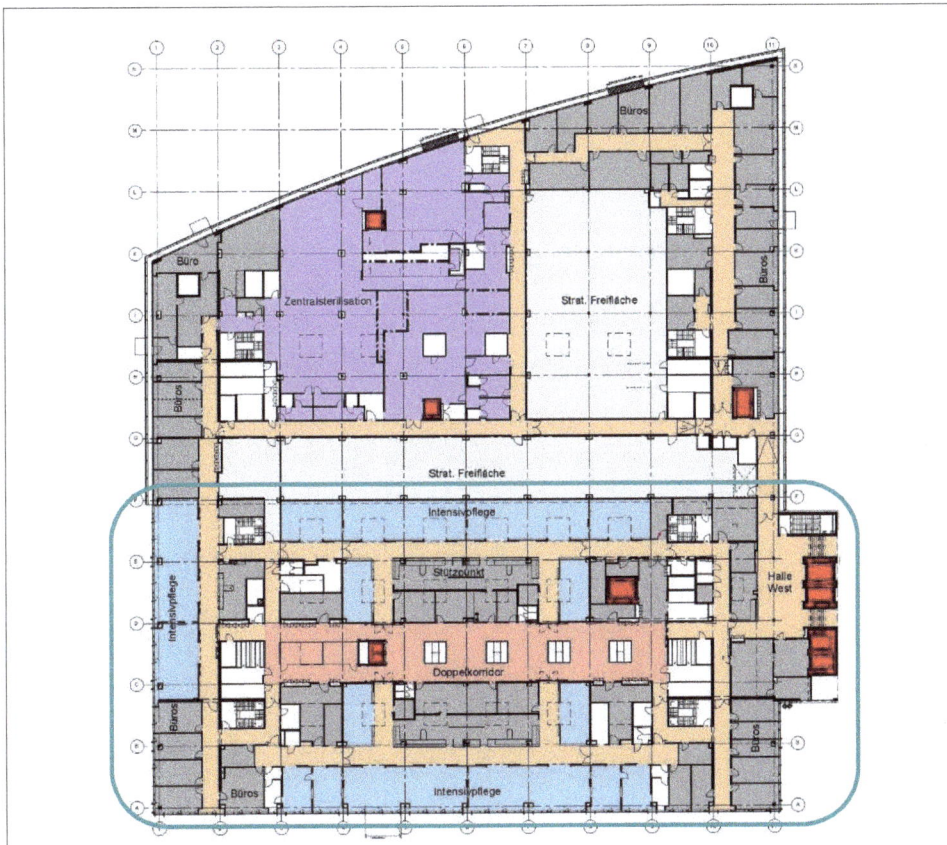

17. *Intensive medicine clinic.*

TESIS Inter-University Research Centre "Systems and Technologies for Social and Healthcare Facilities"
University of Florence, Italy

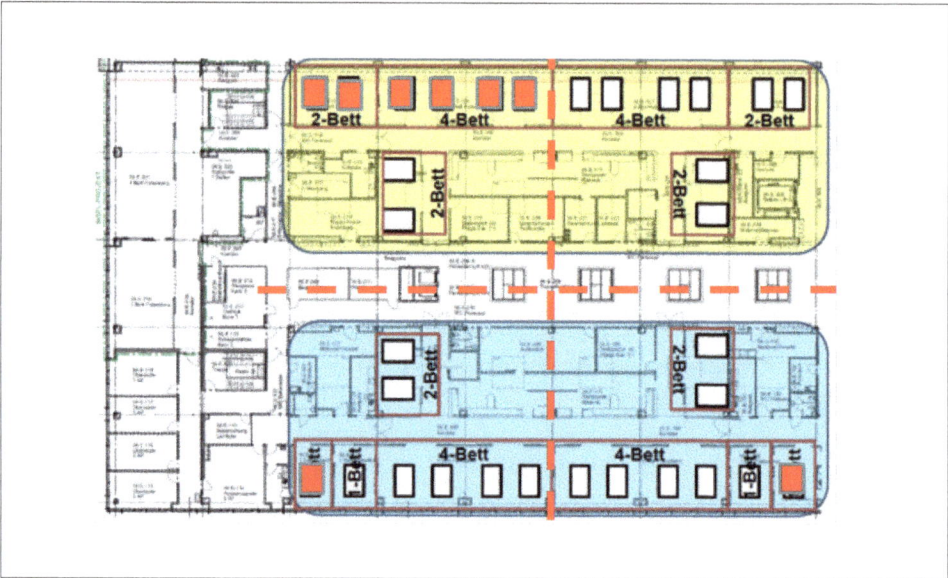

18. In yellow: 16 patients coming from an operation (max. 24 hours). In blue: 16 patients staying for a longer period.

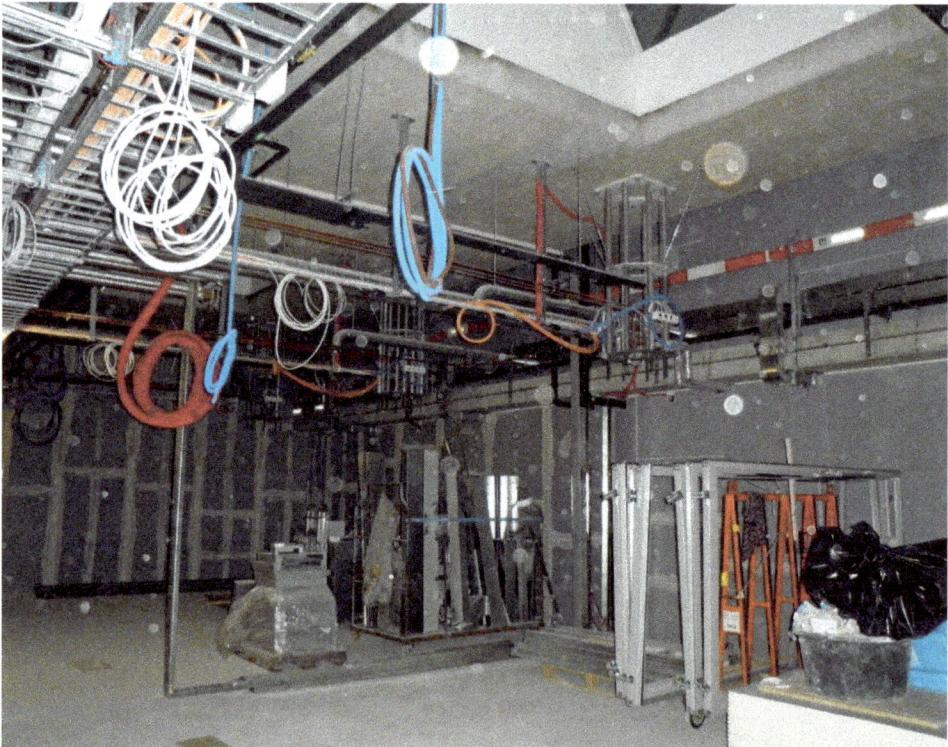

19. Visit in November 2011, all the equipment is suspended from the ceiling.

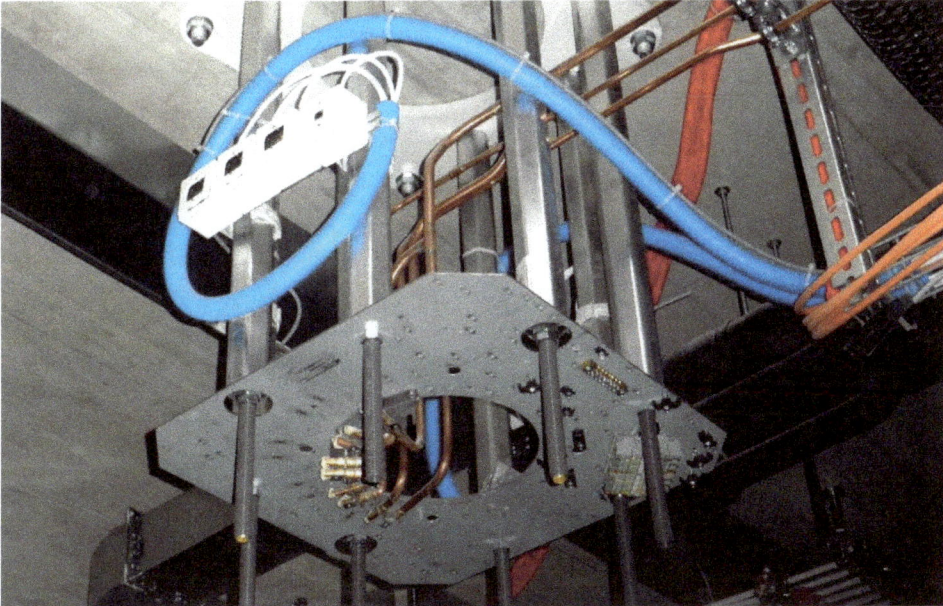

20. Visit in November 2011, detail of the suspended equipment.

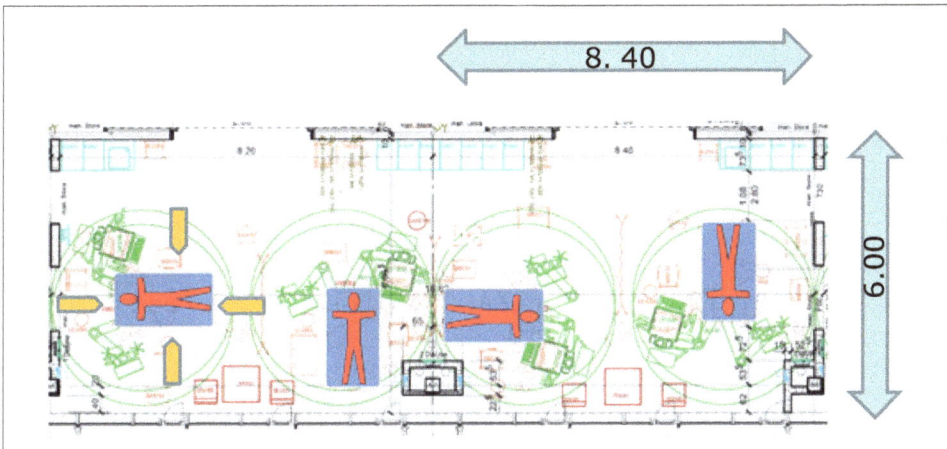

21. ICU design: free choice in the position of the bed, free access for doctors and nurses and benchmark control for quality.

facility, which will open in a few months, and this will be a very complicated procedure.

The author was interested in comparing the Swiss ICU standards with other international standards concerning room sizes and the total square metres.

Image 21 shows an American example which was presented as one of the best at the European Congress Healthcare Planning and Design in Rotterdam in 2010 by Charles D. Cadenhead, FAIA, FACH. The space allocated to patients is more or less the same. One big differ-

178

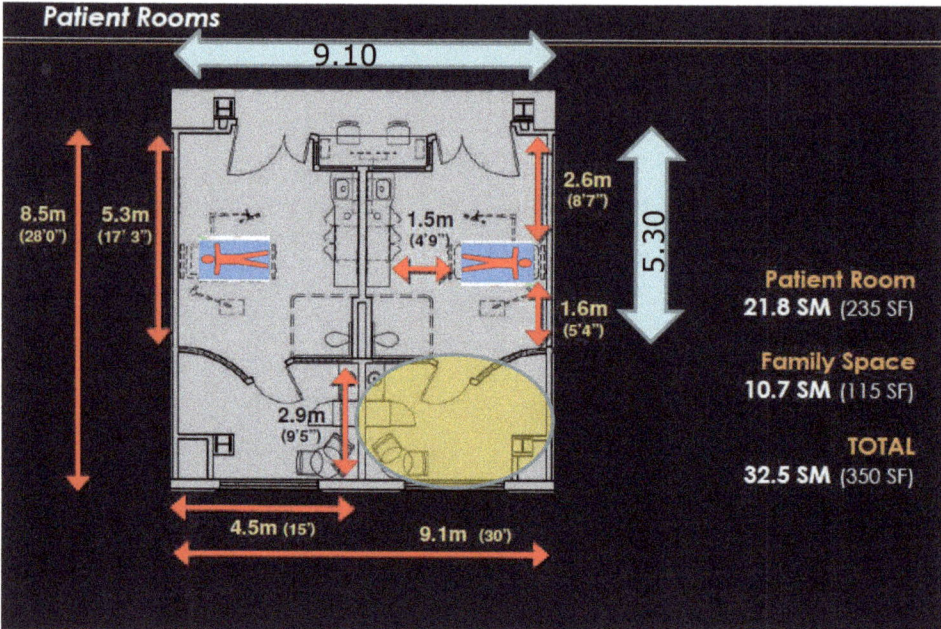

22. American example of ICU by Charles D. Cadenhead.

ence is that in Switzerland family rooms are not placed directly adjacent to the patient; the understanding is that they are not required there.

It would easily be possible to subdivide the larger rooms into smaller units, however priority is given to staff having free access to take care of patients and this also reduces the number of staff. Cost is an important factor in the benchmark comparison.

Itten+Bechbühl have placed the family room in the centre of the ICU. Clearly though if someone wants to sit directly adjacent to the patient this can be organized. This large room will be subdivided into different zones but it was not yet furnished in November 2011.

A particular aspect that makes the ICU very efficient and reduces costs is that the client has developed a logistics con-

cept with a special logistics team in order to assist the nursing staff. Approximately 1800 different items need to be available over a 24-hour period at all the critical points of the ICU and placed as near to the patient as possible. A logistics team is responsible for ensuring that the items are in place at any given moment.

This leaves the nursing staff free to concentrate on providing care.

Here are some details (image 24):

- The central storerooms and cupboards for materials are shown in green;
- The free access space to the storage is shown in light brown;
- The two rooms shown in dark red are the central staff working areas.

Image 26 shows two teams sharing a symmetrical room with individual working places for all the different activities:

- The central storage for disposable ma-

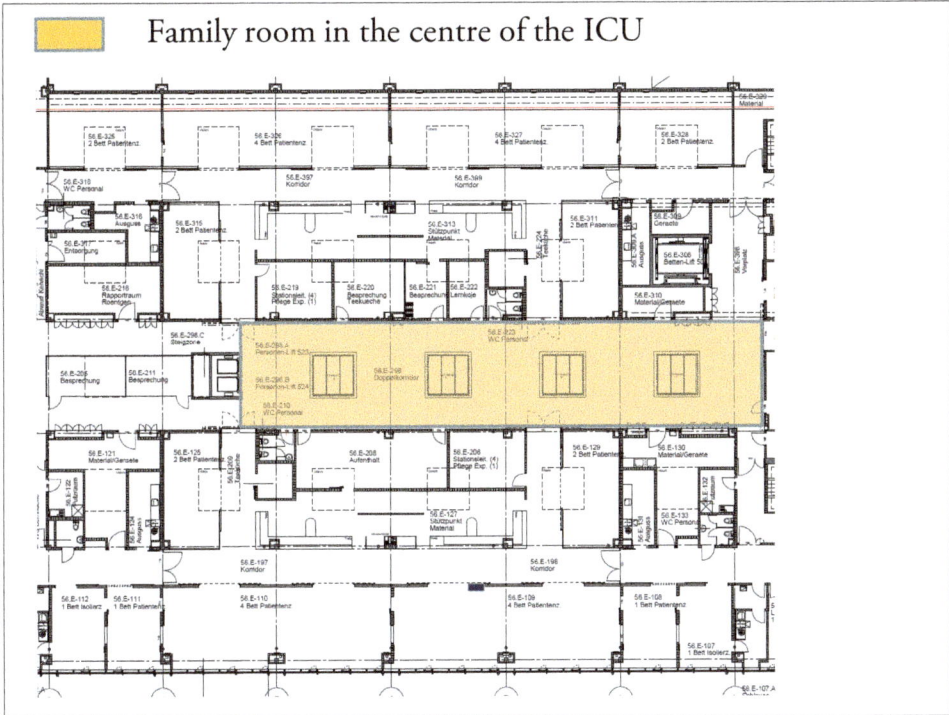

Family room in the centre of the ICU

23. *The family room in the centre of the ICU is shown in yellow.*

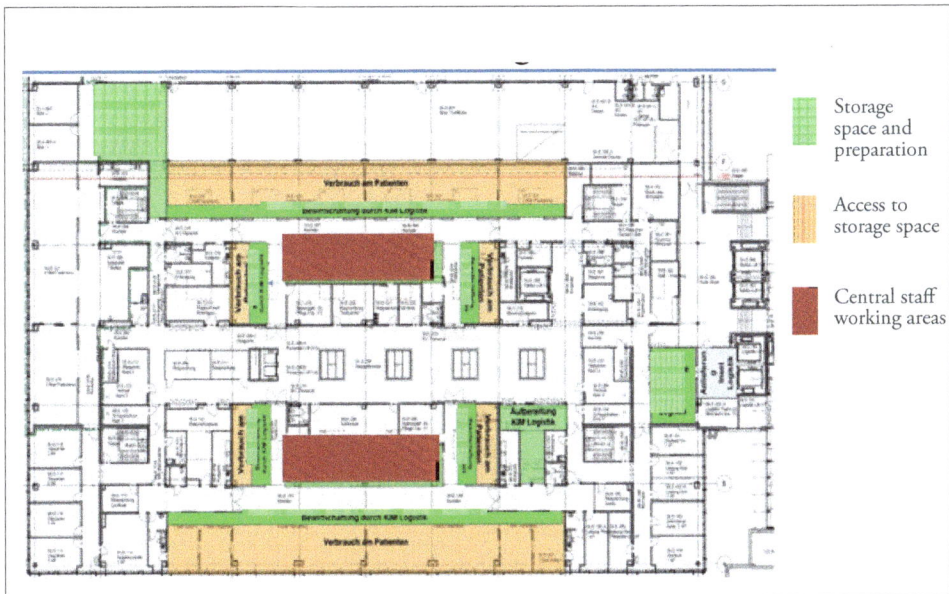

Storage space and preparation

Access to storage space

Central staff working areas

24. *The functioning of the intensive medicine clinic: logistics.*

TESIS Inter-University Research Centre "Systems and Technologies for Social and Healthcare Facilities"
University of Florence, Italy

180

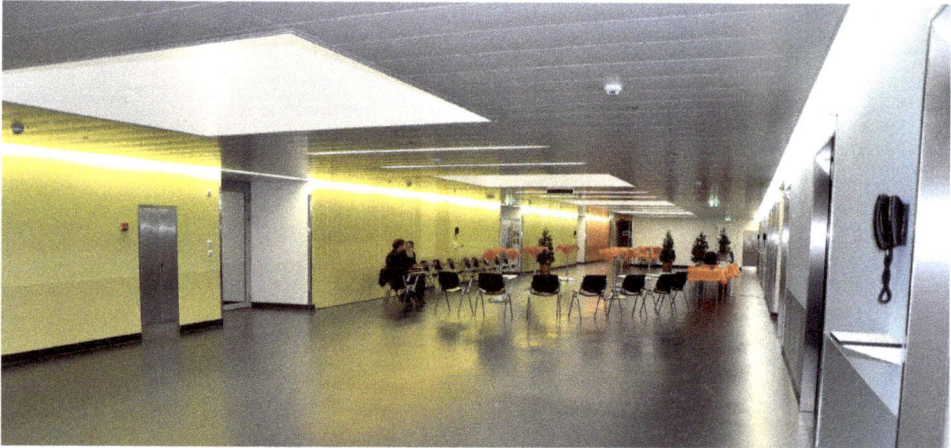

25. *The centre of the ICU.*

terial is shown in yellow;
- The syringe preparation area is shown in red.

An automatic laboratory analyser, capable of making an immediate quick check, is available in the ICU. The central laboratory for the whole University hospital is just one floor above but sometimes a quick result is important in order to make a decision.

1-bed units within the ICU can be used for normal patients but the rooms are technically prepared for cases where patients must be isolated. The multidisciplinary intensive medicine clinic has full responsibility for all its patients and re-

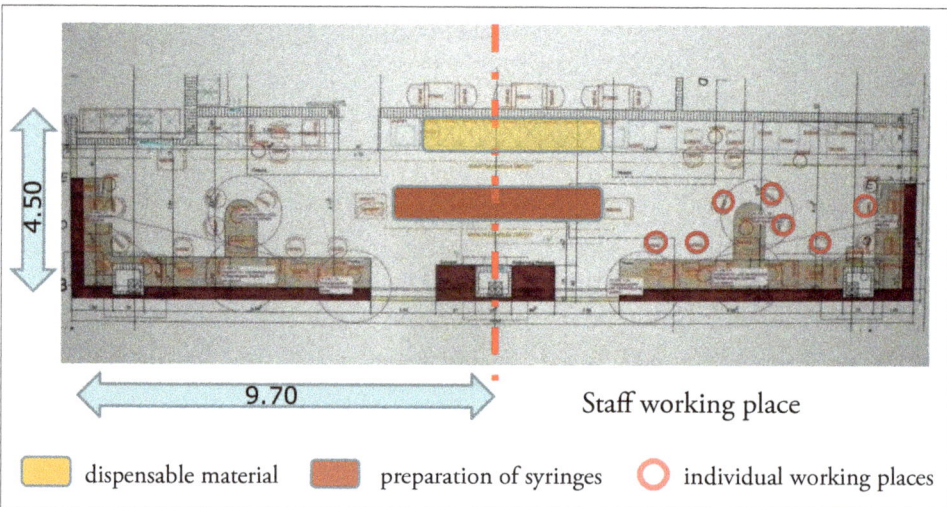

4.50

9.70

Staff working place

dispensable material   preparation of syringes   individual working places

26. *Central staff working areas.*

27. *Automatic analyser.*

28. *1-bed room prepared as an isolation room.*

29. *Intensive medicine clinic: special staff are required.*

ceives the most critical ones. Sometimes infectious diseases are also involved. In this case the room can be closed leaving only one access with two sluices. The air conditioning system can be changed with a single switch providing an air pressure flow towards the patient only. All the air is filtered separately.

To conclude, for the ICU it is possible to state that qualified staff are required in an intensive medicine clinic. The care is intensive which means that staff members work very close to the patients controlling all their data and the results are cross-checked with actual benchmark results from other university hospitals. Operational costs can be reduced with the logistics concept and a corresponding layout.

181

Summary

The INO Building, with 49,000 m2, will be constructed for around CHF 300 million or USD 326 million (or approx. NOK 1860 million). This treatment building is however only a small part of a university hospital. It can be estimated as only 10% of the total investment for a complete university hospital, which nowadays would cost up to around CHF 3000 million or more.

If all the parties on the client's side responsible for the cost would accept that there is an enormous effort and huge amounts invested in the university hospital campus they would have a different attitude. The university hospital will always remain here because there will never be enough money available to design and construct a complete new university hospital on another site.

1. *Composition of images of osar projects.*

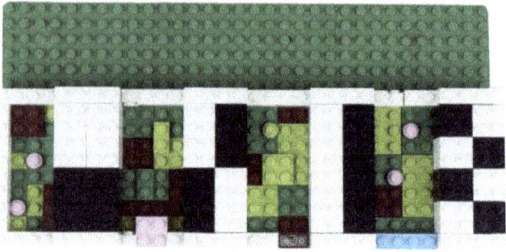

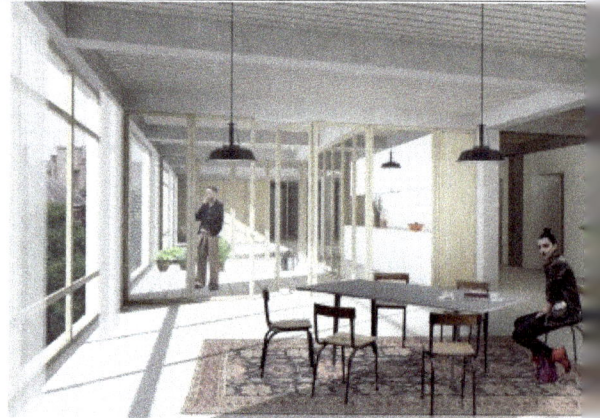

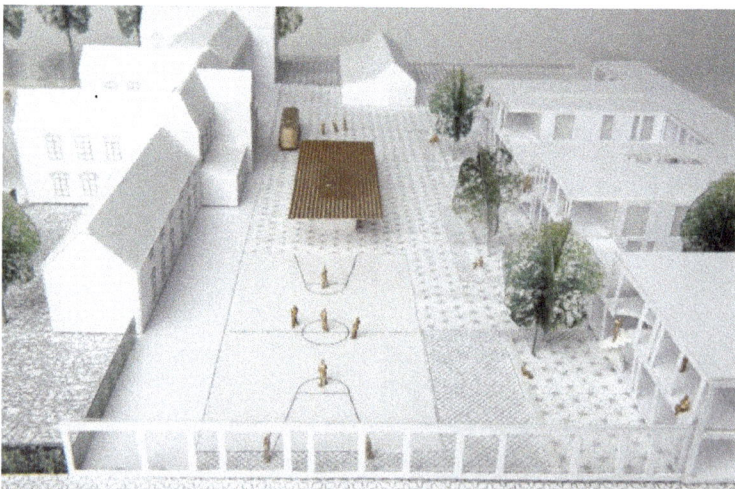

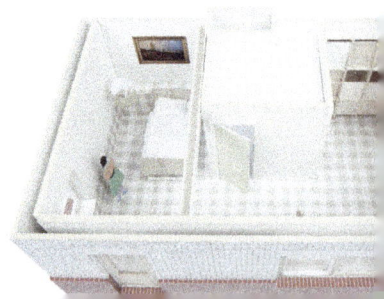

Keeping Up Quality: Research as a Base for Qualitative Architectural Design

Hilde Vermolen (1), Margo Annemans (1,2)

(1) osar architects nv, Jan Van Rijswijcklaan 162/10, 2020 Antwerp, Belgium, hilde.vermolen@osar.be
(2) KULeuven, ASRO, Kasteelpark Arenberg 1/2431, 3001 Heverlee, Belgium

183

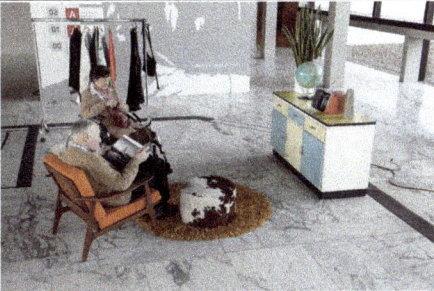

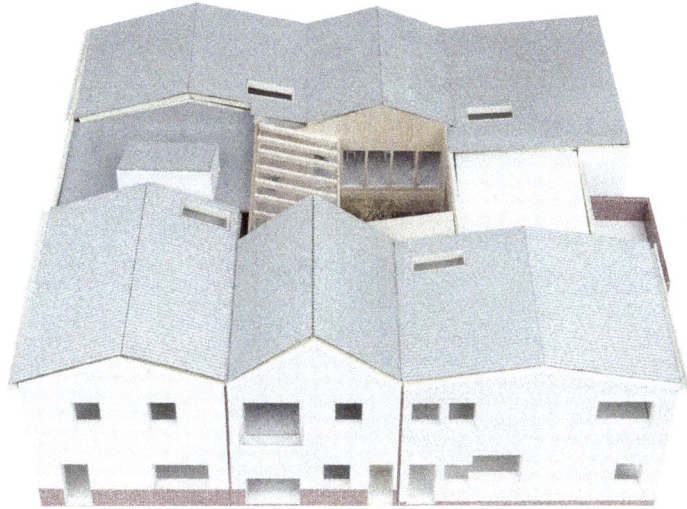

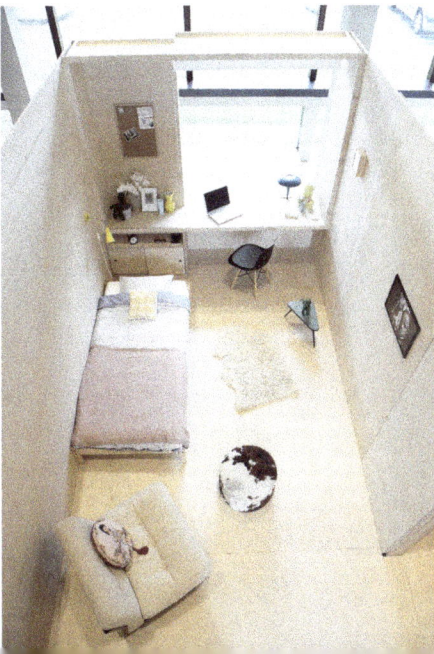

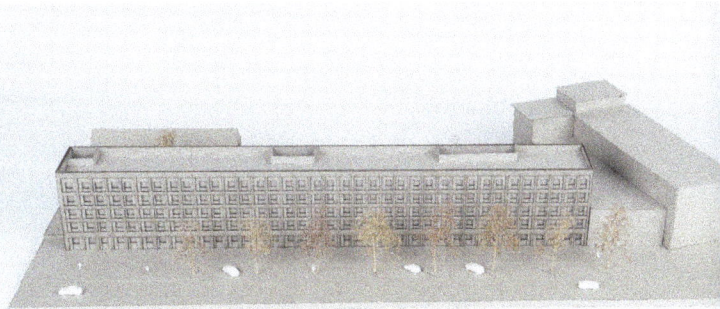

184

Abstract

Hospital quality starts with quality hospital design. Although the actual building phase of a hospital only takes up a minor part of the time and budget consumed over its lifetime, its impact reaches further. The building influences both the exploitation cost and the cost related to the organization. This puts a great responsibility in the hands of the architect and the client. To meet these expectations a profound knowledge of state of the art evidence is essential. For this reason osar decided to conduct her own research on the topic. By questioning the future meaning of the hospital in society and the core business of a hospital, we build up a critical reflection on flexibility and the impact of acute services. Topics such as patient safety and quality already indicate the importance of the user. However, to satisfy all users, we should broaden our view. Designing a healing environment cannot only contribute to the patient experience, but will also influence the well being of staff and visitors, reflecting in organizational matters. In this perspective, research in architecture does not only increase the quality of the build environment, but also can respond to pounding questions about financial problems and cost control.

Keywords: 1:5:200-rule, architecture, costs, informed design

Introduction

The term "architecture" is generally associated with the planning, design and construction of a building. However, what is decided and realised during these phases will have a sincere impact during the further life of the building. In this context, the ratio 1:5:200 (1 as the construction cost, 5 for the exploitation of the building, and 200 as the organizational operating cost) is frequently mentioned. The ratio first turned up in a paper concerning office buildings [1], but soon became a more broadly accepted assumption in various fields (e.g. [2],[3]). Although more recent publications doubt the original data and discuss the credibility of the numbers [4], the basic idea remains. The cost on the organizational level is far bigger than the initial building cost. Especially in the context of hospital buildings, the cost of the personnel should not be underestimated. Although the ratio could let you presume that one should go for the cheapest design, in reality there is a strong connection between the three. When the original building cost is unconsciously reduced, this can trigger a rise in exploitation and organisational cost [3][5]. A simple example of this is how a reduction of the insulation level results in a higher energy cost during the lifetime of the building. The layout of a hospital building can have an important impact on the functioning of both the people working in the building, i.e. walking distances of nursing staff, and the experience of patients and employees.

Keeping these considerations in mind, it is clear that the responsibility of the architect is far bigger than often as-

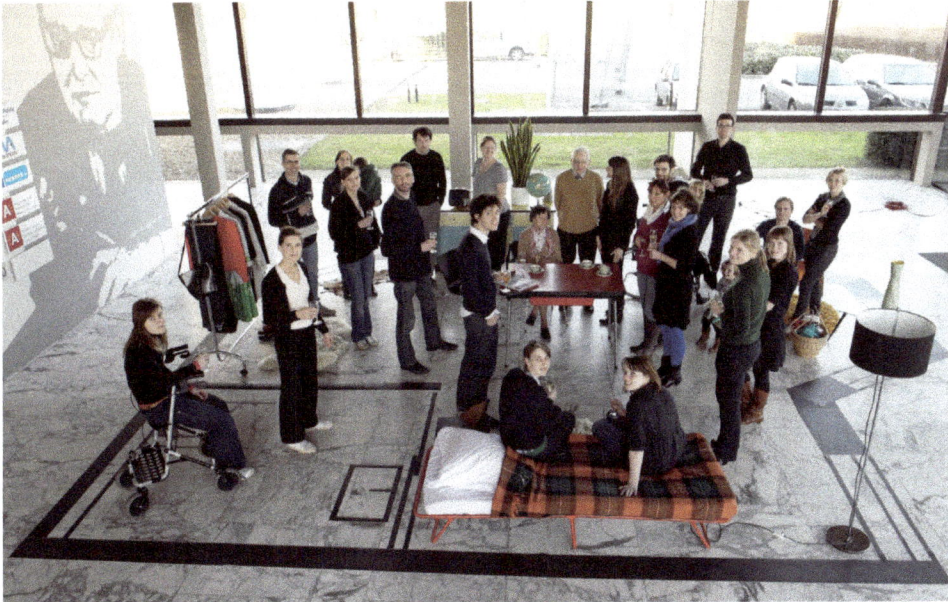

2. Osar, staff of architectural firm.

sumed. As such the architect should be well informed about the impact of his or her decisions on the future functioning of the building. Therefore knowledge about both the exploitation as the organization should be a key element in the design process. However finding and using this information does not always appears to be so easy. As osar architects aims to develop an extremely logical model for each building, based on a profound research on the program, to live up to this ambition, we, at osar, decided to start our own research unit. With the conducted research we try to initiate and contribute to studies in different fields, which add to a base of knowledge about the topics stated above.

Research for design

For years, architects have been designing buildings. Starting from a -some- times- vague description of what a client wants, it is their imagination that provides a physical form and structure for these abstract ideas. What defines them as professionals is mastery of art and technology [6]. Since the 1980's, however, evidence based design (EBD) gained importance, especially in the design of hospitals [2][3]. Although this term mostly relates to spatial elements influencing the healing or well-being of patients [9],[10][11][12] recently the meaning is broadened towards general knowledge needed and used in the design process [6]. As Robert Brandt states [6]: "Evidence-based design is slowly changing how the design is practiced by design professionals and valued by their clients. It can improve the quality of design, especially in ways that benefit the clients." He adds to that, that EBD is also frequently misunderstood by architects who think it is mostly prescriptive,

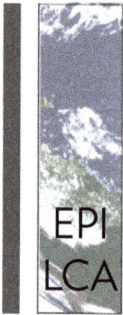

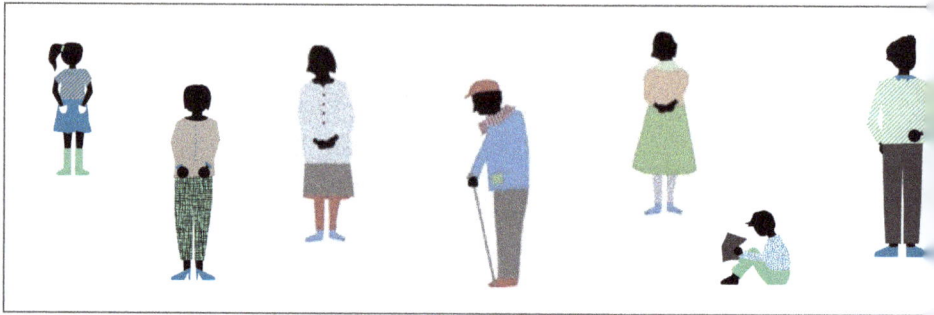

3. Quality design = informed design, necessity of research.

rather than informative. By doing our own research, we try to overcome this burden and find and supply exactly the information needed at each stage of the design process without limiting the creative freedom our architects need.

Building up this knowledge base is not always easy. In the first place you need to develop a solid network of partners from different backgrounds to provide support in various fields. When the information we look for is simply not available, profound research has to be done. In this case cooperation with universities or knowledge centres is essential, while the close connection with the design process and the life at the office should not be overseen. In this respect a PhD about the spatial experience of hospital patients from a lying perspective, is being conducted at osar. In other cases we are rather looking for knowledge specifically about our projects, which might already be available for other programs and were already existing data and methodologies can be used to gain insight in a particular case. Here we think of the life cycle analysis we did of a retirement home to obtain knowledge about the energy demand and materials for fu-

ture designs within this specific context. Furthermore, a good design needs to be made to the background of an environmental and societal vision on the current and future context. To build up this vision, workshops with various actors in the field are being organised.

To obtain good architecture, from the first line of a design to the realisation of the building on the construction site, everyone involved in the process needs to base his or her decisions on the same shared knowledge. Because of the initial restraint of some designers towards information-based design, we know from our own experience that communication is a key issue. At osar we aim to point all heads in the same direction by investing in frequent knowledge sharing. Under the title barosar lunch meetings are organised on a regular base were everyone is invited to participate and present their work. By doing so mutual understanding and dialogue is created which results in a shared idea about what our architecture should look and feel like.

Finally the results of our research are brought to a bigger audience. In the first place through our architecture, we strive for a buildings that can speak for

User Centered Design
Elderly living
Patient Oriented Hospitals

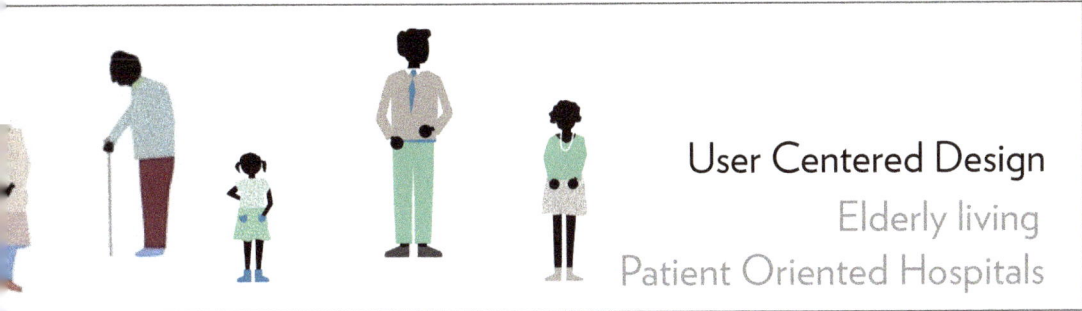

themselves. However, also a vision or an intermediate step can benefit from external interaction. For this reason we reach out beyond what could be called our initial target group. By broadening out horizon, looking beyond the building industry, and listening various actors in fields related to ones we build for, we learn to reach further and start with an open mind which, we believe, adds to the value of the created architecture.

Research in practice

Independent of the actual ratio, the fields addressed by the 1:5:200-rule formed the foundations of the different research tracks at osar. Being architects, in the first place, we need to be informed about the building process, its organisation and the materials used during the construction. All of these things relate to the initial investment. During the design phase decisions are made that impact the maintenance and energy efficiency of the building, both relating to the exploitation cost. However, all of these fields are intertwined and making a division between them is obviously a simplification compared to the reality of hospital building.

The investment in the building

A wide range of elements adds to the realisation of quality architecture. Although it all starts with a well thought-out concept, more technical disciplines like stability and building physics should not be overlooked. Especially when designing a hospital, the incorporation of the technical equipment can make or break the design. All of this has its price. Concerning this financial aspect, managing and controlling the actual building cost during the design and construction phase is obviously an important task of the architect. Given the wide range of aspects that determine the final design, it is important to gain insight in how these different aspects influence each other and what their impact is over the lifetime of the building. To do so, we need to understand both the building as the design process.

In the past osar took the initiative for a research project in which we looked deeper into the architectural process (calculating, describing the project, and drawing) and even more important how knowledge could be shared along the way from the first lines of a design till

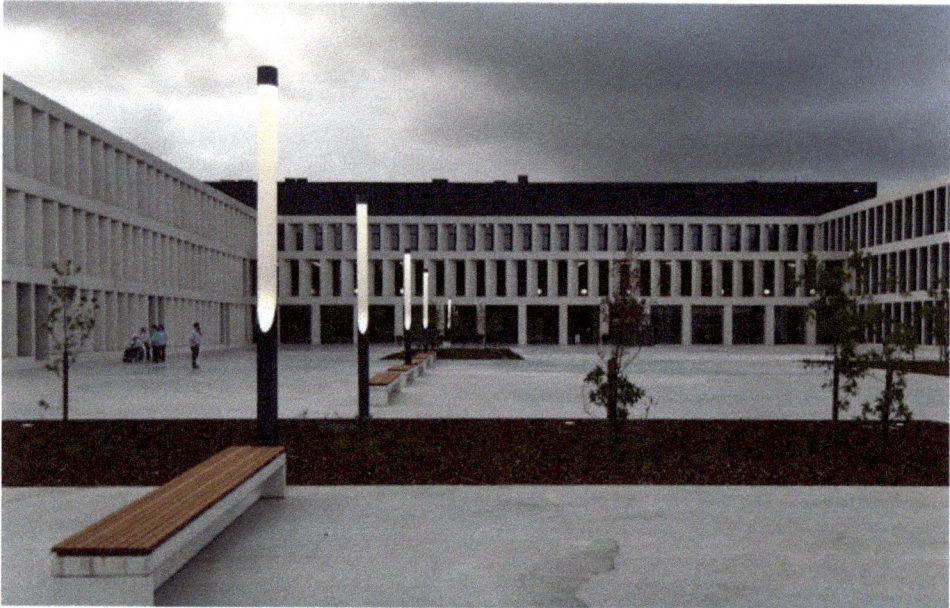

4. AZ Groeninghe, Kortrijk, Belgium, osar architects nv - Baumshlager-Eberle.

188

the finishing of the building.[1] Although this research indeed gained insight in how different parts of a building influence the cost and how they relate to each other, translating the results to the general practice appeared to be quiet hard. Partially for this reason we took a step back and decided to focus on the more practical level in the next research projects.

In this respect, a recent study, which we conducted together with VITO[2], is based on a case study. Starting from a specific building, a 'typical' retirement home, we investigated the impact of a

zero-energy variant on the used materials and did a life cycle analysis. Although the material aspect could be considered part of the investment cost, using more material logically costs more, making this decision obviously influences the exploitation cost of the building you construct [13].

Consequences on the exploitation cost

For now the studies related to the exploitation cost all relate to the strict meaning of sustainability. In 2008, we took part in a study from the Flemish government in which the energy demand in retirement homes was calculated [14]. In 2010 we tried out the calculation tool that came out of the follow up study [15]. Because of the very specific demands of care buildings this kind of studies are essential to gain understanding of the context and be able to design

---

1 Architectural Technology, KMO innovationproject from the Institute for the Promotion of Innovation through Science and Technology in Flanders (IWT-Vlaanderen) nr. 080354

2 VITO is the Flemish Institute for Technical Research (www.vito.be)

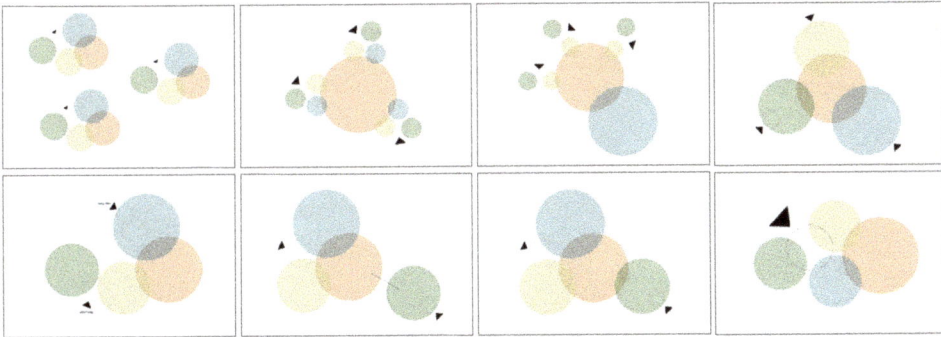

5. (De)Centralisation, future hospitals.

according to the needs and possibilities. For hospitals this kind of data do not exist (yet), definitely a field in which more research should be done.

As said, also the materials, chosen during the design and building phase, and as such part of the investment cost, have a severe impact on the later exploitation.

By making conscious choices in the first phase, not only the energy demand can be seriously reduced, even towards a zero-energy building [13], but also the maintenance costs can decrease. As illustrated in [5], a well thought-out design with attention for disassembly and deconstruction, provides the opportunity to decide for each building component separately whether it needs to be replaced without impacting or degenerating other building components.
No need to say, considering these things during the design influence the entire life cycle cost of the building.

When also adaptability and versatility is taken in mind, we are not only making decisions concerning the exploitation but also keep the door open for different organisational interpretations.

Influence of architecture on the organisation

As the Brundtland Commission defined in 1987 [16]: "Sustainable development is development that meets the needs of the present without compromising the ability of future generations to meet their own needs." Starting from this definition, we cannot limit ourselves, or our fields of interest, to these aspects strictly related to the construction of a building. Indeed, the design and conception of a building will have its impact on how the building will be used, now and in the future.

If we opt to design buildings that we provide the ability for future generations to adapt them in such a way that they suit their own needs, we need a better insight in how our architecture influences the organisation and appearance of inter-human processes going on in a building and vice versa.

Notwithstanding the great importance of a fluid organisation and the impact on the cost factor, little research is being done in this field. Insight in the user experience related to architecture can be

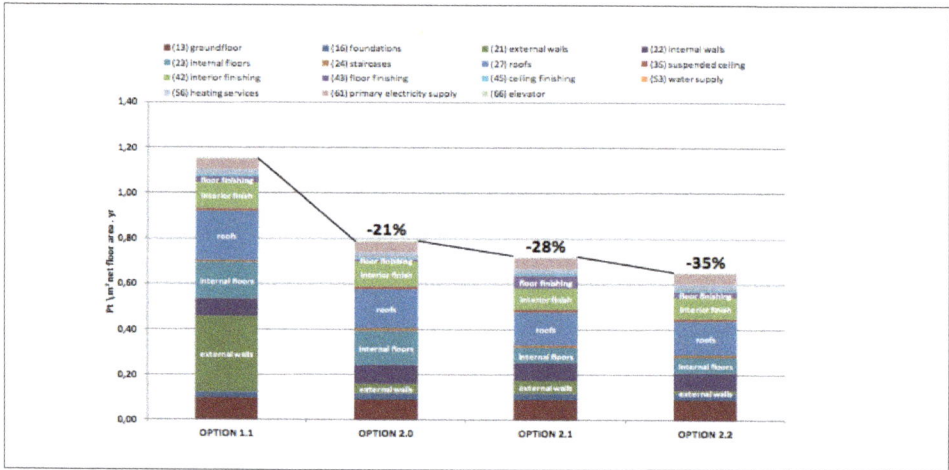

6. LCA Analysis, environmental impact - energy consumption and impact of building materials.

the base of interventions, both material and organisational, that anticipate on the organisation (cost). A first research project at osar[3], aims to gain insight in which aspects that influence the spatial experience of patients lying in a hospital bed [17] [18] and how the gained insights can be used in the design process.

In the near future we plan to look deeper into the impact of the building on the general organisation e.g. logistics and personnel. A similar track is being followed considering elderly care.

Discussion

Although the 1:5:200-rule can serve as

a source of inspiration, its value should not be overestimated.

The numbers are not exact and the division between the three is not always clear. Mutual influences make it hard to define each of the factors, which needs to be done if you aim to do the actual calculations.

Especially defining the organisational factor holds a great challenge, not only has this one the biggest financial influence, it is also the most tricky on to define and it holds the greatest potential to inform architects and inspire them to create innovative architecture.

As illustrated, to realise qualitative, sustainable and cost efficient (hospital) buildings, a profound knowledge on various terrains further or closer related to architecture is essential.

In certain cases this knowledge is directly available or can be easily generated. In other cases profound research is neces-

3 The project "The experience of lying: designing architecture for a wholesome hospital environment" is conducted in close collaboration with the AIDA research group at KU Leuven (www.asro.kuleuven.be/aida) and funded by a PhD grant from the Baekeland program from the Institute for the Promotion of Innovation through Science and Technology in Flanders (IWT-Vlaanderen).

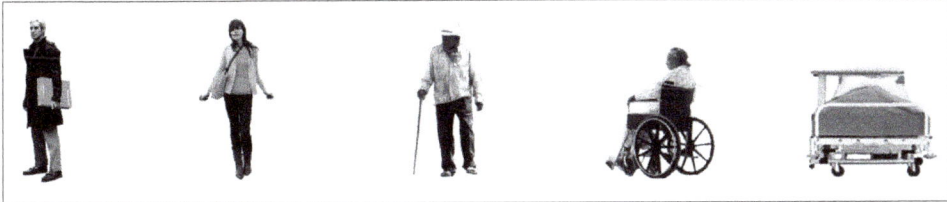

7. User Experience, future hospitals.

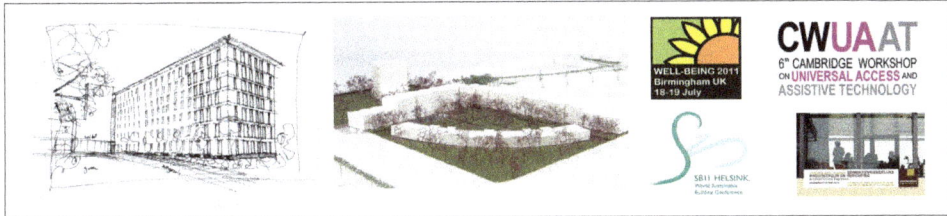

8. Communication towards external parties: architecture, presentations and publications.

sary. As an architecture firm you can stay at the sideline and wait till the academic world picks up the need.

However, you can also take the initiative for new research tracks and as such take up an active role in what is being research. By doing so, the generated results do not only fulfil your needs but also provide you with the needed information from the start, which, we believe, reflects in the final quality of our designs.

When basing your design on new insights from research, only a limited amount of realised projects can be given as a reference. This undeniably holds a (calculated) risk both for the architect as for the client. In order to be able to realise these innovative buildings we aim to design, we need clients that share the spirit of knowledge and innovation.

The greatest challenge for architects can be found here. Finding the combina-

tion of a supportive client and a suitable funding to be able to consider the exploitation and even the organisation in the calculation of the investment cost is definitely a key concern.

Acknowledgements

The authors would like to thank everyone at osar who has been involved in the ongoing research and innovation projects.

Our sincere thanks also goes to the different organisations without which we could not have done the research we manage to do now.

In this respect we think in the first place of the AIDA research group of Prof. A. Heylighen at the KU Leuven, and the people of the Unit Transition Energy and Environment at VITO, but also people from various engineering offices and other institutions should not be overlooked.

TESIS Inter-University Research Centre "Systems and Technologies for Social and Healthcare Facilities"
University of Florence, Italy

References

[1] R. Evans, R. Haryott, N. Haste, en A. Jones, The long term costs of owning and using buildings. London: Royal Academy of Engineering, 1998.

[2] College bouw zorginstellingen., "LCC, life cycle costing, lucratief en crystal clear!", In Perspectief, 15-okt-2006.

[3] College bouw zorginstellingen, Levensduurkosten: kapitaalinvesteringen in gezondheidszorgvoorzieningen. Utrecht: College bouw zorginstellingen, 2006.

[4] W. Hughes, D. Ancell, S. Gruneberg, en L. Hirst, "Exposing the myth of the 1:5:200 ratio relating intitial cost, maintenance and staffing costs of office buildings", in Khosrowshahi, F (Ed.), 20th Annual ARCOM Conference, 2004, vol. 1, pp. 373–381.

[5] M. Annemans, M. Verhaegen, en W. Debacker, "Life Cycle Assessment in Architecture Practice: The Impact of Materials on a Flemish Elderly and Care Residence", in Proceedings of International Symposium on Life Cycle Assessment and Construction, Nantes, France, 2012.

[6] R. M. Brandt, G. H. Chong, W. M. Martin, en American Institute of Architects, Design informed driving innovation with evidence-based design. Hoboken, N.J.: John Wiley & Sons, 2010.

[7] R. Ulrich, "The psychological benefits of plants", Garden, vol. 8, nr. 6, pp. 16–21, 1984.

[8] R. Ulrich, "View through a window may influence recovery from surgery", Science, vol. 224, nr. 4647, pp. 420–421, apr. 1984.

[9] H. Rubin en Center for Health Design., "An investigation to determine whether the built environment affects patients' medical outcomes", Center for Health Design, Martinez Calif., 1998.

[10] R. Ulrich, C. Zimring, X. Quan, A. Joseph, en R. Choudhary, "The role of the physical environment in the hospital of the 21st century: a once-in-a-lifetime opportunity", The Center for Health Design, Martinez Calif., 2004.

[11] K. Dijkstra, M. Pieterse, en A. Pruyn, "Physical environmental stimuli that turn healthcare facilities into healing environments through psychologically mediated effects: systematic review", J Adv Nurs, vol. 56, nr. 2, pp. 166–181, okt. 2006.

[12] College bouw zorginstellingen., "Kwaliteit van de fysieke zorgomgeving : stand van zaken omgevingsvariabelen en de effecten op de (zieke) mens", College bouw zorginstellingen, Utrecht, 2008.

[13] KU Leuven, Daidalos Peutz, en FDA Architecten nv (osar architect nv), "Eindrapport: ontwikkeling van specifieke energieprestatie-indicatoren (EPI) voor rusthuizen", Vlaamse overheid departement Welzijn, Volksgezondheid en Gezin, Brussel, 2008.

[14] Daidalos Peutz, KU Leuven, Universiteit Gent, en Ingenium, "Studieopdracht voor de ontwikkeling van specifieke energieprestatie - indicatoren voor woonzorgcentra – II", Vlaamse Overheid Departement welzijn, volksgezondheid en gezin, Brussel, België, mrt. 2010.

[15] W. Debacker, M. Annemans, M. Van

192

Holm, C. Spirinckx, L. Heyrman, en M. Verhaegen, "Improving the environmental impacts of a typical Flemish retirement home: a life cycle approach", in Proceedings of World Sustainable Building Conference, Helsinki, Finland, 2011.

[16] World Commission on Environment (Brundtland Commission) and Development, "Report of the World Commission on Environment and Development: Our Common Future", United Nations, http://www.un-documents.net/wced-ocf.htm, Annex to document A/42/427 - Development and International Co-operation: Environment, jun. 2012.

[17] M. Annemans, C. Van Audenhove, H. Vermolen, en A. Heylighen, "Lying Architecture: Experiencing Space from a Hospital Bed", presented at the Well-Being 2011, Birmingham, 2011.

[18] M. Annemans, C. Van Audenhove, H. Vermolen, en A. Heylighen, "Hospital Reality from A Lying Perspective: Exploring a Sensory Research Approach", in Designing Inclusive Systems: Designing Inclusion for Real-world Applications, Cambridge, 2012.

193

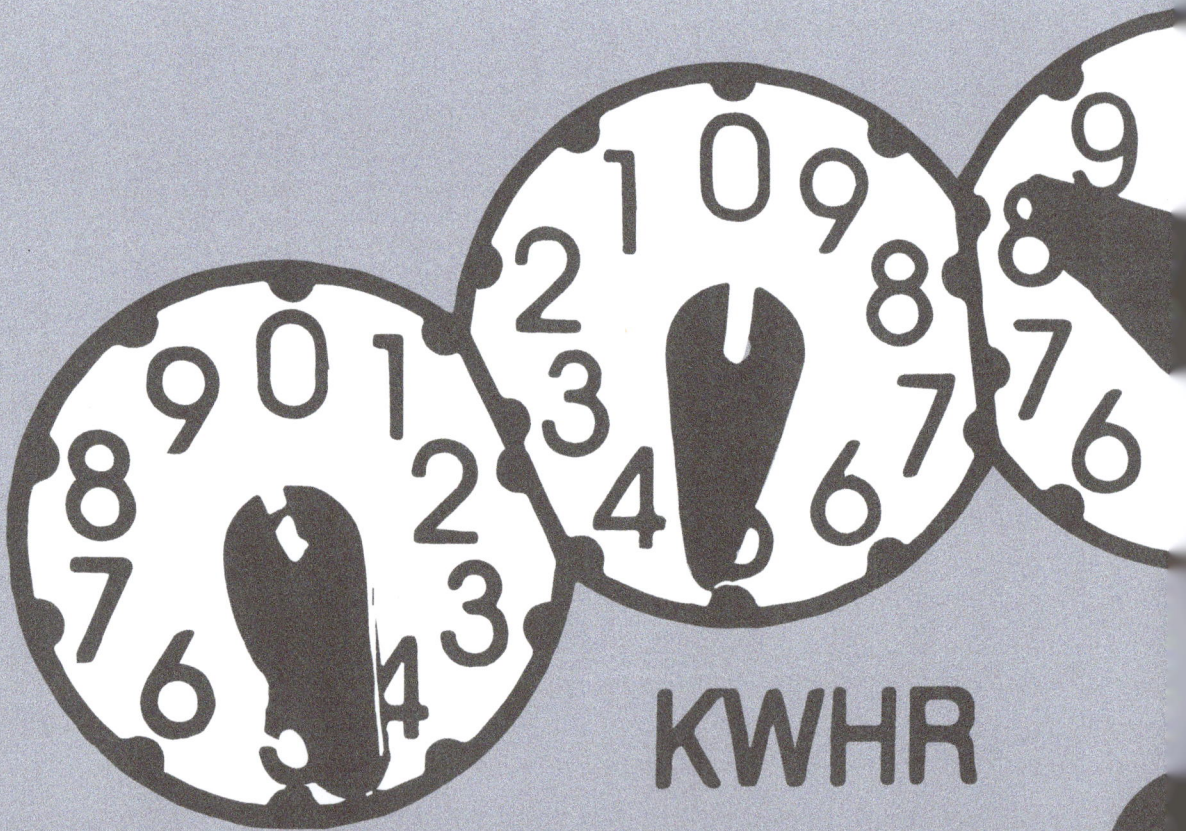

Swiss Healthcare Building
Quality – Quantity – Cost

Karin Imoberdorf
Dipl. Architect EPFL SIA
Master of Public Health

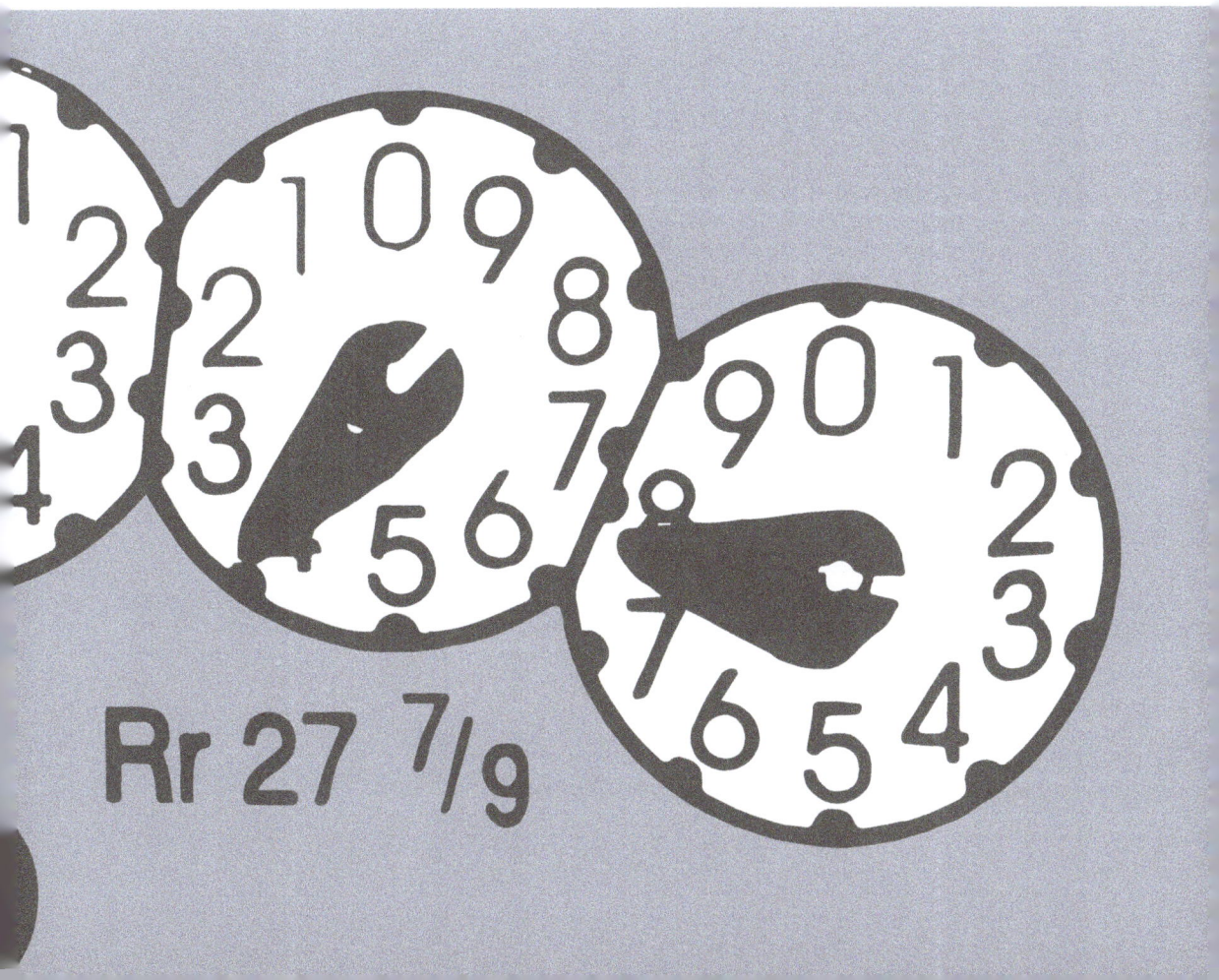

195

Abstract

Is cost more important than quality in hospital planning and building?

The Swiss healthcare system — one of the world's best and most expensive — underwent a fundamental change process.

One consequence of the new financing system is that the hospital infrastructure will not remain a secure part of the annual budget.

From this year on, building managers will get their money from the DRG financing system. While an additional 10% income is assured an unknown amount is required.

Often a gap between "must have" and "how to pay" will open up. The result is that new or further developed tools are required to better define and decide the requirements of the hospital of the future: performance modeling, process simulation, programming and master planning.

How can this vision become reality? The Lead Consultants benchmark system is a systematic tool that combines operating revenues with the values of the existing "Hardware", the entire building complex, from land to hospital beds. In short, the first decision is that costs are more important than quality. But only the right quality — defined through architecture and materialization, process orientation and the long-term ability to develop — will result in the necessary performance and efficiency.

The presentation examined the most recent developments in Swiss healthcare planning and introduced some tools to support this change process.

196

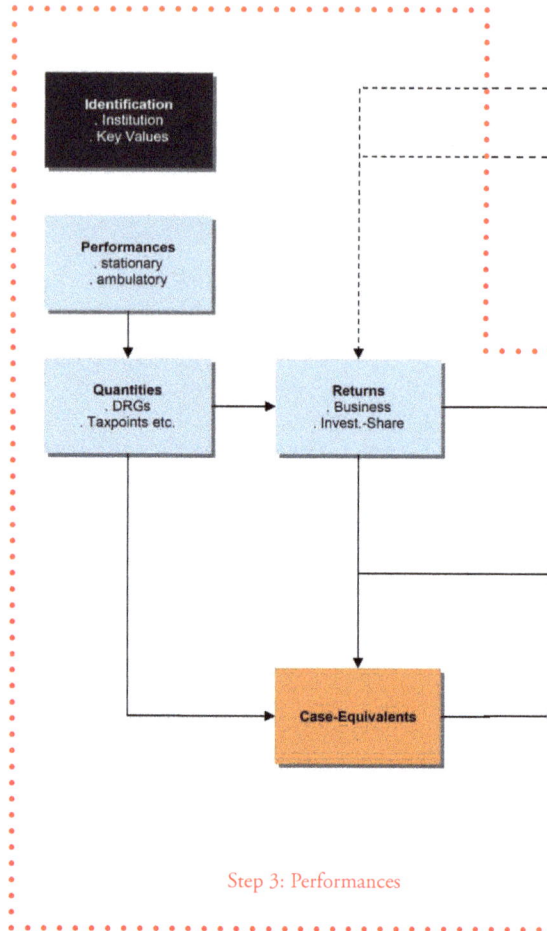

Step 3: Performances

1. *Lead Consultants Benchmark System.*

Introduction

Facts & Figures 2008 / 2009 / 2011
The Swiss healthcare system represents a significant economic sector. The volume of business is briefly represented in the following figures:
- 41,000 m2 – 7.8 million people – 297 hospitals – 38,728 beds;
- or 3.8 hospitals / 100,000 people (hos-

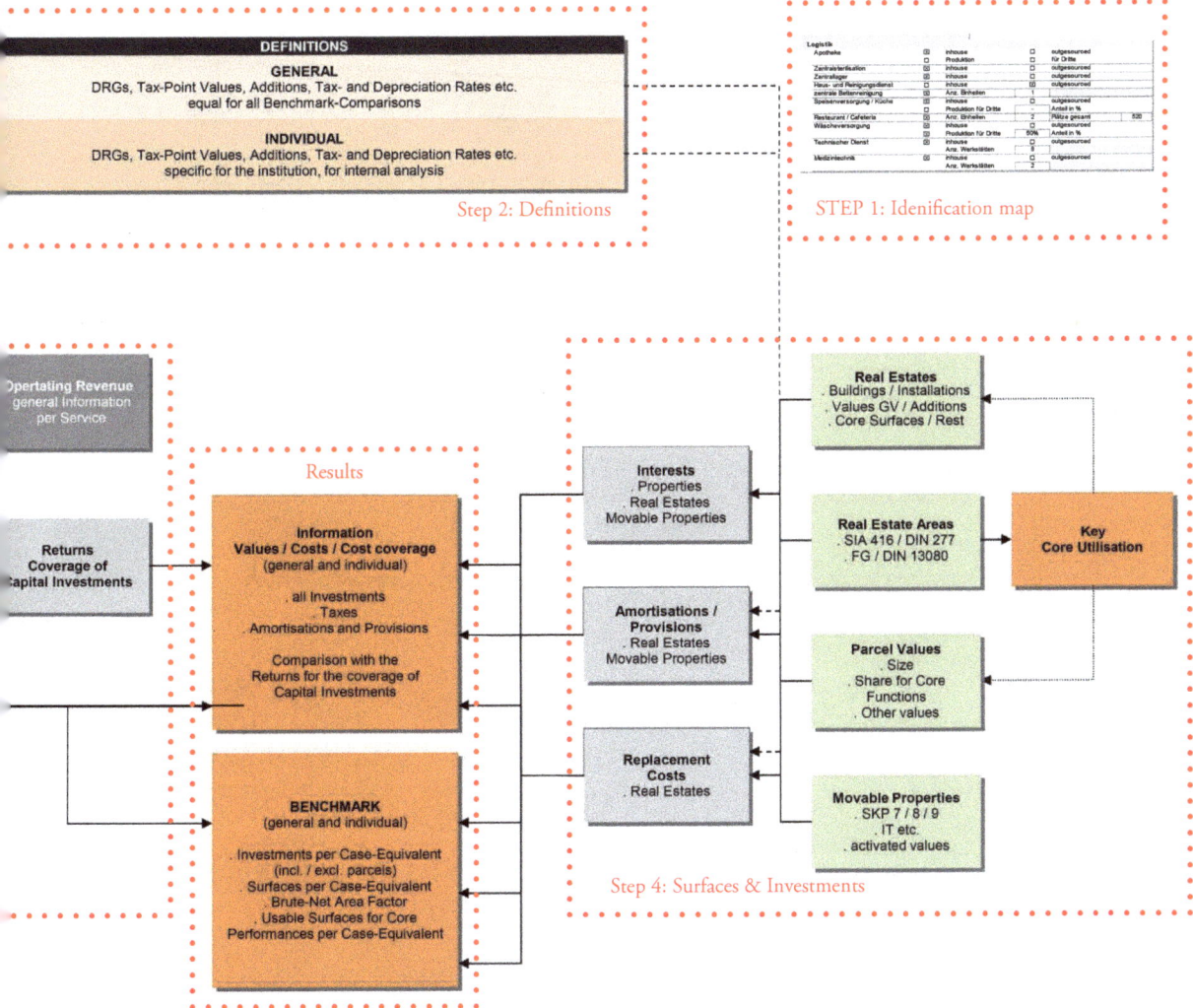

DEFINITIONS

GENERAL
DRGs, Tax-Point Values, Additions, Tax- and Depreciation Rates etc.
equal for all Benchmark-Comparisons

INDIVIDUAL
DRGs, Tax-Point Values, Additions, Tax- and Depreciation Rates etc.
specific for the institution, for internal analysis

Step 2: Definitions

STEP 1: Idenification map

Opertating Revenue
general information
per Service

Results

Returns
Coverage of
Capital Investments

Information
Values / Costs / Cost coverage
(general and individual)

. all Investments
. Taxes
. Amortisations and Provisions

Comparison with the
Returns for the coverage of
Capital Investments

BENCHMARK
(general and individual)

. Investments per Case-Equivalent
(incl. / excl. parcels)
. Surfaces per Case-Equivalent
. Brute-Net Area Factor
. Usable Surfaces for Core
Performances per Case-Equivalent

Interests
. Properties
. Real Estates
Movable Properties

Amortisations /
Provisions
. Real Estates
Movable Properties

Replacement
Costs
. Real Estates

Real Estates
. Buildings / Installations
. Values GV / Additions
. Core Surfaces / Rest

Real Estate Areas
. SIA 416 / DIN 277
. FG / DIN 13080

Key
Core Utilisation

Parcel Values
. Size
. Share for Core
Functions
. Other values

Movable Properties
. SKP 7 / 8 / 9
. IT etc.
. activated values

Step 4: Surfaces & Investments

pital and specialized clinics);
- or 4.9 beds / 1,000 people (hospital and specialized clinics);
- employer of 483,300 people, which represents 12% of the working population in Switzerland and is the biggest employer in all sectors.
Costs: CHF 61 billion = 11.4 % of GDP; CHF 19.2 billion Ambulatory Care; CHF 27.8 billion Stationary Care.

Consequences and new financing system

In 2012 a new financing system for hospitals was implemented in Switzerland.

Regulated competition will lead to greater transparency for all (patients/players/performers); new hospital planning criteria, quality and efficiency; and better cost control.

TESIS Inter-University Research Centre "Systems and Technologies for Social and Healthcare Facilities"
University of Florence, Italy

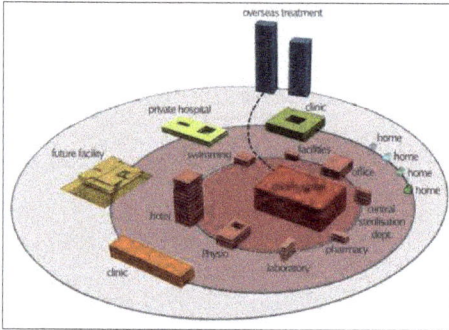

2. *Core hospital Concept.*

198

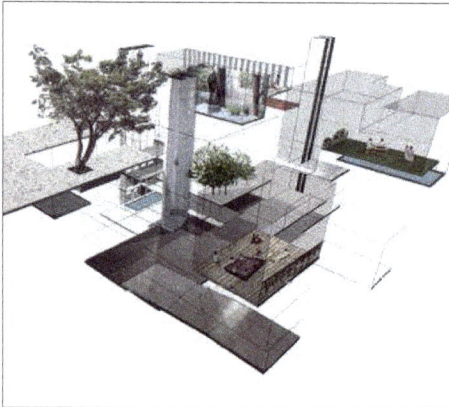

3. *Collaboration with Venhoeven CS and BM Managers, NL.*

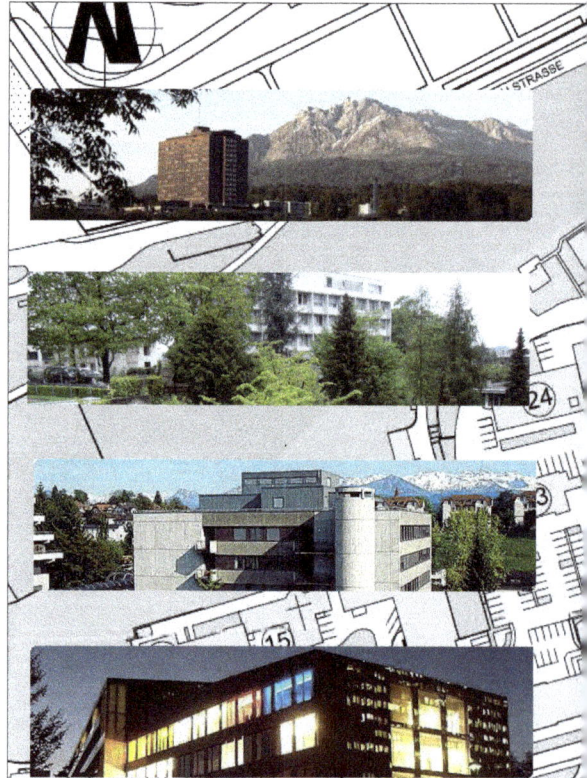

4. *Recent examples: LUKS – Intercantonal Masterplanning.*

The Swiss DRG includes treatment and therapy, and stationary care includes the cost of medication, the cost of education (excluding university), building infrastructure costs and medical equipment costs.

This gives rise to new questions such as:
- what comes first – quality, quantity or costs?
- CHF / NOK / EUR per bed – is this the right value?
- renovation or new construction?
- how to proceed and how to decide?

Decisions are necessary before planning and building. The LC benchmark system helps provide security and therefore the ability to decide.

FOCUS: Lead Consultants Benchmark System

The Lead Consultants Benchmark System delivers clear statements. It is based on simple and normally available figures, it can be employed at a very early project stage, it shows how future investments are covered (or not covered), and it allows variations as the project goes through simulations. This makes it easy to evaluate whether the room plan is realistic (or whether users wished for more than is necessary) and whether the building project is optimized. It supports decision-making and project development.

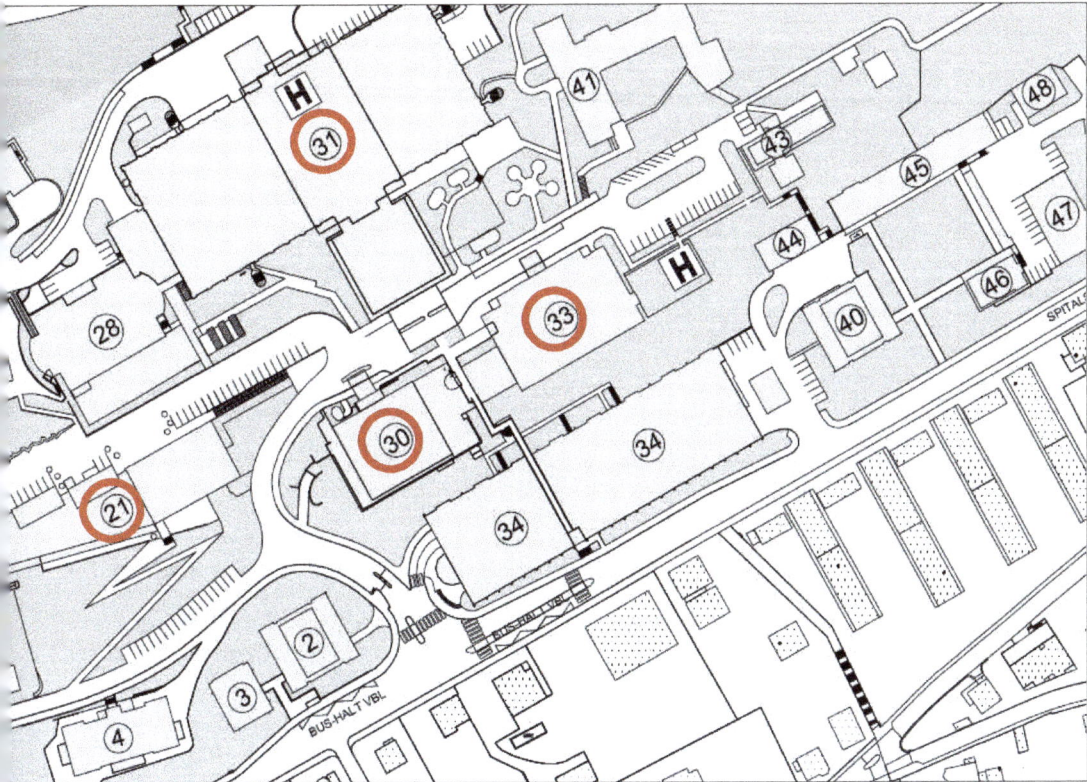

Statements

The Benchmark system must be able to answer the following questions:
- can the total investment (for the building, movable goods and replacement costs) be paid through contributions made to the new financing model (Swiss DRG 2012)?
- are the total surface areas provided to meet future skill requirements realistic compared to other measurement variables (case equivalents)?

Measurement variable

First we need measurement variables to make projects and capital investments comparable.

The measurement variable must consider all the specific features of the respective institutions (basic hospital versus university hospital, etc.).

Furthermore it must be able to follow the development of medicine. Finally the measurement variable must be simple and available.

The measurement variable was found using the case equivalent (the sum of all the income obtained through medical performance divided by the base rate).

200

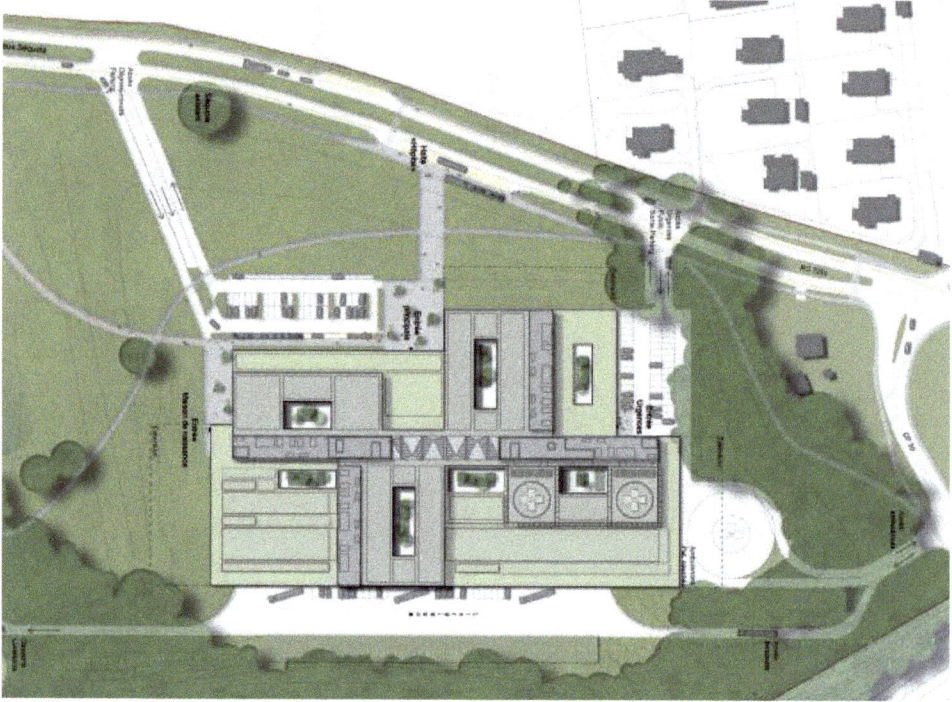

5. Recent examples: Hôpital du Chablais – Competition.

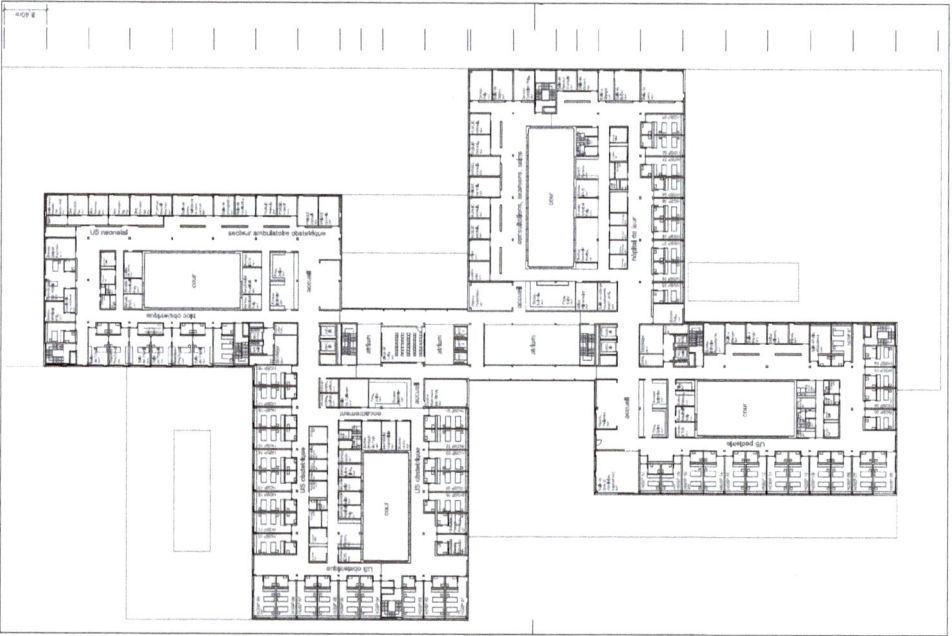

6. Recent examples: Hôpital du Chablais – Competition.

Benchmark System – STEP 1: Identification Map

Despite case equivalents institutions differ from each other. This is taken into account within the overall and the detailed identification map.

Benchmark System – STEP 2: Definitions

General definitions: central, equal for all. Individual definitions give specific values for the institutions such as: flat rates, based surcharges, DRG-values, integrated and extra contributions to cover investments, amortization records, tax rates, etc.Spectrum: acute care for adults, children, rehabilitation, long-term care, psychiatry, etc.

Benchmark System STEP 3: Performances

Numbers of medical performances. All other connected performances are based on their definitions. Calculation of:
- the expected income of the institution;
- the share to cover the investment costs;
- definition of the case equivalent;
- amount of the coverage share from stationary and ambulatory performances.

Benchmark System STEP 4: Surface Areas & Investments

Parcels of land are evaluated as follows:
- properties (separation into buildings and installations);
- replacement values of the properties (activated values);
- calculation of amortizations, provisions and replacement costs and parcels. The replacement values for buildings and movable goods are listed, the surface areas per function are analyzed and core

201

7. Recent examples: Hôpital du Chablais – Competition.

202

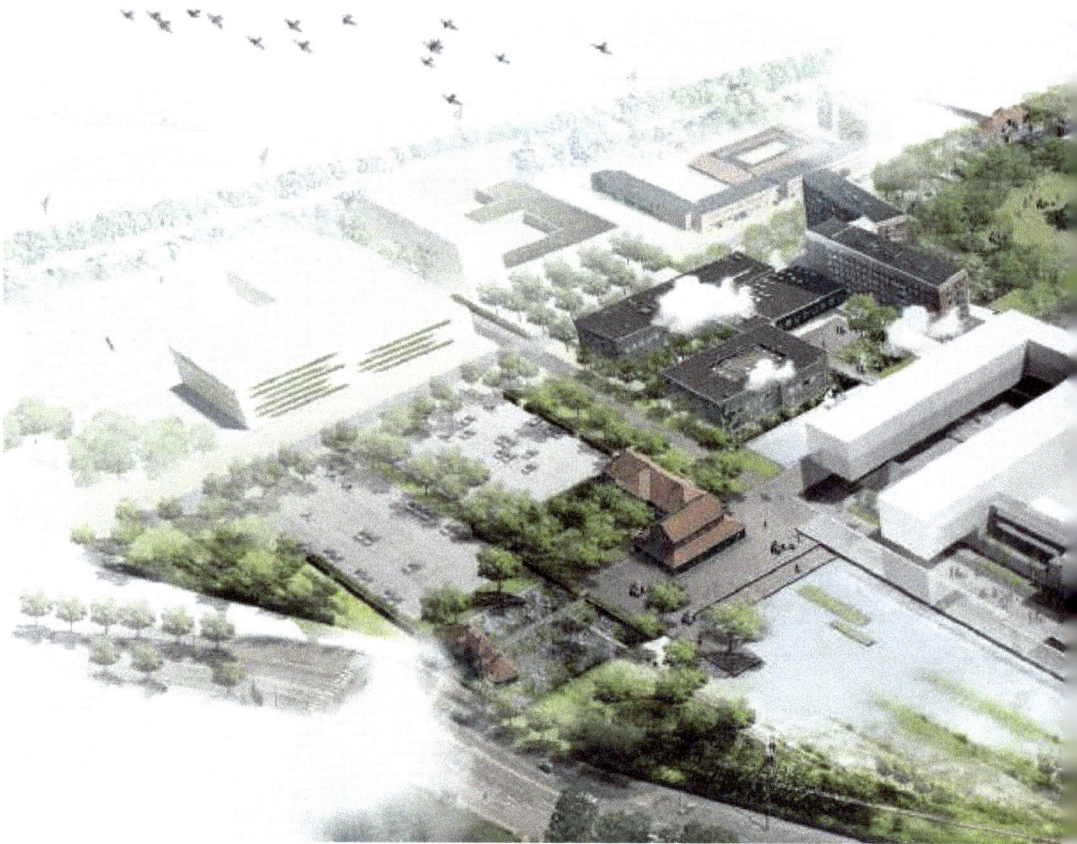

8. Recent examples: Bispegjerg Healthpark, Copenhagen.

functions (i.e. functions that are necessary to fulfill the defined performances) and additional services are grouped.

Earnings and Comparison

The share for stationary and ambulatory investments does not cover the resulting costs if analyzed by considering all influencing factors.

The Lead Consultants Benchmark

System delivers clear statements:

- it is based on simple and normally available figures;
- it can be employed at a very early project stage;
- it shows how future investments are covered (or not covered);
- it allows variations – the project goes through simulations;
- it makes it easy to evaluate whether the room plan is realistic (or whether users wished for more than is necessary) and whether the building project is optimized;
- it supports decision-making and project development.

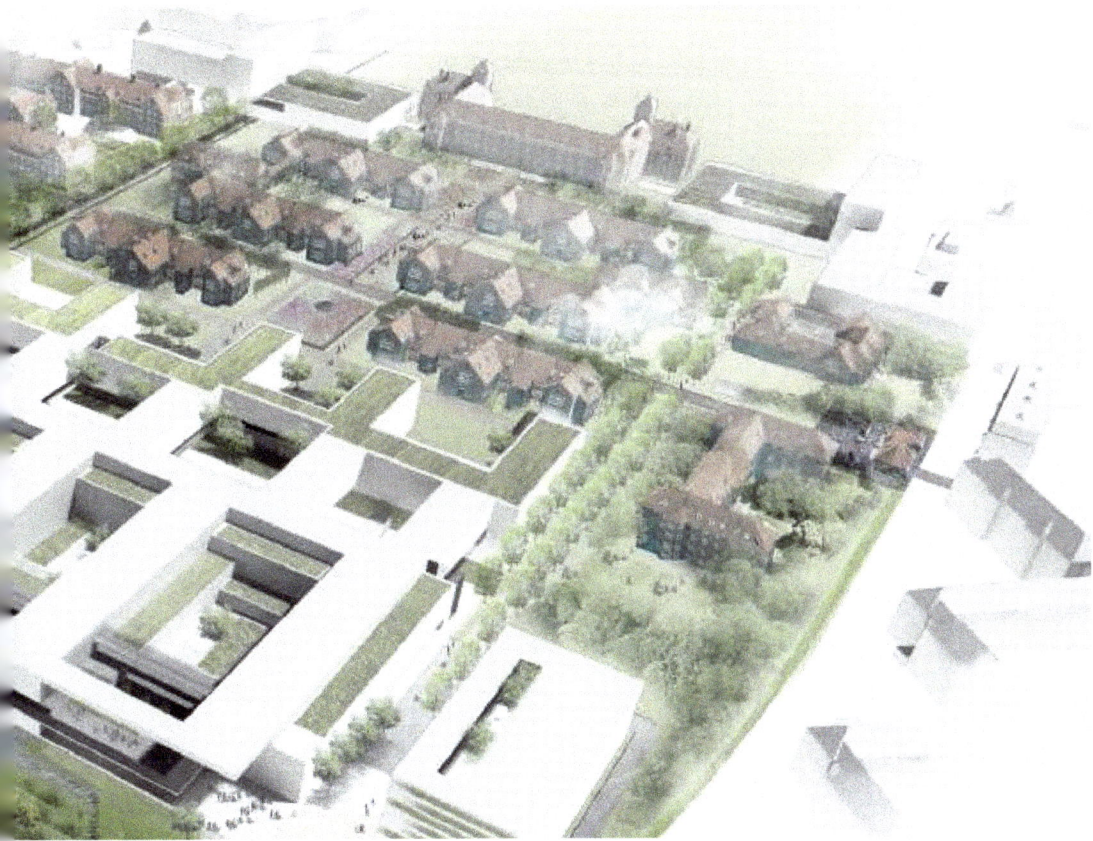

The Benchmark system presented is a simple but meaningful tool that can be employed with reasonable efforts and that delivers clear and comparable results.

Recent examples

Core hospital Concept for the Future hospital – Collaboration with Venhoeven CS and BM Managers, NL
Bispegjerg Healthpark – Master plan competition, Copenhagen, DK

LUKS – Intercantonal Masterplanning, Luzern, CH
Hôpital du Chablais – Competition, Rennaz, CH
BSS – New hospital development for Solothurn, CH
St Claraspital – Master plan for a private hospital in Basel, CH
University Hospital Zurich – Development of planning modules for intensive and standard care, Zurich, CH
Rehabilitation Clinic Bellikon - From Competition to completion, Bellikon, CH.

TESIS Inter-University Research Centre "Systems and Technologies for Social and Healthcare Facilities"
University of Florence, Italy

A Tour Through the Hospital

TESIS Inter-University Research Centre "Systems and Technologies for Social and Healthcare Facilities"
University of Florence, Italy

A Tour Through Akershus University Hospital

At the conference in Oslo on 23-24 March 2012 the UIA/PHG members toured Akershus University Hospital in Oslo. The images in this section were taken on that occasion.

In 2003, the Norwegian parliament gave the green light for the transformation of the historic structure of Akershus into a modern university hospital. Construction work began in 2004 and ended in 2008. The spaces were designed with the aim of increasing well-being through their use by patients, staff and visitors; the hospital's art collection has made a decisive contribution to the pursuit of this goal.

The following description focuses in particular on the program of art works that were photographed during the visit.

Some brief explanations of art works have been selected and included in the text.

Architecture

The new Akersus University Hospital was designed and built by the Danish architectural firm C. F. Møller Architects. The design choices attempted to combine low cost solutions with a high quality environment. The main street is the most important functional artery of the building, and the glass cover ensures the presence of natural light which interacts harmoniously with the wood used for the structure. The architectural solutions give the environments an appearance that is non-institutional, accessible and user friendly for patients, family members, visitors and staff alike. The presence of transparent surfaces guaran-

207

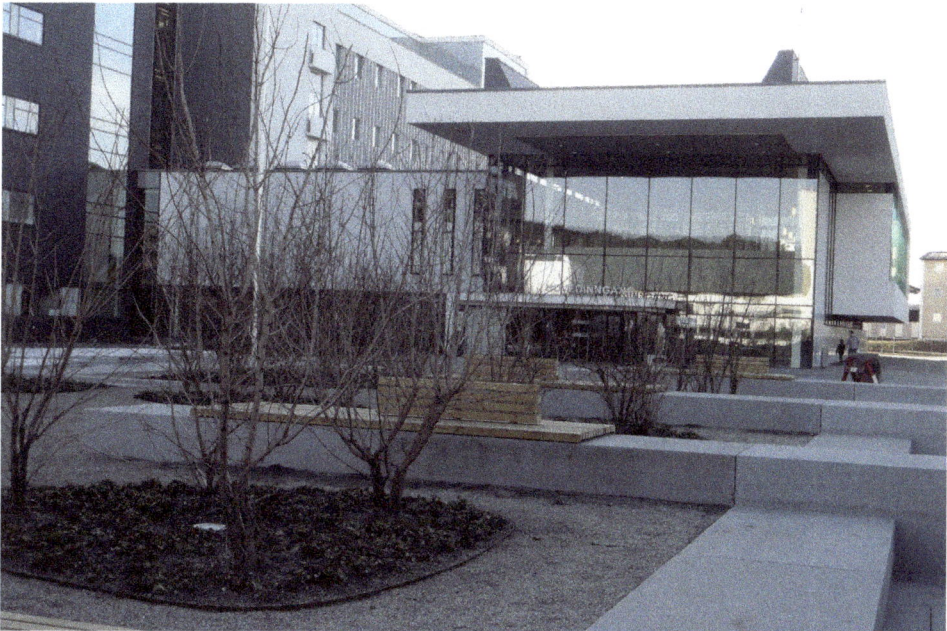

1. Garden facing the main entrance.

TESIS Inter-University Research Centre "Systems and Technologies for Social and Healthcare Facilities"
University of Florence, Italy

TESIS

tees the possibility of observing the surrounding environment and landscape. The departments are differentiated by size and shape thereby creating different visual experiences for users, which can improve orientation within the structure.

Art in the hospital

208

The new Akersus University Hospital is characterized by the presence of an important art collection. The program of art work installations within Akershus was curated by Claes Soderquist and Anne Beate Hovind. The works integration project was carried out during the hospital construction process, and the budget for the art program was 2.3 mil-

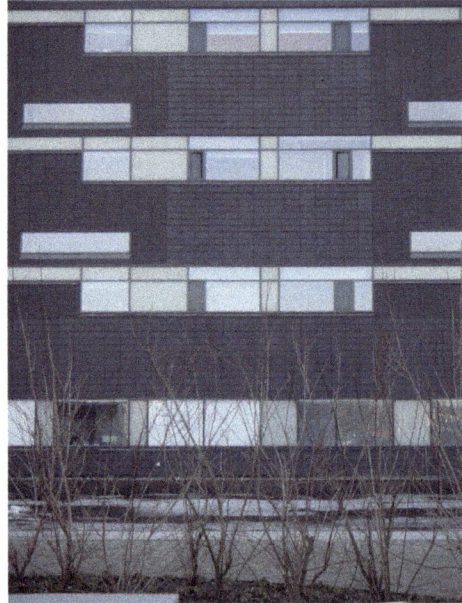
2. Detail of façade.

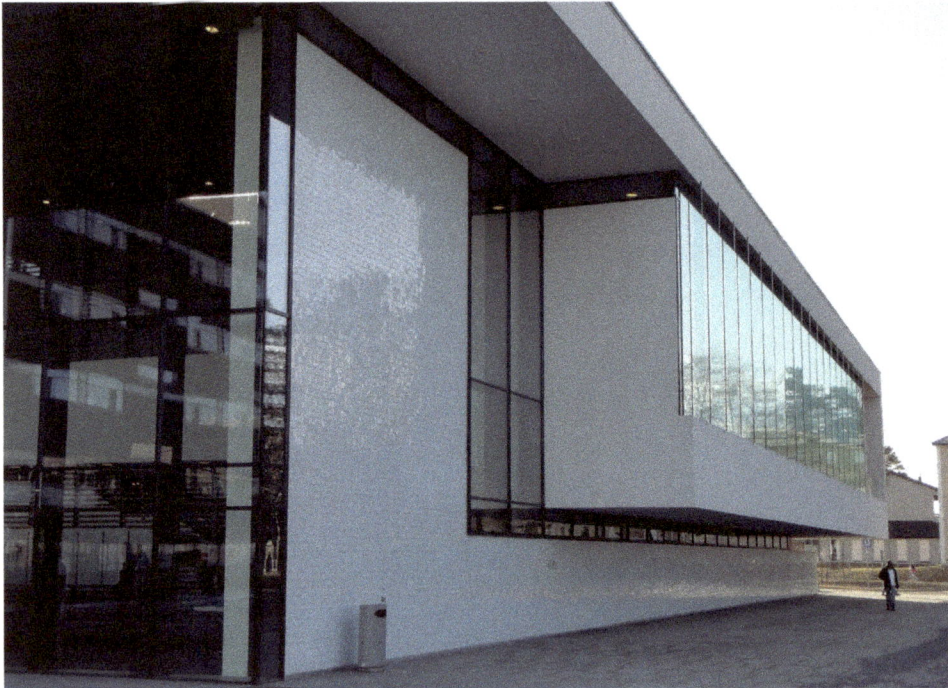
3. Petteri Nisunen and Tommi Grönlund 2009, interactive sound installation outside, along the main entrance: auditory artwork with nine sources.

lion euros. In this case the art collection was conceived during the construction phase, which meant that the principle of acquiring works already available on the market was overcome.

The intervention has significantly contributed to raising the environmental quality of the public spaces of the hospital, with the art works being spread over a total area of 137,000 square meters. The art works were designed not with the goal of inducing healing but rather with the intention of creating a series of environments that engage the senses and minds of the visitors. "A hospital is a special place to display art. People come there in very different moods and situations - from the highest happiness to the deepest grief. And no one has actually asked to see the art," said Hovind. She believes art's task in the hospital is to activate thought processes and create meaning.

With this collection, the hospital has become not only an art recipient but an important opportunity for artistic innovation, just think of the preliminary work of cataloging the existing art works assigned to the visual artist Beathe C. Rønning. The artist, along with Tone Hansen, was responsible for assessing and analyzing the existing art collection in the hospital in order to understand what worked, considering how products stand out from an artistic point of view and which ones do not. This activity showed the presence of a heterogeneous series of works from various collections with different styles and decorations. This research process has itself become a work of art. The paintings or sculptures were photographed in their original con-

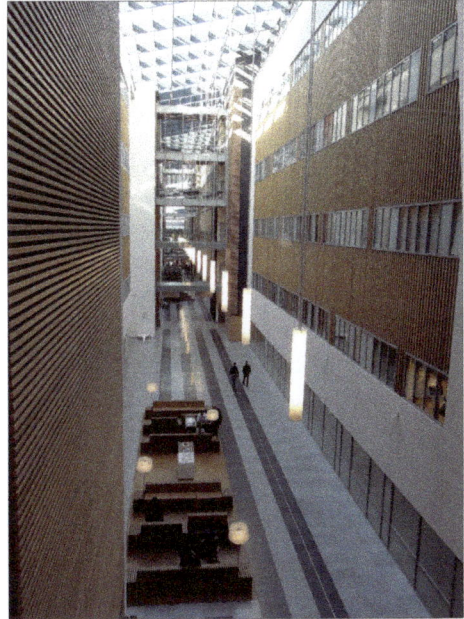

4. *The hospital's main communications artery, the glass street.*

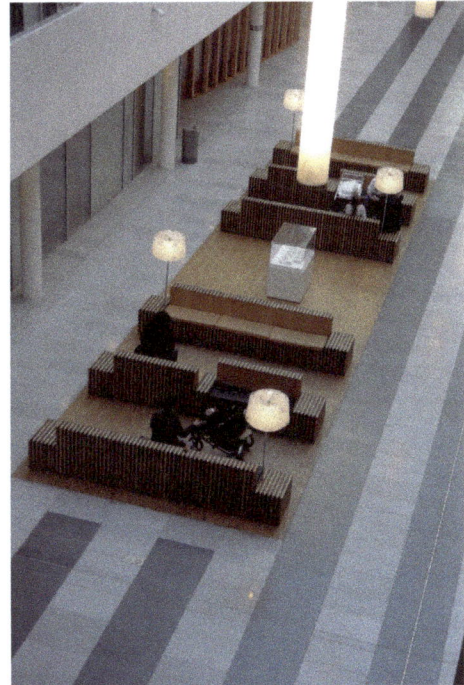

5. *Waiting area in the glass street.*

209

TESIS Inter-University Research Centre "Systems and Technologies for Social and Healthcare Facilities"
University of Florence, Italy

text, and the images were posted on the walls with comments that described the sounds or sensations that the works of art were able to conjure up in their previous location.

This photographic collection allowed the past to be witnessed and documented, and images of the old hospital were projected inside the modern health care centre.

210

The art collection was designed in close relation with the architecture. The public areas were characterized by C. F. Møller Architects through the use of materials typical of the Scandinavian design tradition, such as wood and glass. Likewise the works of art were entrusted to artists from Scandinavia, and this choice was seen as an opportunity for reflection and cultural identity, able to simultaneously stimulate the senses and minds of the observers.

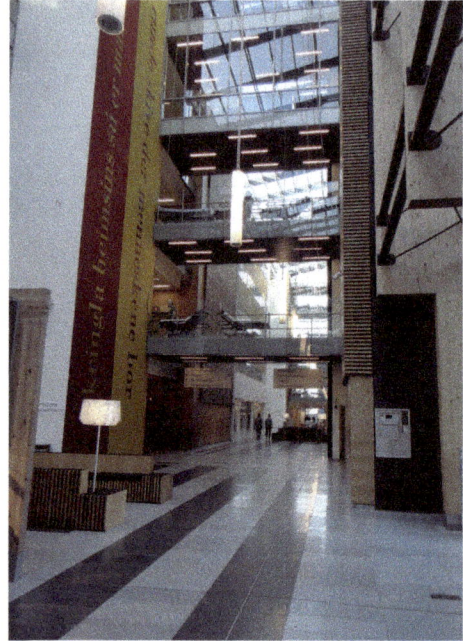

6. Birgir Andrésson 2009: wall mural, four painted wall surfaces. Text in painted aluminum. 25 x 6 feet. The four murals stretch across five floors and accentuate the architectural elevation drawing.

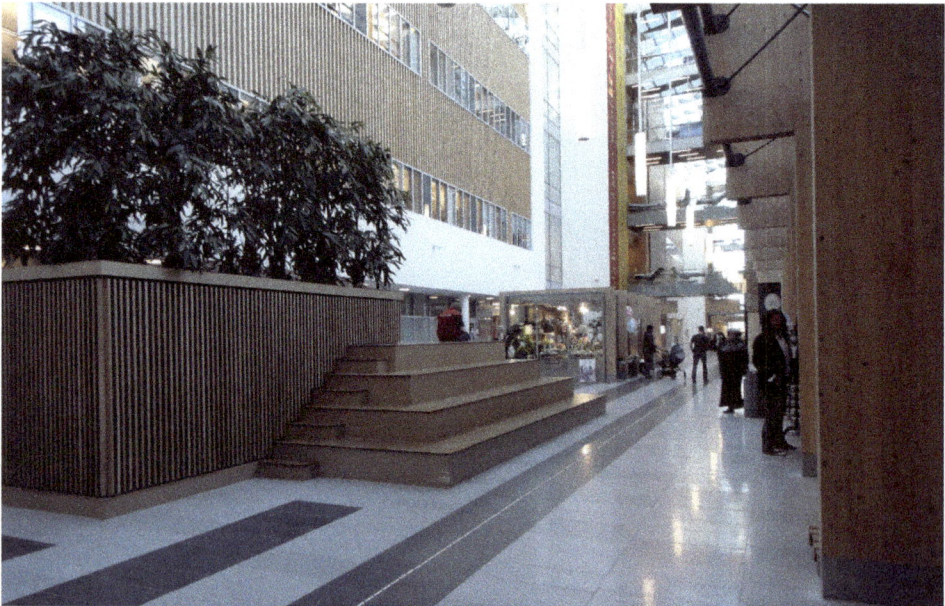

7. Public space.

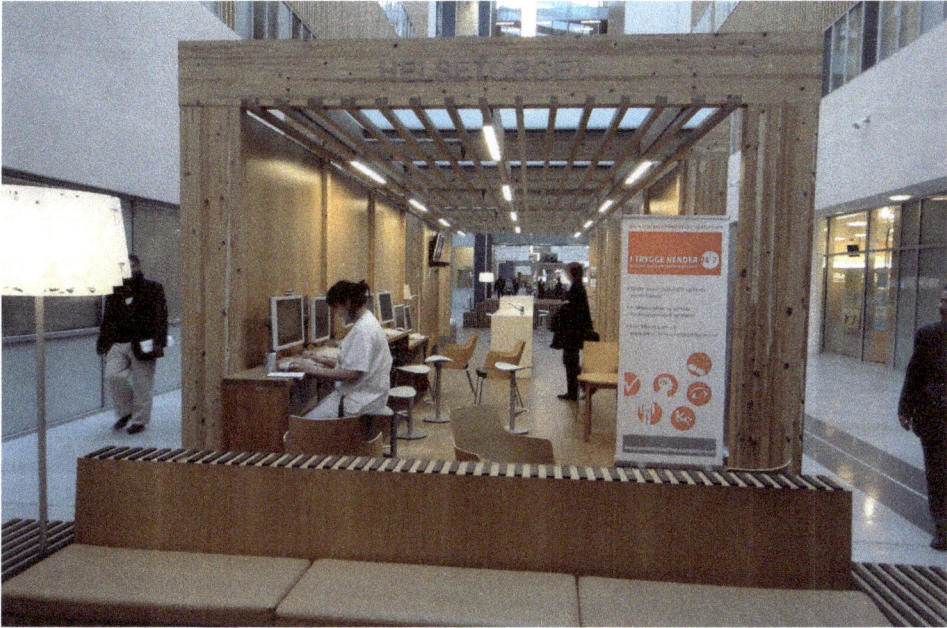

8. *Health square.*

211

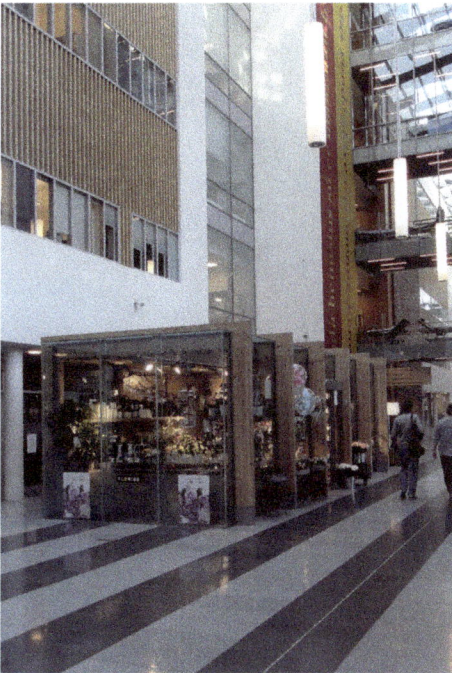

9. *Walkways in the glass street.*

Petteri Nisunen and Tommi Grönlund, born in 1962 and 1967 respectively, Finland (image 3)

Welcoming visitors through the main entrance is a sound installation by Petteri Nisunen and Tommi Grönlund, which extends for about thirty meters. The nine built-in sensors of the overhanging floor are activated by the passage of people, thereby triggering a variable composition of sound files that is broadcast over the speakers. The work is a reflection on the specific sound of the site and the experience of moving through space.

Birgir Andrésson, 1955-2007, Iceland (images 6-7)

The work of Birgir Andrésson is composed of two colored panels that extend

212

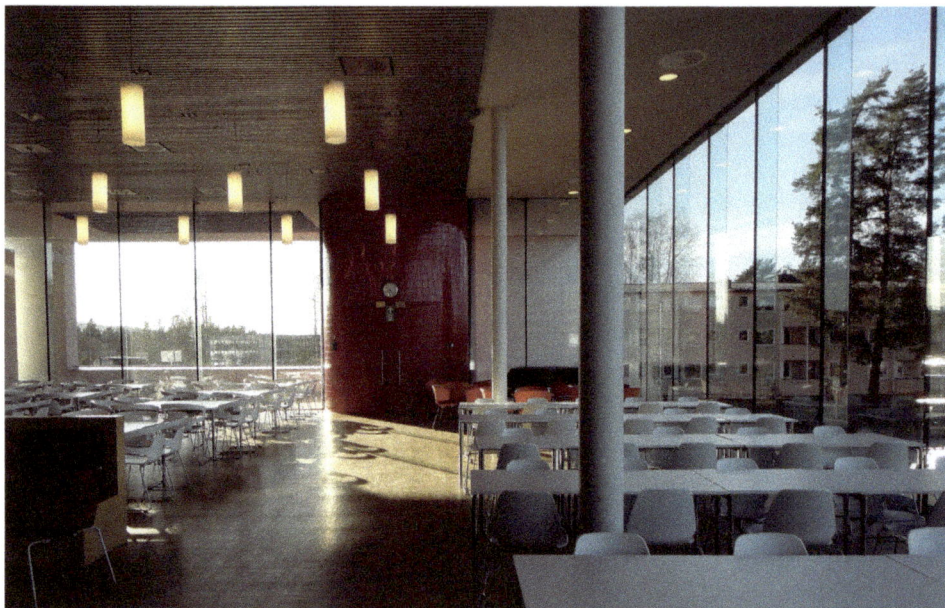

10. *Staff lunchroom: the north side is a glass surface open to the landscape.*

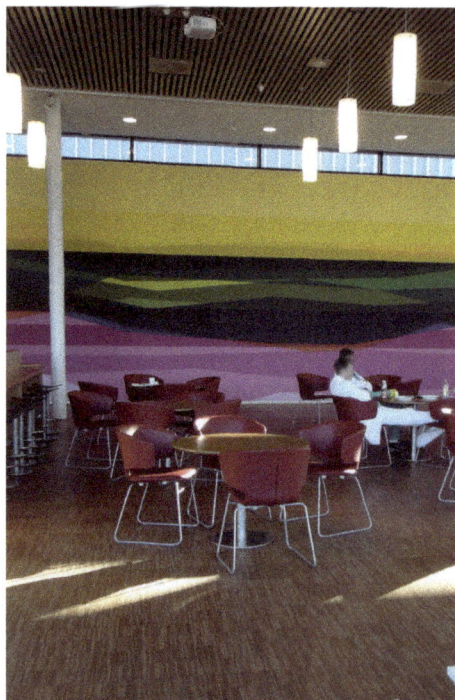

11. *Staff lunchroom. Artwork by Jan Christensen, 2008: wall textile. Printed textile. 4 x 24 m.*

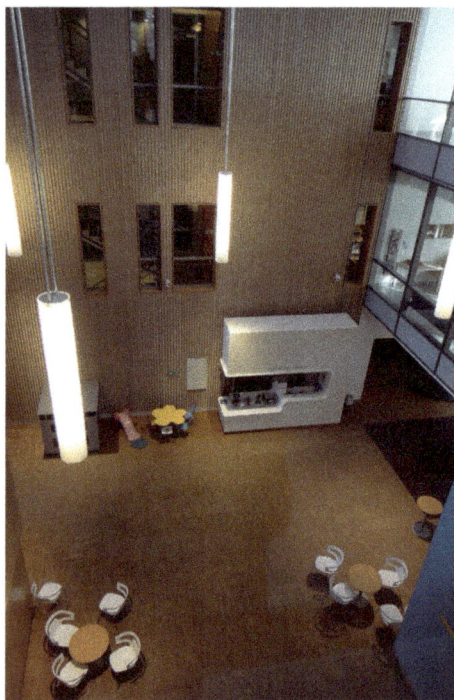

12. *Per Sundberg 2009: 22 hanging lamps in fiber optics and glass cylinders. Height: 16 m.*

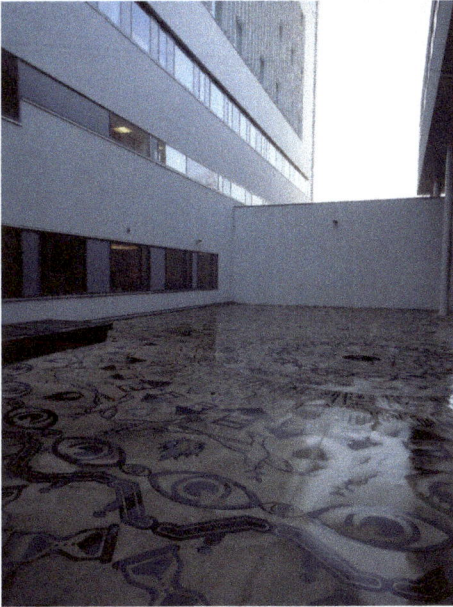

13. *Gunilla Klingberg 2009, the hospital's artwork collection.*

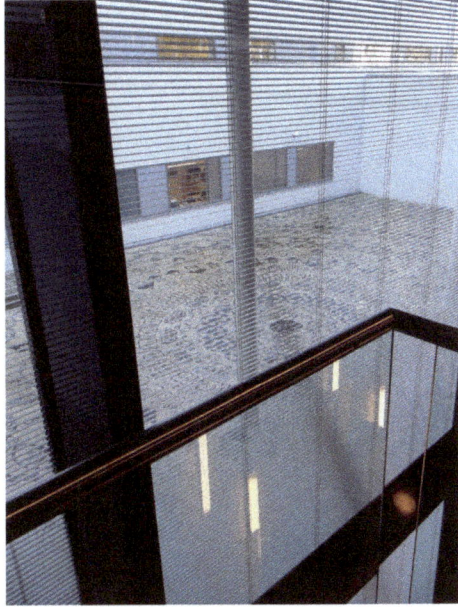

14. *Art and daylight.*

213

in height along the five planes of the main street. The two different coloured backgrounds and the font colours alternate in the two fields containing one phrase in Norwegian and one in Icelandic taken from the text Heimskringla, a saga that represents the cultural heritage shared by the two nations. The installation is therefore a reflection on tradition, history, national identity and language.

Jan Christensen, born in 1977, Norway (images 11-12)

The wall of the hospital staff lunchroom is decorated by the art work of Jan Christensen. It is a canvas that has the same dimensions as the wall, 4 x 24 m, and is supported by an aluminum structure. The subject matter was a stylized landscape coloured with bright hues. The scene is rendered through a figurative language, and in fact there are typi-

cal features that characterize a generic landscape: the horizon, the sky and the ground. The work is very large so it can also be seen from the outside through the glass wall.

Gunilla Klingberg, born in 1966, Sweden (images 13-14)

The installation by Gunilla Klingberg decorates the floor of a courtyard of the hospital. It is a circular representation in which the motifs are repeated and distorted. Ideograms of everyday life alternate with those of oriental symbolism to form a pattern that leads the viewer to reflect on the meaning of the Western civilization of consumption[1].

---

1 *The information provided on the artists and installations was taken from the Akersus University Hospital official website www.ahus.no.*

214

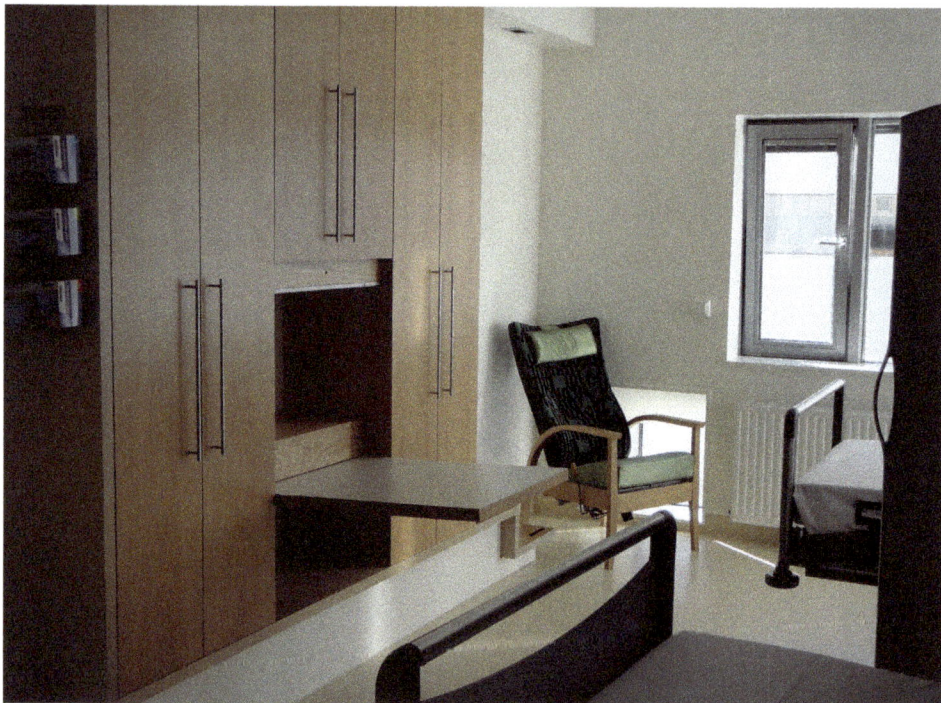

15. Patient room.

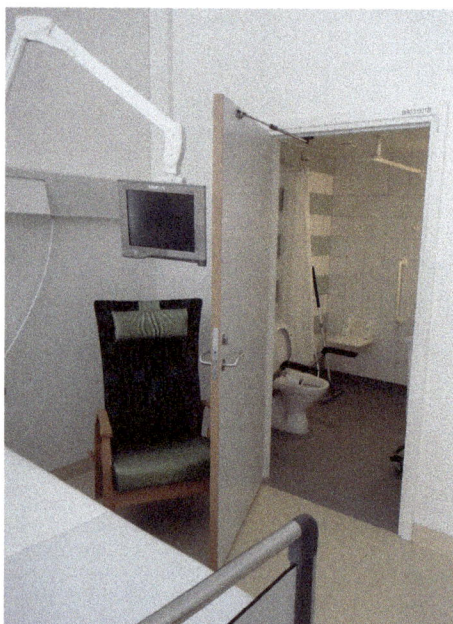

16. Bathroom of a patient room.

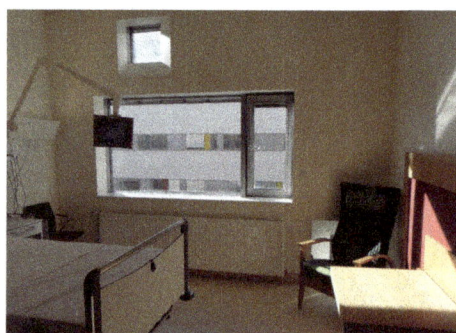

17. Window of the patient room.

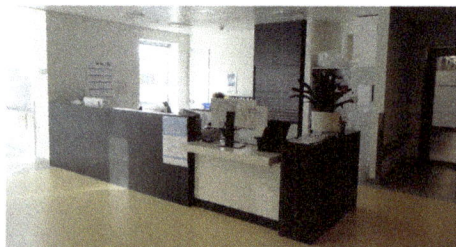

18. Workstation.

A Tour Through Rikshospitalet

At the conference in Oslo on 23-24 March 2012, the UIA/PHG members toured the Rikshospitalet in Oslo. The images in this section were taken at that time.

Oslo University Hospital is a highly specialized hospital in charge of extensive regional and local hospital assignments and the provision of high quality services for the citizens of Oslo. The hospital also has nationwide responsibility for a number of national and multi-regional assignments and has several national centres of competence.[1]

1 From the hospital's official website www.oslo-universitetssykehus.no.

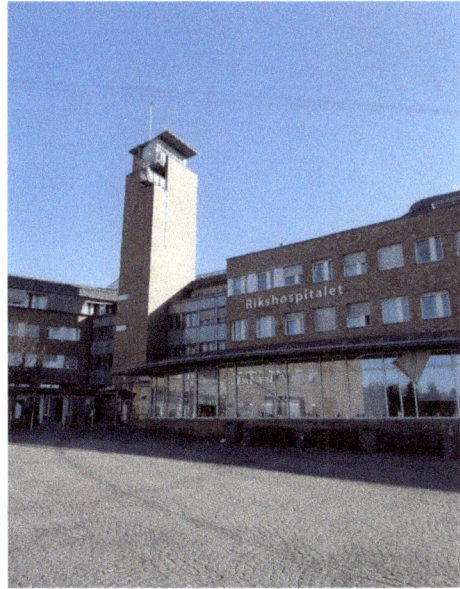

1. The tower, a landmark of Rikshospitalet.

215

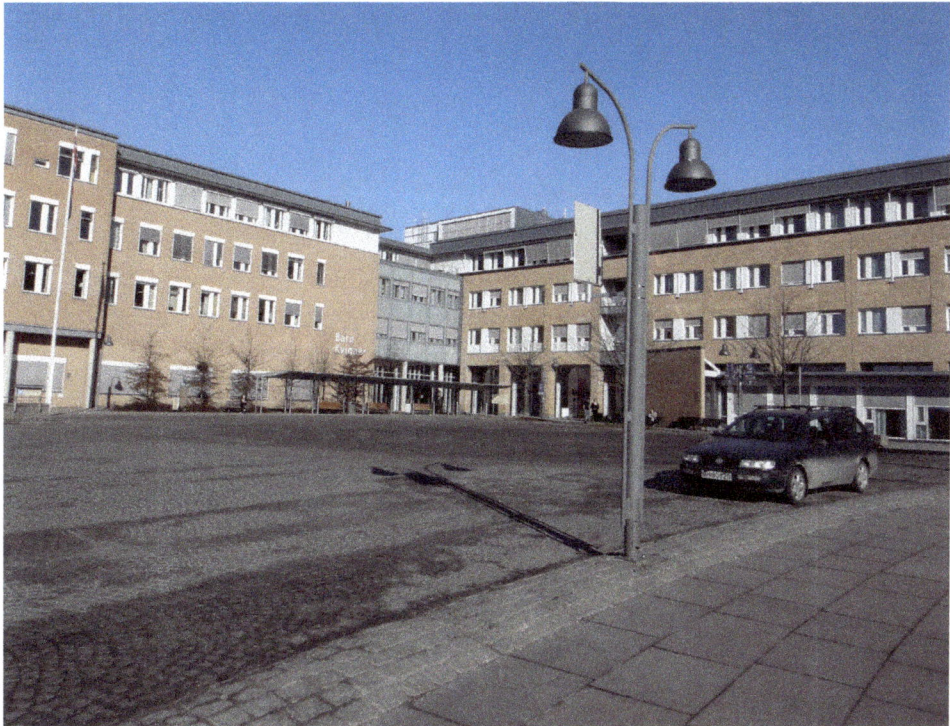

2. The hospital square.

TESIS Inter-University Research Centre "Systems and Technologies for Social and Healthcare Facilities"
University of Florence, Italy

216

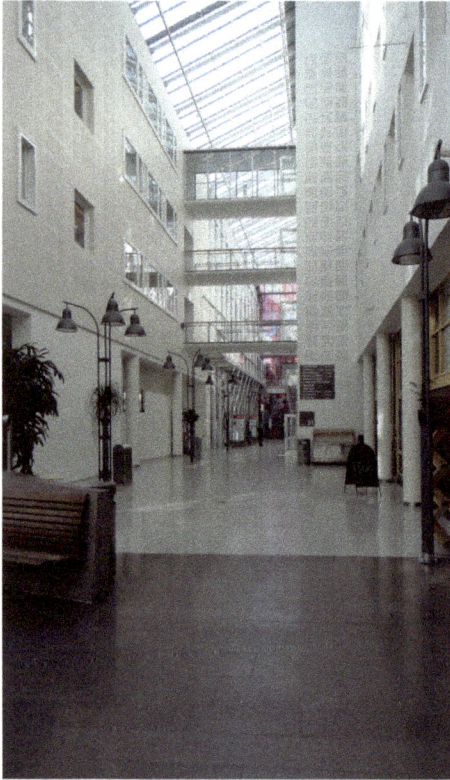

3. Interior main street.

Rikshospitalet in Oslo

The Rikshospitalet was designed by the group Medplan AS architects who won the design competition in 1991. The motive that inspired the project was to place user needs as the central focus of the designed environments in order to create what is known as a "humanistic hospital." "A primary goal was to create a physical environment that inspires the trust and confidence of hospital users, patients, staff and visitors alike. A low construction connected by streets and squares, adapted to the site's bowl shape, was a natural starting point for effective logistics. Building devices with various features such as wards, treatment buildings, laboratories and research units are joined together in an "urban" corridor along a glazed, indoor main street. Glass strips follow the site slope and crossroads lead to the different wings of the hospital"[2].

2 From the website of Medplan AS architects www.medplan.no, updated 20.2.2009.

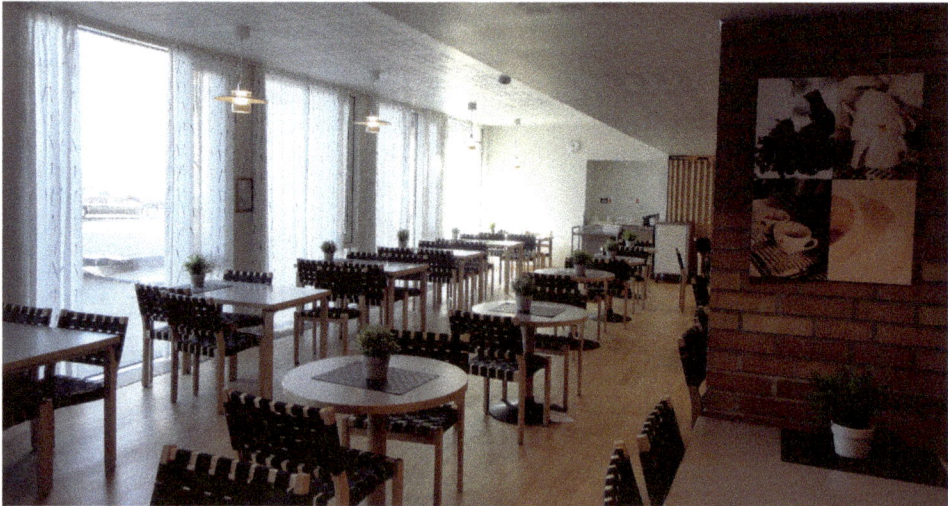

4. Cafeteria.

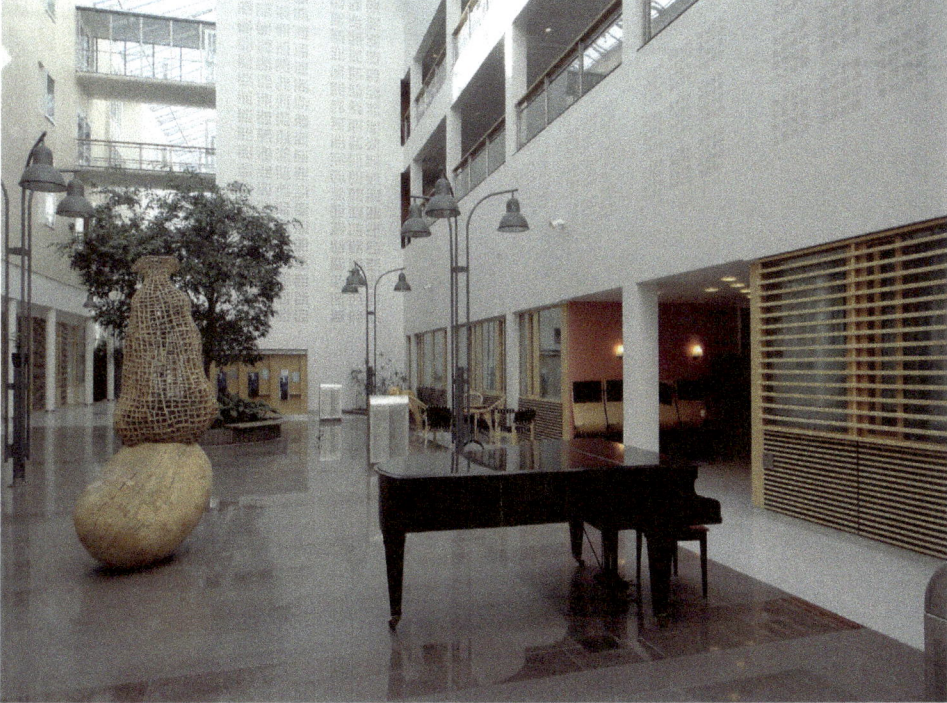

5. *Music and art environments in the ground floor street.*

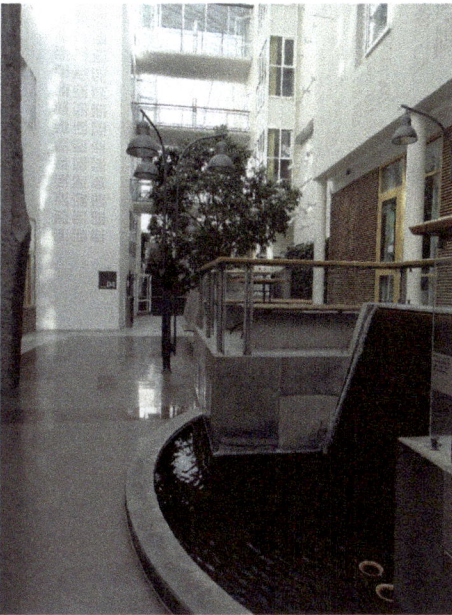

6. *Natural elements in the hospital.*

Integration between care research and education activities

Rikshospitalet is a hospital where patient care is carried out in close connection with education and research. From a therapeutic point of view the latest advanced medicine procedures are used in the hospital. The centre conducts research and provides a point of reference at national level, mainly with regard to clinical research. The hospital includes other centres of research and training activities are carried out giving importance to clinical practice.

These activities are carried out in environments that have distinctive spatial organization: the floors dedicated to nursing staff are open and visually connected with the wards, and as regards

TESIS Inter-University Research Centre "Systems and Technologies for Social and Healthcare Facilities"
University of Florence, Italy

TESIS

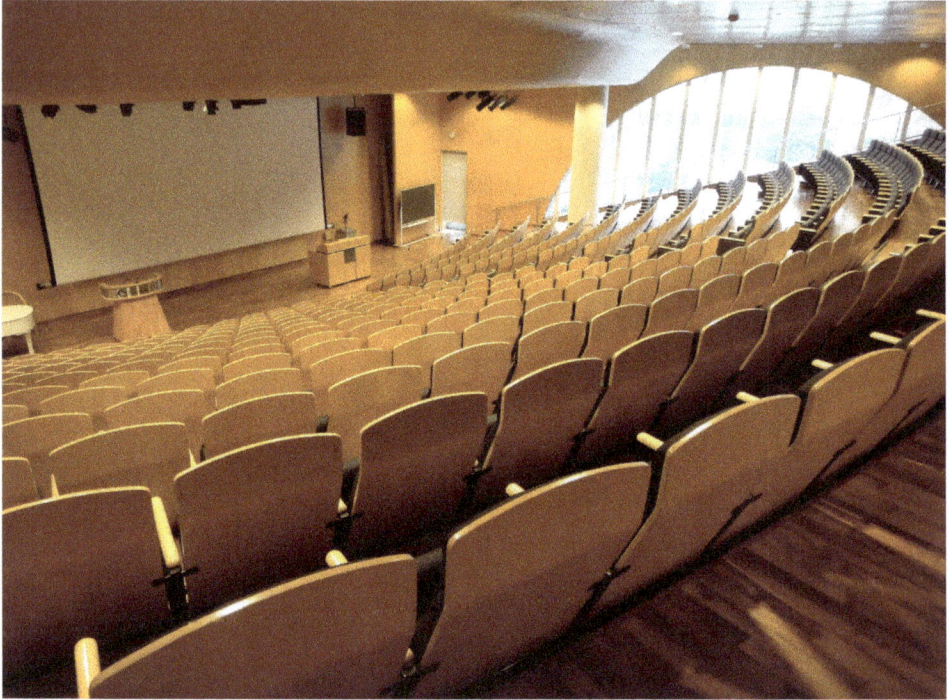

7. Auditorium.

environmental quality importance has been given to natural light, which is present in all work areas. Interaction between patients and staff is facilitated through the construction of a single aisle, which implies a natural division of the flow of people without the need for separate paths.

Architecture for the wellbeing of patients, visitors and staff

The internal passageways are characterized by a well thought-out spatial distribution: in the laboratories the corridor walls were removed on the sides exposed to natural light; the reception is located along the corridors and all the walls dividing them from the relaxation areas were removed; niche spaces were created

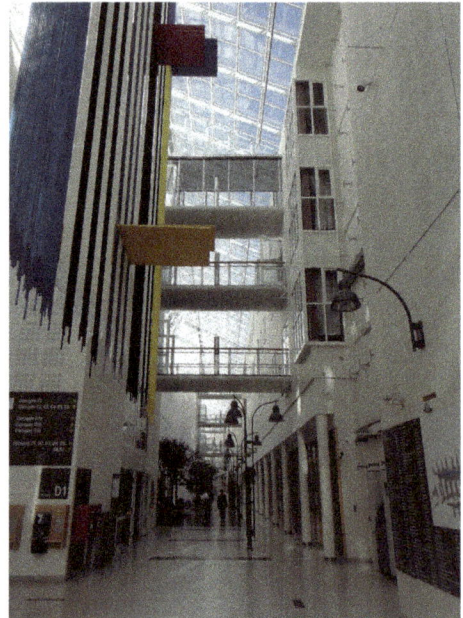

8. Footbridges.

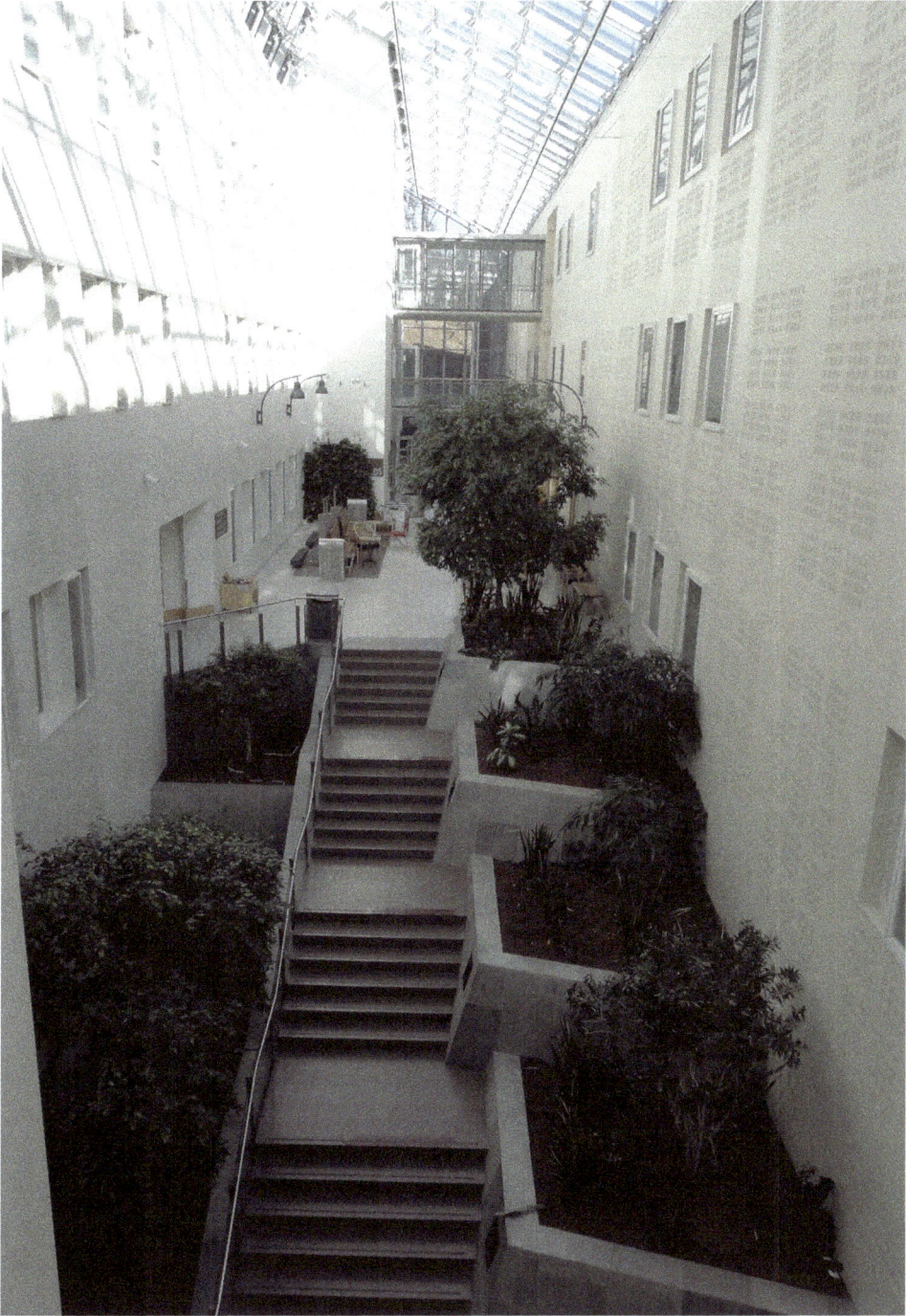

9. *Green terraced steps in the hospital street.*

TESIS Inter-University Research Centre "Systems and Technologies for Social and Healthcare Facilities"
University of Florence, Italy

220

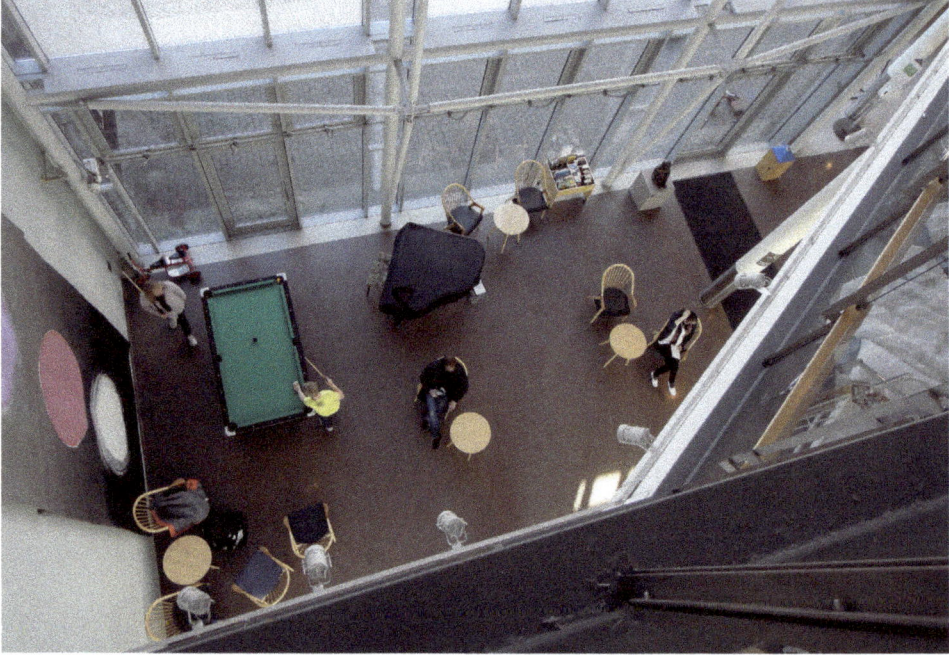

10. Aerial view of the positive distractions area.

in the the heavily frequented areas and they are used as lunch and resting areas. Environments that did not require any particular system solutions were placed freely within the structure, for instance university laboratories pertaining to radiology were placed in the south wing of the hospital, while the psychotherapy laboratories are in the north wing. An area where only offices and clinics are grouped was located south of the ICU units and operating rooms. The wards, clinics, operating theaters and laboratories may in any case be used by different specializations.

Changing the organization of the space and not the built environment

In 1996 the hospital was expanded and there was a need for a new MR and an angiographic laboratory in the radiology department. For this reason the research areas and offices were moved. Molecular pathology was placed in the area where the Centre for Health Administration was located, which in turn was moved.

The expansion of the paediatrics department led to the transfer of two small units to another building.

Subsequently significant organizational changes were made without altering the built environment: Cardiology, Lung Medicine and Thorax Surgery were incorporated within the Heart Clinic, and ¼ of the ICU units were moved from Anesthesia to Thorax Surgery. Neurosurgery was expanded from 33 to 55 beds, and no changes were made to the buildings during these relocation processes.

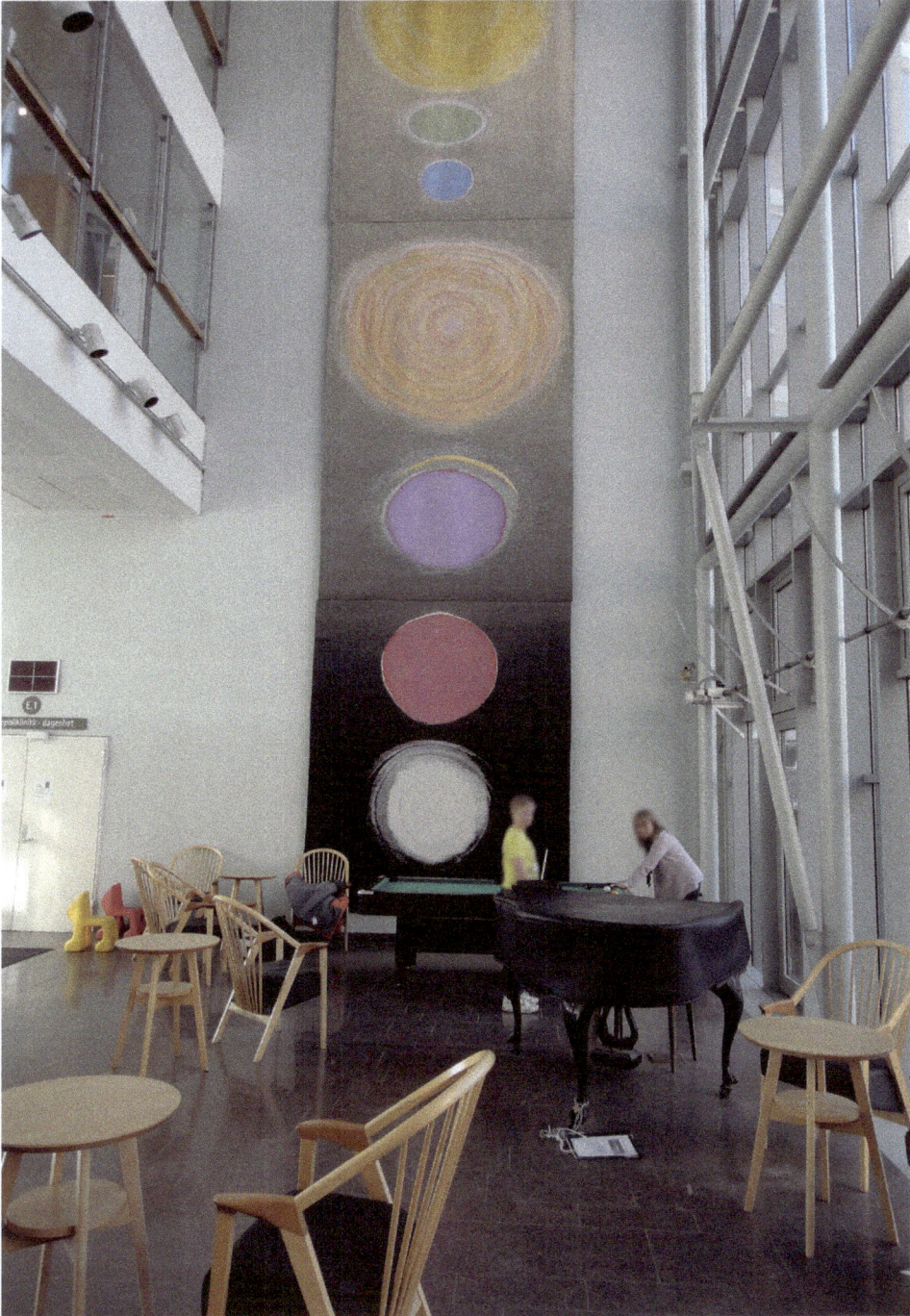

11. Positive distractions area.

TESIS Inter-University Research Centre "Systems and Technologies for Social and Healthcare Facilities"
University of Florence, Italy

222

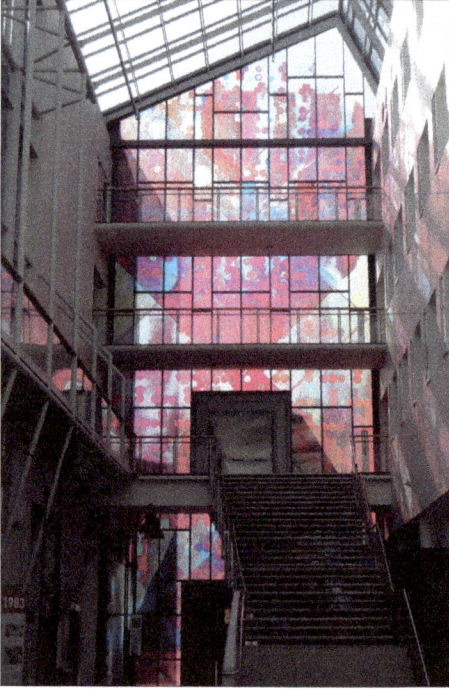

12. Stained glass allows daylight to penetrate the interior.

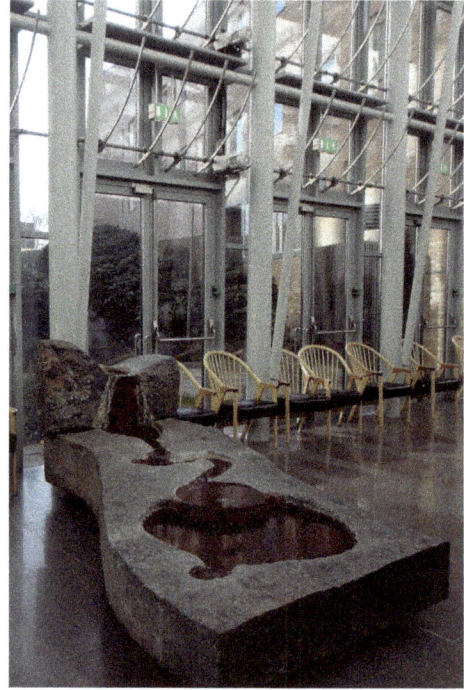

13. Fountain, the sound of water to relax the senses.

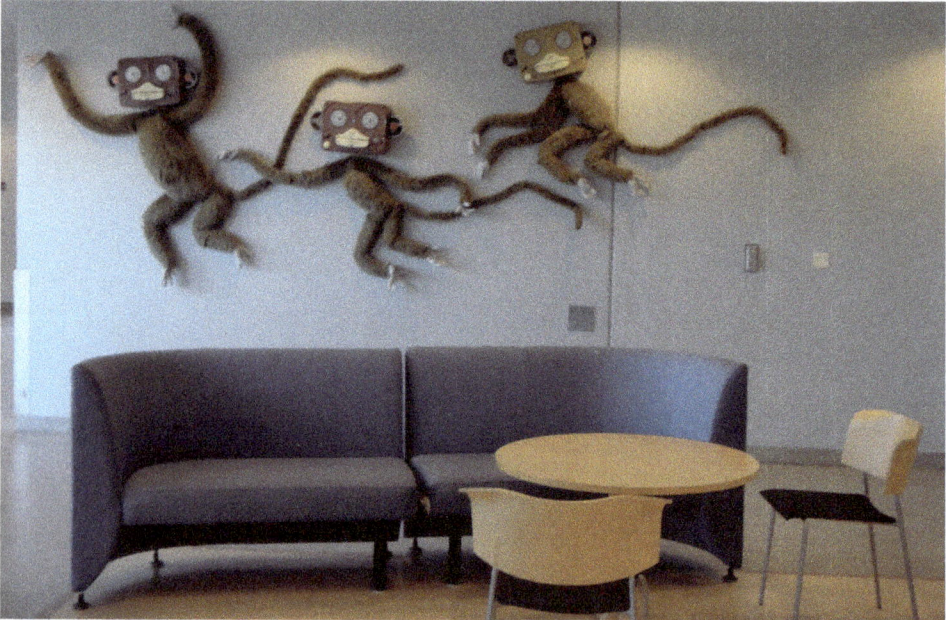

14. Waiting area.